Understanding
Health Inequalities
and Justice

Studies in Social Medicine

Allan M. Brandt, Larry R. Churchill, and Jonathan Oberlander, editors

This series publishes books at the intersection of medicine, health, and society that further our understanding of how medicine and society shape one another historically, politically, and ethically. The series is grounded in the convictions that medicine is a social science, that medicine is humanistic and cultural as well as biological, and that it should be studied as a social, political, ethical, and economic force.

UNDERSTANDING HEALTH INEQUALITIES AND JUSTICE

NEW CONVERSATIONS
ACROSS THE DISCIPLINES

Edited by Mara Buchbinder,
Michele Rivkin-Fish, and
Rebecca L. Walker

THE UNIVERSITY OF NORTH CAROLINA PRESS

Chapel Hill

Jacket illustration: © istock.com/PM78

Library of Congress Cataloging-in-Publication Data
Names: Buchbinder, Mara, editor. | Rivkin-Fish,
Michele R., editor. | Walker, Rebecca L., editor.
Title: Understanding health inequalities and justice : new conversations
across the disciplines / edited by Mara Buchbinder,
Michele Rivkin-Fish, and Rebecca L. Walker.
Other titles: Studies in social medicine.
Description: Chapel Hill : The University of North Carolina Press, [2016] |
Series: Studies in social medicine | Includes bibliographical references and index.
Identifiers: LCCN 2016016536 | ISBN 9781469630342 (cloth : alk. paper) |
ISBN 9781469630359 (pbk : alk. paper) | ISBN 9781469630366 (ebook)
Subjects: LCSH: Medical policy—United States. | Public health—
United States. | Equality—Health aspects—United States. | Justice—
Health aspects—United States. | Health—Social aspects—
United States. | Health—Political aspects—United States.
Classification: LCC RA395.A3 U473 2016 | DDC 362.10973—dc23
LC record available at https://lccn.loc.gov/2016016536

*To researchers and scholars who reach across
disciplines to further health justice*

Contents

Figures

Acknowledgments

Thinking about justice leads one to pose questions of fairness, equality, and duty. The work of academic collaboration involves efforts to both ponder and live out these concerns, joining them with practical expressions of collegiality and reciprocity. We were privileged to be able to devote our energies to both endeavors because of the immense support we received for this project from numerous colleagues and institutions. We are delighted to acknowledge and express our gratitude to them here.

Our focused attention to the production of knowledge around health inequalities and justice began with conversations in UNC's research groups on Bioethics and on the Moral Economies of Medicine, where we were inspired in developing our initial questions. With generous financial support from UNC's College of Arts and Sciences (Award for Interdisciplinary Initiatives), Center for Bioethics, Institute for Arts and Humanities, and Departments of Social Medicine, Philosophy, and Anthropology, we explored these issues at a conference titled "Comparing Approaches to Health Inequalities and Justice: A Dialogue on Theory, Method, and (Inter)-Disciplinarity," held in October 2013 at the UNC Institute for Arts and Humanities. We express our deep appreciation to Ruth Faden for providing our keynote address and for the inspiration that her work on social justice provided to both the conference and this volume. For their openness to pushing beyond conventional disciplinary comfort zones and helping achieve an unusual set of conversations, we thank the conference speakers: Paula Braveman, Paul Brodwin, Debra DeBruin, Sarah Horton, Rosalina James, Carla Keirns, Paul Kelleher, Nicholas King, Eva Kittay, Barbara Koenig, Carolyn Rouse, Jennifer Prah Ruger, and Janet Shim.

We immensely appreciate the ongoing support of Eric Juengst, who helped us envision the conference and work through numerous practical details. We also thank Annie Lyerly and Gail Henderson for their sustained support of the conference, and Laurel Bradley, Warren Whipple, Laura Wagner, Guy Shalev, and the Carolina Undergraduate Bioethics Scholars for helping with the many practical details of the event.

Developing this edited volume enabled us to deepen the debates opened up at the conference. The volume's goal of bridging diverse perspectives required its contributors to explicitly engage one another's chapters, and they proved admirably willing to explore new avenues of intellectual and creative analysis. We also thank our contributors for their indulgence and timely responses to all of our requests. Eric Juengst, Jon Oberlander, and Peter Redfield provided helpful feedback on our introduction and vision for the volume, for which we are sincerely grateful. We thank Dragana Lassiter and Warren Whipple for their assiduous attention to detail and generosity of spirit in their help with preparing the manuscript. We are also grateful for a publication grant from UNC's University Research Council.

Our editors at UNC Press, Joe Parsons and Allie Shay, deserve special thanks for their tireless support in guiding us and ushering this manuscript through the review and publication process. We also greatly appreciate the support and helpful suggestions of the Studies in Social Medicine editors, Beatrix Hoffman, and three additional external reviewers. Finally, we thank each other for the patience, perseverance, and friendship that made this project so intellectually and personally rewarding.

Abbreviations

ACA	2010 Patient Protection and Affordable Care Act
ACMG	American College of Medical Genetics
ACOG	American College of Obstetricians and Gynecologists
AFDC	Aid to Families with Dependent Children
AHRQ	Agency for Healthcare Research and Quality
CBO	Congressional Budget Office
CDC	U.S. Centers for Disease Control and Prevention
CHC	cultural health capital
CHCF	California Health Care Foundation
CHIP	Children's Health Insurance Program
ECC	early childhood caries
ECT	electroconvulsive therapy
FDA	U.S. Food and Drug Administration
GHW	Global Health Watch
HAART	highly active antiretroviral therapy
HHS	Health and Human Services
HIE	RAND Health Insurance Experiment
IHME	Institute for Health Metrics and Evaluation
LBW	low birth weight
NCHS	National Center for Health Statistics
NCMHD	NIH Center on Minority Health and Health Disparities
NGOs	nongovernmental organizations

NIH	National Institutes of Health
ODPHP	Office of Disease Prevention and Health Promotion
OGRRG	Obstetrics and Gynecology Risk Research Group
OHCHR	Office of the United Nations High Commissioner for Human Rights
OMH	Office of Minority Health
ORWH	NIH Office of Research on Women's Health
PCC	patient-centered care
PCORI	Patient-Centered Outcomes Research Institute
PI	principal investigator
PTB	preterm birth
RCTs	randomized controlled trials
SDH	social determinants of health
SMFM	Society for Maternal Fetal Medicine
SSDI	Social Security Disability Insurance
TANF	Temporary Assistance for Needy Families
UKDFID	United Kingdom Department for International Development
UNAIDS	Joint United Nations Programme on HIV/AIDS
UNDP	United Nations Development Programme
UNGA	United Nations General Assembly
UNICEF	United Nations Children's Fund
USAID	U.S. Agency for International Development
USDHHS	U.S. Department of Health and Human Services
WHO	World Health Organization
WHOCSDH	World Health Organization Commission on the Social Determinants of Health
WWWG	What Works Working Group

Understanding
Health Inequalities
and Justice

Introduction

Rebecca L. Walker, Michele Rivkin-Fish, and Mara Buchbinder

Across the globe and within local communities, people suffer from disease, disability, and early mortality at vastly different rates from one another. Some of these differences, such as those that stem from impoverished environmental conditions or a lack of access to health care, strike many observers as unjust; others, such as those that reflect choices to engage in potentially dangerous elite sports, may seem to have little to do with justice. How we understand the relationship between health inequalities and justice is influenced by many factors, including notions of deservingness, choice, vulnerability, luck, cultural and familial practices, and social group membership and status. Digging deeper, health "inequalities" themselves are constructed through choices about how to measure and reflect health differences, and concepts of justice reflect varying ideals of equality and fairness.

This book is about *how* we approach health inequalities and justice, and the relationship between them, and why that matters. Many of the conversations taking place in this volume are focused on issues of particular salience to the United States, but others reach beyond those borders. Consider an example to illustrate the significance of how we approach the interrelationship between health inequalities and justice. In 2012, average life expectancy at birth was almost seventy-three years for girls, while for boys it was just over sixty-eight years (WHO 2014). Is this gap of five years unjust? One relevant question is whether this "inequality" is simply a difference for health-care planners to work around, or whether it reflects an inequity that makes a moral demand on their attention and our shared resources. A related question is whether the statistic itself is as meaningful as it initially appears.

At first, it may seem that boys are at an unfair disadvantage merely in virtue of their sex, as long as we agree that one's sex is not something that should determine one's share of some significant good (here, life itself).

On reflection, an observer may note that whether the difference is unfair or merely unfortunate depends on the cause of the life expectancy gap. Perhaps if the gap reflects a biologically determined difference between the sexes, it is merely unfortunate. However, other potential causes, such as higher rates of men's participation in war or more dangerous employment, might bolster the perspective that boys are actually at an unfair disadvantage. Conversely, if we focus on risk factors associated with adverse health behaviors, like smoking tobacco or drinking alcohol, perspectives about fairness might shift as concepts of choice and deservingness are mobilized. In response, others may emphasize the ways in which health behavior is socially and culturally influenced, and therefore not merely an individual choice. Finally, turning the conversation on its head, we might instead argue that this statistic actually reflects female disadvantage. In Japan, for example, life expectancy at birth in 2012 was eighty-seven years for girls and eighty for boys (WHO 2014). It may be argued that this additional two-year longevity gap more closely reflects women's actual biological advantage, which in other countries is squandered through political, social, and cultural practices that put women at a longevity disadvantage.

Broadening the scope of the conversation, we might consider what statistical information regarding life expectancy really matters, and for what context. For example, the adage that "women get sicker, but men die quicker" seems borne out in comparisons of healthy life expectancy at birth. Worldwide in 2012, women's expectation for healthy life years was only three years greater than men's despite the five-year advantage in terms of total life expectancy. In many countries with particularly low life expectancy for both sexes, girls born in 2012 could expect to live the same number of healthy years as boys (or just one year more), despite their biological advantage. Complicating matters here is whether women have fewer healthy life years simply because they live longer (and the last years of life are less healthy) or whether their relative ill health precedes the end-of-life years.

Others may argue that what is significant is neither mere life nor even healthy life, but a broader notion of human development that also includes access to knowledge and education and a decent standard of living (Lewis and Burd-Sharps 2014). On those indicators, within the United States, for example, the widest gaps are those between different racial and ethnic groups, not the sexes. Further, gaps in all indicators are widely divergent by location. In Mississippi, an African American worker can expect to make $17,000 less per year than someone of the same race in Maryland, and a white baby born in the

District of Columbia can expect to live almost nine more years than a baby of the same race born in West Virginia (Lewis and Burd-Sharps 2014, 24).

In sum, a seemingly simple statistic regarding sex differences in worldwide average life expectancy at birth does not, in itself, tell us much about how to answer questions of fairness or justice about this difference. The information we might think is important in answering these kinds of questions, or even in understanding what a health "inequality" consists in, may differ depending on what we value (life itself, healthy life, well-being). In fact, a global life expectancy measure says very little in terms of the expectations for (healthy) life of a baby girl or boy born in any particular community. This illustrates a central theme of this book: that in addressing issues of health inequalities and justice, it matters a great deal *how* we approach and consider those questions.

The book pursues this theme in three ways through its main sections: theoretical perspectives on health inequalities and justice, case studies illustrating the productive interplay of theoretical and empirical factors, and the interrelationships among science, ethics, and policy that structure how we view and act on health justice and inequality. Informing all three sections, moreover, are broader reflections regarding how interdisciplinarity may contribute to new, useful conceptualizations of health inequalities and justice.

CHANGING THE CONVERSATION ABOUT
HEALTH INEQUALITIES AND JUSTICE

Questions of health inequalities and justice have long captured the interest of scholars in the social sciences, humanities, medicine, and public health. Yet interdisciplinary conversations have been hampered by background theoretical and methodological assumptions about the purpose, scope, and requirements of good research. Explicit attention to what different perspectives alternately clarify and obscure is essential for rigorously analyzing problems of health inequalities and offering possibilities for health justice. To pursue this challenge, we invited researchers and scholars from contributing fields to imagine how they might combine their skills and sensibilities to promote a richer understanding of health equality and justice. Their efforts open up new channels for conversation about the intersections and relationships between justice and health inequalities among people from different backgrounds.

This book thus represents multiple scholarly perspectives, including voices from medicine, public health, anthropology, sociology, history, philosophy, and bioethics. It also puts contributors from various fields in conversation with each other to illustrate how different vantage points and starting assumptions can complicate widely accepted views on health inequalities and justice. For example, much work in public health assumes that social determinants—that is, the structural conditions in which people are born, grow up, work, and age—are the causes of specific health inequalities.[1] This assumption has gained a strong foothold with scholars interested in promoting health justice, leading to such influential publications as *Is Inequality Bad for Our Health?* (Daniels, Kennedy, and Kawachi 1999).

However, Nicholas King (chapter 8, this volume) questions whether this assumption is empirically misguided and, further, whether it is ethically appropriate to argue for social equality as a means to promote health equality. King asks: Shouldn't we change the conversation and promote social justice independently of its effects on our health? Yet Paula Braveman (chapter 1, this volume) argues that the connection between social inequality and health inequality is not only empirically sound, but critical to promoting the social right to health. In particular, she argues against those who would offer an individual, rather than group-based, approach to the measurement of health inequalities. Her reasoning is that the individual approach obfuscates inequalities that are profound at the social group level. One type of exchange in this volume, then, shows how a seemingly noncontroversial starting place for relating social inequality to health inequality obscures not only empirical complexity, but also embedded assumptions about the political and moral value of particular methodological approaches to measuring health inequality.

In another conversation, Eva Kittay (chapter 4, this volume) and Janet Shim and colleagues (chapter 9, this volume) both address a similar healthcare phenomenon while using different theoretical and methodological lenses. Kittay considers the unintended ways in which a key bioethical principle, "respect for patient autonomy," reinforces and deepens problems of social and distributive justice. Shim and colleagues demonstrate how the well-intentioned goals of "patient-centered care," a key feature of President Obama's Affordable Care Act, inadvertently reinforce social inequalities. Drawing on rich ethnographic data, Shim et al. make a compelling case that patient-centered care relies on a specific, idealized model of the patient as an autonomous individual who is activated, engaged, and health literate. Kittay, for her part, describes the theoretical legacy of the concept of autonomy and draws out the ethical implications of how dominant ways of valuing autonomy may undermine goals of justice. In this volume, then, the reader is presented with varying theoretical and methodological perspectives regarding significant, but underrecognized, problems for health justice and inequality.

A third example of the type of new conversation that this volume promotes is illustrated by the exchange between Paul Kelleher (chapter 3, this volume) and Sarah Horton and Judith Barker (chapter 5, this volume). While Kelleher is a philosopher concerned with examining the theoretical contours of justice, and Horton and Barker are social scientists working to reframe the causal narrative for a specific set of oral health inequalities, these chapters creatively engage one another and consequently expand their respective boundaries. Kelleher illustrates his theoretical analysis by considering the specific health disparity addressed by Horton and Barker, thus reaching beyond typical philosophical routines of engaging more generalized cases or hypothetical examples. Horton and Barker, for their part, push their considerations to include questions of justice frequently left out of, or left implicit in, social science accounts of health inequalities. Taken together, these new kinds of conversations illustrate the ways that attention to how we variously conceptualize health and justice can enrich analyses and open up new channels of dialogue.

BEYOND DISCIPLINARY DIVIDES

Interdisciplinary work is not easy. Changing the kinds of conversations that we can have in cross-disciplinary forums is even more challenging, given the propensity for scholars trained in different conventions to sometimes talk past each other in intellectual exchanges. Disciplinary training provides the comfort of a set of presuppositions that scholars can take for granted in conversations within the field. Bridging across disciplines means bracketing, questioning, and justifying these presuppositions, or at least making background assumptions explicit. Of course, interdisciplinary fields like bioethics and medicine frequently bring together scholars and researchers from different backgrounds and perspectives, but they may not always think reflexively about the value that particular approaches bring. As editors, we came to this project with deep intellectual curiosities about other disciplinary traditions, but also with our own sets of biases and methodological and theoretical assumptions.[2] Because characterizing disciplinary trends entails the possibility that generalization will turn into caricature, we begin cautiously, by focusing on our own fields: anthropology and philosophy.

Philosophical inquiries regarding health inequalities and justice frequently examine when inequality is or is not an indicator of injustice, and when and to what degree particular individuals, groups, or political bodies have an obligation to try to change the given inequality. The logical steps in a scholar's reasoning, including the adequacy with which she defines her terms and clarifies her distinctions, are all key to an argument's persuasiveness and felicity. Yet, not infrequently, philosophical discourses are abstracted from the empirical details of social life, and they may involve imagined scenarios designed to elicit a distilled vision of the key ethical issues at stake.

Cultural anthropologists, by contrast, tend to focus their research on describing what inequality looks like, empirically, in its material and symbolic manifestations. They may ask how specific inequalities get perpetuated or ameliorated, how society comes to accept particular inequalities as natural, or, on the contrary, how certain kinds of inequalities become problems demanding redress. Cultural anthropologists often work with the assumption that inequalities are, per se, unjust, leaving aside the hard work of precisely defining what constitutes the injustice at hand.

Sometimes disciplinary differences amount to differences of perception rather than substantive disagreement. For example, *Lancet* editor in chief Richard Horton incited a great deal of disciplinary animosity with his recent declaration that contemporary medical history is "a corpus of activity lying moribund on its way to the scholarly mortuary" (Horton 2014, 292). Horton particularly decried what he viewed as the field's failure to attain contemporary public relevance. However, in a thoughtful rejoinder, the medical historian Carsten Timmermans (2014) noted that much recent work in his field invites readers "to engage in a dialogue with the past to understand the present of medicine and draw attention to historical alternatives that are difficult to conceive without such dialogue." In this case, then, the difference appears to lie in different perceptions of how the past may help to explain the present.

While these simplified accounts crystallize the difference that a disciplinary perspective can make, differences can also play out within disciplinary boundaries. Both philosophy and cultural anthropology have amassed legacies of dissent over how to integrate empirical and conceptual questions and evidence, or data and theory, in research and scholarly work. In the context of this book, then, changing the conversation about health inequalities and justice means moving beyond simplistic frames for categorizing research—qualitative versus quantitative, theoretical versus empirical, prescriptive versus descriptive[3]—to think more holistically about the potential gains, both practical and analytical, of integrating diverse perspectives.

Another key set of differences among the contributors to this volume concerns whether their primary entry point into this interdisciplinary dialogue is from the literature on justice or that on health inequalities. As previously noted, many social scientists—and health professionals, too—may begin with the assumption that health inequalities are inherently unjust and spend less time delineating precisely how such inequalities raise questions about justice. Likewise, philosophers and bioethicists may employ data on health inequalities in the service of arguments about justice without critically examining how the data were collected, analyzed, and interpreted. Here, changing the conversation entails pushing scholars to consider their background assumptions, standards of evidence, and the broader implications of their research, issues about which they might not have given much previous thought—or which they may not have reflexively questioned.

To ensure that this volume changes the conversation on health inequalities and justice, we have asked all of the contributors to address in some way the following organizing questions for the volume:

1. How do scholars variously approach relations between health inequalities and ideals of justice? What are the *methods*, broadly construed as the analytic toolkit, brought to bear on these questions?
2. When do justice considerations bear on questions about how to address health inequalities, and how do specific health inequalities affect our perceptions of injustice?
3. In what specific ways can diverse scholarly approaches contribute to better health policy?

To create a conversation that is engaged and coherent within the confines of this volume, each chapter also directly and substantially engages the content of at least one other chapter. In this introduction, we both reflect on the exchanges that occur within specific chapters and indicate and create points of connection and contrast beyond what the authors themselves address. By weaving these crosscutting discussions and focal points throughout the volume, we illustrate the potential for diverse perspectives to advance interdisciplinary dialogue and move the conversation forward.

PART I: INTERROGATING NORMATIVE PERSPECTIVES
ON HEALTH INEQUALITY AND JUSTICE

In addressing health justice and inequalities, a critical philosophical question is: What counts as justice and injustice? And, relatedly, if justice is our goal, how shall we know when we have achieved it? This core issue has been a matter of lively debate since at least Plato's presentation of justice in the *Republic* as the governing virtue of individuals (and societies) that organizes other ethical responses and promotes individual and social harmony. The notion of justice as a virtue echoes through contemporary discussions as well, with John Rawls positing justice as the "first virtue of social institutions" (1971, 3). At the same time, theorists today do not tend to think of justice as a moral concept that overlays all others, but as one distinctively (though not exclusively) related to matters of distribution and deservingness. Modern constructions also focus less on the state of those who obtain justice as a character trait and more on how justice is manifested in terms of social arrangements and individual actions. And, of course, to the modern ear, how justice is *made* manifest may have less to do with political and personal harmony than with social struggle and recognition.

One significant question about justice particularly salient to liberal democracies is how socially recognized and produced benefits (for example, health care) and burdens (for example, taxation) are distributed, which has given rise to debate over adequate allocation principles. Some suggestions have been, for example, "(1) to each person an equal share, (2) to each person according to individual need, (3) to each person according to individual effort, (4) to each person according to societal contribution, [or] (5) to each person according to merit" (National Commission 1979). The first and second of these models of distribution are *forward-looking* in aiming to enact some sort of equality between persons, either by dividing up social goods and resources equally or by addressing individual welfare deficits in order to bring everyone up to some basic level of well-being. Such forward-looking views feature among some broadly *egalitarian* models of distribution, a general framework that has been enormously influential in moral and political philosophy and that we shall discuss in more detail later in this section. Another forward-looking framework for the allocation of resources is *utilitarianism*, which typically aims to maximize the collective welfare of all those affected by an action or policy. As Carla Keirns's contribution to this volume reflects (chapter 11), utilitarian thought has been highly influential in the health-care arena generally, both in the policy evaluation of potential health-care interventions by means of cost-effectiveness (getting the biggest "bang for the buck" in terms of advancing a population's health utility) and also in the increased focus on efficiency within health-care institutions.

The third, fourth, and fifth models of distribution listed above, on the other hand, are *backward-looking* in viewing justice as relative to some past action or deservedness. *Libertarian* views, which envision justice as whatever distribution arises from the free exchange of goods and services between politically equal individuals, are similarly backward-looking. They evaluate not the shape of any distribution, but only the process whereby distribution took place.[4] While libertarianism and other backward-looking perspectives frequently have a minority voice within contemporary philosophical approaches to distributive justice, such views echo throughout the political and social landscape of the United States—particularly in notions of just deserts, individual responsibility, and moral merit, and these threads are taken up in different ways throughout this volume.

While egalitarian, utilitarian, and libertarian perspectives provide broad philosophical frames delimiting a range of acceptable approaches to the distribution of social benefits and burdens, other views of justice take no stand on the acceptability of particular distributive mechanisms. One such perspective is the arguably dominant moral framework in the field of bioethics, the *principles-based* approach developed in Tom Beauchamp and James Childress's *Principles of Biomedical Ethics* (now in its seventh edition).[5] According to this view, practical ethical problems in biomedicine are addressed by specification and balance, in context, of the various relevant (and sometimes competing) principles, including justice, beneficence, nonmaleficence, and respect for autonomy (Beauchamp and Childress 2009, 12–22). Because such specification and balancing require a background context, the principles approach explains and illustrates various theories and components of distributive justice, but takes no overall theoretical stance regarding competing distributive mechanisms (Beauchamp and Childress 2009, 240–81).

It is against the backdrop of the principles-based approach to biomedical ethics that Eva Kittay (chapter 4, this volume) enters the arena as "a philosopher who is concerned with issues of justice and care [and who has] become suspicious of a notion that plays a key role in political and moral philosophy, in bioethics and in medical practice, the concept of autonomy" (114). Connecting with Shim et al.'s discussion of cultural health capital (chapter 9, this volume), Kittay proposes that this valuation of autonomy reinforces already existing stratifications of social status and (dis)advantage. To illustrate her argument, Kittay analyzes an example of three patients from different socioeconomic, cultural, and ethnic backgrounds, each experiencing a heart attack in New York City. She shows that when autonomy is privileged as an overriding value in health care, each patient's actual course of illness and recovery depended on how well that autonomy was shored up by the patient's preexisting financial and social resources, including choice of health-care facility, geographic location when emergent care was needed, extent and status of social network, and availability of family supportive care.

By arguing that "many medical practices that suppose and crystalize around the concept of autonomy serve as one pathway by which inequalities in socioeconomic status result in unequal health outcomes" (114), Kittay changes the predominant bioethical conversation on respect for autonomy. Within a principles-based approach to biomedical ethics, respect for autonomy is rarely seen in tension with justice, but primarily as rubbing up against the requirement to benevolence (a physician's obligation to promote their patient's welfare, potentially despite the patient's own preferences). Further, Kittay argues that the dichotomy set up between the autonomous and the nonautonomous patient is deeply problematic. Those not considered autonomous are viewed as incompetent to make significant medical decisions, but that designation may also disengage those patients as individuals with hopes, wishes, and relevant preferences to be taken into account in the course of their medical care.

In the principles-based view of biomedical ethics, justice must be specified and balanced in context, meaning against the demands of other contextually relevant moral principles. As we have seen, this approach avoids the need to align itself in advance with a theory of justice. In some contrast, the *human rights* view of justice finds its roots in a particular (and distinctively modern) theoretical narrative regarding the demands of human equality in the legal, political, and moral promulgation and protection of human rights (see, e.g., Moyn 2010). Human rights are deployed differently in law, policy, and ethics but in general represent a set of agreements (or attributions) regarding the claims of individuals and groups for the protection and/or promotion of certain spheres of human activity and welfare and the correlative obligations of individuals, institutions, and nations with regard to those claims. A human right to health care, for example, is a positive right that people should be guaranteed a resource promoting a particular core aspect of human well-being (health). It carries an obligation on the part of identifiable individuals and institutions (including particularly governmental institutions) to provide such care.

While in an ethics context we can debate whether such a right to health care exists, in a political and legal context we might look to international and regional human rights treaties regarding a *right to health* as "the highest attainable standard of health" (WHO 1948) and consider matters of national enforceability. Paula Braveman (chapter 1, this volume) enters this discussion as a health disparities researcher with training in both medicine and public health who aims to bridge the divide between measurements of health inequality and conceptions of justice. Braveman argues that those health disparities negatively affecting groups identified as deserving special protections within the human rights tradition should be viewed as matters of justice, independently of our capacity to show a causal link between certain forms of social disadvantage and health inequality.

As a health disparities researcher, Braveman has focused intently on the significance of how we measure, define, and label various health inequalities. Her chapter thus offers clear and helpful distinctions between health inequalities or *disparities*, which are defined as health differences that are "unfair because they put an already socially disadvantaged group at further disadvantage" regardless of their cause, on the one hand, and health *inequities, on the other*, which is a term that she reserves for those health disparities which can be shown to have been caused by social disadvantage (34). Most significantly, however, her chapter offers a model for measuring health inequality that explicitly embeds considerations about the justice or injustice of those health differences. It is in this way that Braveman's chapter bridges conversations between theorists concerned with honing plausible conceptions of justice, and health inequalities researchers who aim to accurately measure health differences.

The essential insight of human rights, that all human beings are moral equals, is shared broadly among Western (post-Enlightenment) accounts of justice. The sticky issue between these accounts is what human moral equality demands in terms of justice. This question has been particularly taken up within egalitarianism, beginning with interrogation of what it is that ought be equally distributed. On a narrow account of *equality of opportunity*, for example, the demands of egalitarianism may be met by a society in which all are free to pursue political and economic positions in line with their talents and interests. This perspective, compatible with the backward-looking view of merit-based justice, need pay no attention to whether people in fact have equal shares of some particular social good. At the same time, larger differences in distribution will appear depending on whether equality of opportunity is formal, thus allowing for inherited wealth advantage and other forms of privilege (though denying rigid caste systems), or substantive in aiming to achieve a more radical equality of opportunity for all regardless of socioeconomic class or heritage.[6]

Perspectives on justice that adopt the moniker of "egalitarianism," however, are frequently interested to specify some particular type of good that ought to be equally distributed. Here the question "Equality of what?" has been intensely debated between several camps of theorists. One group, promoting equality of social *resources*, follows the theoretical legacy of John Rawls's notion of primary goods (Rawls 1971), which are resources that may be socially distributed and are desirable whatever particular conception of a good life one may have (examples, arguably, are income and wealth).

Rawls took his view as competing with a utilitarian conception in which *welfare*, rather than resources, is the appropriate measure of value. While classical utilitarians aimed to maximize collective welfare, but did not attend to its distribution, such views are egalitarian insofar as each person's welfare contributes with equal weight to the total collective. However, others have been interested to put forward a more thoroughly egalitarian perspective in which welfare ought to be equally distributed between individuals.

Positioning itself as critical of both welfarist and resourcist views, the equal *capabilities* approach first promoted by Amartya Sen (1979) argues that what is important to equalize is the effective freedom to achieve significant human functions (freedoms for people to "be and do" what they value). Sen views the capabilities approach as responsive to the shortcomings of a "fetishistic" focus on goods (resources) that may ignore how individuals engage with these resources (i.e., the choices they make with respect to them), as well as focus on welfare as an individual's "mental reaction" (or utility) while ignoring individuals' actual capabilities (1979, 218). To put it simply, neither providing people with resources that they do not value nor counting as beneficial their satisfaction with substandard situations does them any good. The capabilities view instead promotes that people are enabled to pursue their valued ends within the confines of a shared norm of human well-being. Some have been critical of the capabilities approach because it prioritizes freedom over outcomes, sidesteps issues of personal responsibility, and relies on a shared norm of human flourishing (Arneson 2013).

In chapter 2, Jennifer Prah Ruger enters these debates as a political economist trained in law and international relations who is interested in developing an account of global health justice that can address issues of both health inequality and national and international policy. Despite a plethora of recent activity in the global health arena, which she describes, Ruger bemoans the lack of a theoretical framework to mobilize concern for global health inequalities as unjust and around which to organize health policy. For example, recognition that infectious diseases easily travel the world has given "new urgency to addressing health on a global scale" (67) yet global health governance lacks any clear structure, and "disease surveillance and control, despite their global implications, depend on the capacity and decisions of national governments" (67). What is needed in this situation, Ruger argues, is a theoretical framework that calls on us to address infectious diseases as a matter of justice and not simply self-interest (or national interest) and that unifies our global health priorities around improving individual health capabilities.

Ruger's theory, "provincial globalism," is "global" in that it takes an individual capabilities approach to health equity and thus focuses on the individual as the "moral unit" of concern over and above states. It is "provincial" in that it acknowledges the important role of states and communities in global health governance. In Ruger's view, the capabilities approach offers a perspective that foregrounds health as critical for human flourishing, including what she calls individual and collective "health agency," but also promotes particular approaches to measurement and policy that she believes best promote global and local health.

For example, in addition to promoting a capabilities approach to *what* should be distributed to achieve global health justice (e.g., capability to achieve health functioning), Ruger also weighs in on whether the goal of health justice should be health *equality* or some other distributive pattern. We have already considered how distribution according to backward-looking criteria such as merit or desert does not necessarily promote health equality. However, even if the aim is to distribute according to forward-looking goals of welfare, resources, or capabilities, equality may not be the most desirable option. Indeed, the moral problem with global health inequality may be less the fact of *inequality* in health and more the devastating levels of ill health and early death among the world's poor. Instead of prioritizing health equality, we might focus instead on *raising the condition of the least-well-off* members of a society (or global community) or providing some basic *sufficient* level of a distributed good (a resource, healthy condition, or capability). Attending closely to Braveman's focus on disadvantaged groups and health rights, Ruger proposes that global health justice should rely on how much of a "shortfall" disadvantaged groups and individuals have against a sufficient threshold level of health functioning and should prioritize health achievement for the most disadvantaged groups and individuals.

While questions of *what* to distribute, and at which *level*, focus on both individuals and groups as in some sense disassociated units of comparison (how much to individual or group *x, y, z*, and of what sort of good), another line of thought within egalitarianism is concerned precisely with matters of the relationships between different individuals and social groups. These considerations are taken up as *relational egalitarianism* by Paul Kelleher (chapter 3, this volume), a philosopher whose work engages the intersection of theories of distributive justice and health policies. Kelleher positions relational accounts of egalitarianism in contrast to philosophical views holding that inequalities resulting from the responsible choices of individuals are not unjust. According to those views, unjust inequalities result in some way from "bad luck," which could be as mundane a matter as where a person is born (e.g., in an impoverished country).

The interest in accommodating notions of human responsibility runs deep in philosophical thought and is apparent in the ideal of equality of opportunity, as well as in libertarian views and in the promotion of distribution according to merit or past social contribution. Even theorists holding views of distributive justice that do not easily accommodate intuitions about personal responsibility, such as capability or utilitarian views, may see this as a flaw in their theory which they aim to rectify.[7] At the same time, accounting for individual responsibility within distributive justice is a notoriously fraught exercise. What choices are truly autonomous and belong to the individual as opposed to being problematically shaped by social, cultural, economic, or political forces? How do we disentangle the intersection of bad luck and systemic disadvantage?

In his chapter, Kelleher describes three different types of relational egalitarianism that "share the conviction that if an ideal of equality is morally important for distributive justice, it must be reinterpreted as something other than mere similarity of condition between individuals who bear no further distinctive relation to one another" (94). He then argues that all three types of relational egalitarianism (*equality of treatment, equality of concern*, and *social egalitarianism*) can work together, as exemplified in his analysis of material from Sarah Horton and Judith Barker's work examining oral health disparities (chapter 5, this volume).

The chapters in part 1, "Interrogating Normative Perspectives on Health Inequality and Justice," share modern political philosophy's overarching focus on matters of distribution and desert. In this discussion, the Platonic idea of justice as a virtue of the harmonious soul and polis has largely been replaced with questions linking justice to the promotion of human moral equality. Yet these chapters also demonstrate the multiple (and sometimes competing) ways of pursuing that goal. The chapters in part 1 examine matters of principle, capability, rights, and equality with respect to health inequalities. They aim to provoke and promote conversations between perspectives on justice and health inequalities that do not usually take place—between principles of respect for autonomy and justice, measurement of health inequality and human rights, international health policy and obligations to promote human flourishing, and versions of egalitarianism and qualitative descriptions of inequality.

PART II: DISRUPTING ASSUMPTIONS AND EXPANDING PERSPECTIVES THROUGH CASES

Beginning with normative frameworks about justice offers one way to open debate and analyze health inequalities. Other approaches begin from a more grounded perspective, seeking empirical evidence that includes local, cultural perspectives on well-being and fair distribution, often in the form of a particular case or example. The recognition of cultural diversity in health-related values and goals raises an interesting dilemma for scholars of health inequalities and justice. Respect for diversity calls into question claims about the universality of normative principles or values; yet in contexts of vast health inequalities, attention to culture alone is clearly inadequate for understanding why certain groups' health status is relatively worse or better than others.[8] Case study approaches guard against the problems that can result from the unquestioning reliance on normative models, by introducing the multiple dynamics of culture, political economy, and historical disadvantage that shape specific health inequalities. Yet case-based research generally does not make explicit the ethical reasons regarding why certain inequalities should (or should not) be considered unjust. Part 2 of this volume offers examples of work that brings together empirically based insights about cultural values and stratification patterns with normative analyses of the reasons certain inequalities should be considered unjust and in need of amelioration.

We find inspiration for combining these approaches in Madison Powers and Ruth Faden's *Social Justice: The Moral Foundations of Public Health and Health Policy* (2006). Powers and Faden begin with the premise that a just society is one in which social policies and social institutions aim to establish the conditions for all persons to attain well-being. They offer a carefully devised definition of well-being as comprising six fundamental human needs: personal security, cognition, attachments, health, respect and equal standing, and self-determination. Moreover, Powers and Faden also establish a societal obligation to aim for "structural fairness," which involves recognizing and combating actual forms of social disadvantage as they appear in society, even when these do not affect a particular individual's well-being. Importantly, this paradigm is based on Powers and Faden's perceptions of the needs of persons given the specific vulnerabilities they face within particular institutional settings. As such, this approach leaves room for policies to address culturally variable forms of attachment, respect, and health, and to ameliorate locally specific forms of disadvantage.

When viewed in comparison with other normative approaches to justice we have described, Powers and Faden's paradigm can be characterized as a threshold view, establishing what is adequate for a decent human life. Yet their justification for this approach reveals it to be far more than a threshold view of human well-being. Powers and Faden ground their vision of justice in a recognition that the conditions for human well-being interrelate, building cumulatively on each other in ways that benefit or disadvantage people in multiple dimensions. They argue, "Failures of the social structure to provide for or respond to needs for preserving health through health care, or needs for developing capacities of reason through education, not only affect health or reason, but can cause additional injustice associated with lack of respect, which is an insult to one's dignity" (Powers and Faden 2006, 23–24).

This argument resonates with social science and public health findings regarding the ways social structures create and reinforce inequalities.[9] As a foundation for conceptualizing justice, this framework opens up an analytical space where empirical research on institutional policies and their effects on specific populations can be joined to the theoretical analysis of justice. By identifying the overlapping, holistic character of well-being and, conversely, demonstrating that social hierarchies structurally position some people at a *systemic disadvantage*, Powers and Faden present a framework for undertaking sociologically inflected studies of the justice of various public policies and social arrangements. This vision of justice is the basis of their claim that addressing processes of systemic disadvantage is a matter of "moral urgency" (Powers and Faden 2006, 8).

Joining empirical and philosophical analyses highlights questions regarding the dynamics between cases and theory. While theoretical frameworks set up the terms of debate and the questions that matter for a given scholarly conversation, the analysis of specific cases can work to develop or challenge theoretical paradigms: they may yield examples that seem emblematic of broader trends, anomalies that prove the rule, or perhaps anomalies that lead us to question our starting assumptions (Berlant 2007; Ragin and Becker 1992). And although the use of cases is a common practice in all scholarship, dialogue across fields is often difficult precisely because the theoretical foundations that scholars hold may differ and their criteria for assessing adequate evidence, or the purview of a case, frequently diverge. One scholar's disciplinary training may cause her to doubt the foundational presuppositions that mobilize another scholar's project, from their method of forming cases, to relating cases to broader theoretical concerns, to deriving conclusions. Such skepticism may be expressed through questions such as: Is the case described truly characteristic of some broader trend? Are the questions being asked the most significant ones? Are the presuppositions embedded in the methodology problematic or infelicitous? The distinct organization of cases, and their composition, use, and evaluation in different fields, expose the challenges of undertaking conversations across disciplines.

The chapters in part II of *Understanding Health Inequalities and Justice* strive to recognize these challenges and proceed toward creative new dialogues across fields. The chapters present cases that concern distinct populations' health-related issues where matters of justice are at stake. Sarah Horton and Judith C. Barker examine oral health vulnerabilities among the children of Mexican migrant workers in California. Debra DeBruin and colleagues explore how American cultural notions of risk and risk management in pregnancy result in gender inequality and harm women's health. Finally, Paul Brodwin investigates the injustice of disrespect faced by those in psychiatric treatment as seen through the account of a survivor and the theories of concerned observers. These chapters thus address a wide range of topics; each combines distinct forms of data in unique ways. Our goal in bringing them together in a section on "cases" serves to foreground the ways each study creatively bridges a set of disciplinary divides. Importantly, all three chapters illustrate how attention to the *making* of a specific case can reveal problems and possibilities for the production of knowledge about health inequalities and justice more generally.

As outlined in Braveman's chapter, the assumptions structuring the human rights framework of justice begin with the fact that health inequalities track long-standing forms of social stratification. Much research in this vein, consequently, aims to expose the systematic effects that certain public policies or institutional arrangements have on various social groups: women,

African Americans, rural residents, persons with disabilities, and so forth. On the one hand, recognizing that social stratification is a product of historical and political dynamics allows one to imagine the possible transformation of existing arrangements in order to establish a more just social organization and, perhaps, thereby create conditions for improving the health of historically disenfranchised populations. On the other hand, as researchers inspired by these goals delve deeply into specific case studies, they often find that the boundaries constituting a socially disadvantaged group are hard to define and/or that the criteria and cause of "disadvantage" may be murky or multifaceted. The chapters in part II illustrate such complexities in their case studies. Taken together, they demonstrate how an adequate understanding of the content of social disadvantage and the nature of particular injustice(s) requires moving beyond discipline-specific forms of theory and data. They provide fascinating examples of how cases are both important in their own right and essential for refining theoretical presuppositions.

Sarah Horton and Judith Barker are anthropologists with expertise in studies of health inequalities in vulnerable populations. Their contribution (chapter 5) begins with an identifiable minority group, the children of Mexican migrant farmworkers in California, documenting both their relative poor oral health compared to other groups and the social policies behind this inequality. But the chapter does more than measure and reaffirm that a group recognized as ethnically and politically marginalized suffers systemic disadvantage. First, it exposes the multiple consequences of their poor oral health, which include both immediate biological vulnerabilities such as infection, pain, and illness, and long-term social consequences such as an inability to conform to the normalized aesthetic standards necessary for social mobility in U.S. society. The policies that compromise the oral health of migrant workers' children place them at risk of facing systematic disadvantages throughout their life course.

Second, methodologically, Horton and Barker demonstrate the importance of bringing together distinct methods and frameworks for studying this issue. While epidemiology can reveal patterns of poor oral health, and policy analysis can explain the limited care opportunities made available to these populations, ethnography can illuminate the ways migrant workers themselves understand practices and choices around infant and child feeding. The use of multiple methods for analyzing migrant oral health enables the authors to identify how social disadvantage becomes physically embodied and understood by this particular social group.

Authoring chapter 6 is a team of scholars with expertise in feminist bioethics and backgrounds in philosophy, medicine, and nursing. The case addressed in DeBruin and colleagues' chapter highlights the fact that justice involves more than issues of resource distribution, demonstrating how cultural norms can underwrite the unfair treatment of pregnant women. Specifically, they are concerned with the ways American cultural expectations for "good mothering" result in the unscientific and even oppressive treatment of women in both popular and medical approaches to pregnancy. They identify specific ways that these cultural norms generate troubling outcomes, including the normative surveillance of pregnant women (in some cases taken to such an extreme that pregnant women have been incarcerated on the grounds of state protection of fetuses); the prevalence of invasive and scientifically unfounded interventions during childbirth in the name of "risk prevention"; and the lack of clinical research on how best to treat women's health issues that are not obstetric-related during pregnancy. These authors' unit of analysis becomes cultural assumptions about gendered risk, not pregnant women as an a priori socially vulnerable group. American culture's management of risk in pregnancy, in other words, is highlighted as an unrecognized, but important, source of injustice.

DeBruin et al. also offer alternative approaches to addressing risk management in pregnancy that broaden attention beyond women's individual lifestyle behaviors—a current preoccupation of clinicians, public policy experts, and popular surveillance. They argue that because risk in pregnancy is closely tied to broader, social determinants of health, achieving justice requires new agendas that include addressing research on nonobstetric health conditions and treatments during pregnancy, and changing society's misconceptions that women's lifestyles contribute the dominant impact on pregnancy risk and outcome. DeBruin et al. insist that such changes are imperative "so that judgments about how to manage risk can be informed by science rather than grounded in sexist norms" (180).

Paul Brodwin is an anthropologist with long-standing research in the anthropology of psychiatry and public sector mental health services, as well as the ethnography of bioethics. In chapter 7, he examines the requirements of justice for those categorized as mentally ill, through a case that is contained within a single memoir—author and advocate Judy Chamberlin's autobiographical narrative of the intense suffering she endured through stigmatization and coerced hospitalizations that followed her being labeled "mentally ill." Inasmuch as Chamberlin richly describes the lack of respect she endured as a significant source of her personal suffering, Brodwin explores what may be gained by examining Chamberlin's memoir together with theoretical work by Axel Honneth and Stephen Darwall on the philosophy of recognition and respect. Can such distinct genres, rhetorical strategies, and modes of knowledge be put into dialogue? he inquires. What would the commensuration of these distinct forms of knowledge require? What are the challenges and promises of such an undertaking? In addressing these theoretical and methodological processes, Brodwin's chapter thus takes on the goals of our volume explicitly, both modeling and articulating the "interpretive generosity" that is essential to undertaking conversations across widely divergent approaches to particular problems of health justice and inequality, whether the differences are disciplinary or genre-based. It details the need for creativity and open-mindedness, the willingness to cocreate "a new shared space of understanding" (190).

Specifically, Brodwin focuses on the question of what a personal account of trauma and recovery may offer to analytical renderings of respect, and, conversely, what might be gained by examining individual narratives in light of theoretical generalizations. Like DeBruin et al., Brodwin understands questions of health justice as escaping the confines of distributive justice and including the impact of both interpersonal and social respect and disrespect. In this way, both chapters also take up the types of concerns relevant to relational egalitarianism as discussed above. Drawing on theories that parse the abstract concept of "rights" into both political and subtler, interpersonal forms of inclusion, Brodwin highlights the ways social processes such as the failure to recognize another, and the communication of disrespect, produce systematic disadvantage and injustice.

There is thus ample support for research that addresses the ways cumulative disadvantages lead to systematic inequalities—a prime example of injustice in the terms of Powers and Faden, in the human rights paradigm, and in the assumptions of sociologists and public health scholars. Interestingly, however, these authors' open-ended use of specific cases also acts as a corrective to preexisting assumptions about what constitutes systemic inequalities and disadvantages and what kinds of injustice result. The cases examined here demonstrate Powers and Faden's argument that well-being is much more than a matter of formal access to health care, even as Horton and Barker's study unquestionably demonstrates that access to certain kinds of medical care can be very important to prevent illness and long-term suffering.[10] DeBruin et al. and Brodwin (and Rouse, chapter 10), however, reveal how, at times, the use of medical care can itself be a source of dis-ease, resulting in stigma, surveillance/control, loss of self-determination, and lack of respect—additional forms of injustice in Powers and Faden's terms.

In sum, the chapters in part 2 demonstrate how cases, as theoretical and methodological products, can reveal generalizations from the particular and also serve to catalyze the intellectually valuable work of disrupting assumptions and presuppositions. In studies of health inequalities and justice, they can help scholars refine implicit ideas about who is disadvantaged and how, find new paths for understanding how disadvantage manifests itself in health-related terms, and imagine the kinds of policy interventions possible for reversing inequalities that constitute injustices.

PART III: RETHINKING EVIDENCE AND THE MAKING OF POLICY

Our goal of promoting metareflection on knowledge production about health inequalities and justice is particularly salient for analyses of public policy. Health policies are undergirded by a range of hidden assumptions and value judgments about the kinds of people, practices, and institutions that societies want to cultivate (cf. Horton 2014; Kaufman and Fjord 2011; Mulligan 2014; Oberlander 2003; Storeng and Béhague 2014). In part 3, contributors highlight how critical perspectives on health inequalities and justice and the relationships between them can bring such previously hidden assumptions to the foreground and thereby change the conversation about specific health policy concerns in productive ways.

In chapter 11 of this volume, Carla Keirns—a palliative care physician, historian of medicine, health services researcher, and clinical ethicist—brings her unique set of disciplinary lenses to bear on the problem of health-care reform. Keirns argues that recent proposals for payment reform in U.S. health care are implicitly based on utilitarian models, which privilege the maximization of benefits for the greatest number of people. Drawing on the case of health reform in Massachusetts, Keirns shows how such proposals for payment reform can cause unexpected harms to vulnerable populations even as they benefit society at large, thereby exacerbating disparities. In Massachusetts, Keirns illustrates, a set of reforms enacted in 2006 served its intended purpose of increasing coverage of the uninsured but had devastating economic consequences for both safety-net hospitals and the poorest patients. Thus, whether policy makers prioritize boosting population-level measures of health and well-being (a utilitarian model) or closing the gap between individuals (an egalitarian goal) has critical ramifications, both for the welfare of the most vulnerable members of society and, on a more theoretical level, for how we think about justice.

Where Keirns draws important historical and philosophical lessons from the unexpected challenges to Massachusetts's experiment with health-care reform, sociologists Janet Shim, Jamie Chang, and Leslie Dubbin (chapter 9, this volume) employ a critical sociological lens to examine an aspect of the Affordable Care Act that has received little public attention: its institutionalization of a set of medical values and practices known as patient-centered care. They do so through the concept of *cultural health capital*, which highlights how health behavior is more an outcome of people's socioeconomic resources and opportunities, and less a matter of "autonomous" decisions, insights that resonate with Kittay's chapter. In concert with recent social scientific critiques of patient-centered care which point out that "patient-centeredness" may fly in the face of patient expectations and does not necessarily improve health outcomes (cf. Grob 2013; Pilnick and Dingwall 2011), the authors question the notion that patient-centered care necessarily promotes more equitable health care. They ask: What kind of a person does this model of "virtuous" patienthood presuppose? And what are the health-care consequences of such assumptions? They argue that if patient-centeredness provides the metric by which health-care encounters are evaluated, it may set up patients who are already activated, engaged, and health literate (i.e., patients from more privileged socioeconomic backgrounds) to be judged as better patients and receive more optimal care.

While it may seem obvious that health policies are shaped by the values of policy makers and the constituents they represent, less self-evident is the notion that the scientific evidence on which many policy shifts are justified is likewise far from value-neutral. Historically, a changing scientific evidence base and the introduction of new biomedical technologies have shaped many shifts in U.S. health policy, from mass immunization to cancer screening. Often, new policies are rhetorically framed as inevitable outcomes of scientific progress, suggesting that ethical debates are to a certain extent moot. For example, some observers of the moral controversies surrounding whole-genome sequencing suggest that it is not a matter of *if* but *when* these technologies will become widely clinically available. This can in turn lead to the conclusion that policy makers should embrace such technologies regardless of the ethical challenges they pose—for example, what might constitute adequate informed consent and how to handle disclosure of incidental findings.

The recent expansion of state-mandated newborn screening in the United States provides an instructive example of how value judgments are always already embedded in the scientific process. In 2006, a task force of the American College of Medical Genetics (ACMG) appointed by the Health Resources and Services Administration issued a report recommending a standardized panel of screening targets that greatly expanded the number of disorders screened for by most states (Watson et al. 2006). However, experts in preventive and evidence-based medicine criticized the criteria used to evaluate potential screening targets because they overlooked established standards of evidence for the preventive efficacy of screening, such as the stipulation that screening targets be treatable and their incidence and natural history well understood (Moyer et al. 2008). Instead, experts were compelled by the persuasive arguments of parent advocates that society could ill afford to wait to set "lifesaving" policies until the research gaps were filled in (Buchbinder and Timmermans 2014). Seen from this light, the scientific process that drove the ACMG recommendations reveals the workings of a host of hidden biases and value judgments regarding the urgency of "saving babies" from rare disorders.

Yet moral values enter the policy arena even earlier than considerations about what types of technologies and interventions society ought to invest in. They also suffuse every aspect of the scientific process, from decisions about which research projects deserve funding priority to issues of design and measurement and the interpretation of results. For example, breast cancer receives far more research funding than lung cancer because of moral judgments regarding personal responsibility for each disease, even though lung cancer kills more people on an annual basis, including growing numbers of nonsmoking women (Klawiter 2008; Jain 2013; see also Best 2012).

Likewise, when a recent sociological study found that there was no effect of breast-feeding on several health and behavioral outcomes among discordant sibling pairs (Colen and Ramey 2014), popular media outlets were quick to mobilize the study to challenge the biological benefits of breast-feeding (e.g., Grose 2014). Yet scientists in the academic blogosphere were just as quick to critique the design, statistical analyses, and interpretations of results (Cassels 2014; Martin 2014; Quinn 2014), suggesting that the authors may have been swayed by the moral commitments underlying their policy conclusions—namely, that we ought to change the societal structures that make it difficult for so many American women to follow breast-feeding recommendations rather than demonize individual women for failing to meet these demands. The firestorm of controversy that followed this publication keenly demonstrates how difficult it may be to separate scientific research from the moral values and political goals that animate it.

Nicholas King, in chapter 8 of this volume, argues that health inequalities researchers often falsely assume that measurement is an objective process. Trained as a historian of science, King currently directs an interdisciplinary research collaborative focused on ethical issues in scientific measurement. This background motivates a thoughtful critique in his chapter of the ways in which normative judgments about injustice shape the selection of measures and statistical strategies. For example, King shows that the choice of absolute versus relative inequality measures to track changing mortality rates following the introduction of antiretroviral therapy for HIV/AIDS can lead researchers to come to very different conclusions about the same data. Using recent research on the structural determinants of health as a case study, King raises a critical challenge to policies promoting social or economic resource redistribution on the grounds that health inequalities are caused by social inequalities. Namely, he argues that scholars may overreach in marshaling evidence about the relationships between social and health inequalities toward policy solutions. The corrective, from King's perspective, is a more careful, critical engagement in multidisciplinary discussion about methods.

Carolyn Rouse, an anthropologist with expertise in critical race theory and social justice in health care, similarly destabilizes ideas about the value-neutrality of science in its relationship to health policy (chapter 10, this volume). Rouse traces key rhetorical shifts from the 2010 to 2020 versions of "Healthy People," a set of U.S. policy initiatives aimed at improving national health outcomes through rigorous scientific investigation, from disparities-specific goals toward a more inclusive (if diluted) vision of achieving health equity. By illustrating the methodological politics inherent in health disparities research debates about whether to target the health of vulnerable minority groups or the health of the nation more broadly, Rouse implicitly builds on the conceptual foundation laid out by Paula Braveman's discussion of the univariate versus the human-rights-based approach to health disparities research (chapter 1, this volume) with a detailed analysis of the policy implications of these approaches. Ultimately, Rouse concludes that the rhetoric of Healthy People 2020 shifted away from racial and ethnic disparities because of methodological weaknesses and design flaws in the health disparities evidence base, such as casting race as an independent variable without accounting for the interrelated roles of income and geography.

The four chapters of part 3 thus bring together analyses of U.S.-based health reform with examinations of the research-policy nexus to demonstrate how cultural values and moral assumptions embedded in certain kinds of knowledge production enter policy making, often with unanticipated outcomes.

CONCLUSION

In sum, the purpose of this volume is not to propose a single, authoritative approach to understanding health inequalities and justice; rather, it is to illustrate how a comparative understanding of the range of approaches used in scholarly research can inspire important conjunctures and novel analyses as well as offer significant implications for health policy. This introduction has outlined some of the main normative approaches to justice and empirical approaches to assessing health inequalities. It has also offered reflections on the theoretical and methodological strengths and limitations of these diverse approaches. Our goal in foregrounding these comparisons is to provide readers access to the taken-for-granted assumptions and structuring concerns of diverse scholarly traditions, so that dialogue across fields concerned with health and justice can flourish.

It is our hope that empirical researchers might find their work enriched by normative debates regarding what constitutes justice, what justice requires, and where (on whom) various moral obligations lie. The chapters that follow investigate broad aspects of justice, from distributive processes of material resources, access to services, and opportunities, to forms of recognition that include respect and equal moral standing. Similarly, we open up the question of how diverse scholarly approaches identify, measure, and categorize health inequalities including their relationship to justice. Measurements of inequality are themselves implicitly shaped by values, including about how society works or should work, assumptions that the individual or specific social groups should be the unit of analysis, and the roles of merit, deservingness, choice, and evidence in evaluations of justice.

Many of the chapters in this volume undertake a critical analysis of commonly held assumptions about justice (DeBruin et al.; King, Kittay, Ruger, Shim et al.) or intervene in debates about the constitution of health inequalities (Braveman, King, Rouse). Others are structured to analyze normative approaches along with cases and policies (Brodwin, Keirns, Kelleher, Kittay) in creative ways that push the conceptual boundaries of these approaches. Similarly, attention to methodological pluralism enables Horton and Barker and Rouse to layer ethnographic data onto quantitative findings in order to contribute new kinds of insights.

In bringing to the table a set of scholars who are preoccupied with similar kinds of problems but who otherwise may not engage each other in conversation, we needed a special set of participants who would bring both an open mind to reflecting on limitations of their own paradigms, and a spirit of generosity necessary for learning from others. Our hope is that such conversations enlarge the scope of questions considered relevant and the kinds of data that are brought together. A core question for us has been what precisely it takes to build bridges across disciplines and schools of thought. We eagerly invite our readers to continue this conversation.

NOTES

1. While social determinants of health are theorized as encompassing a wide range of conditions, including geographic location and type of employment, they are typically measured solely in terms of income, education attainment, and race.

2. This project was born from our fortuitous experiments in cross-disciplinary exchanges between scholars in the Departments of Social Medicine and Anthropology at UNC–Chapel Hill, our departmental homes. Our collaboration began as a working conference that we hosted at UNC–Chapel Hill in October 2013, with generous funding from the Center for Bioethics, the School of Medicine Merrimon Lectureship, the College of Arts and Sciences, the Institute for Arts and Humanities, the Moral Economies of Medicine Working Group, the Center for Health Equity Research, the Parr Center for Ethics, the Carolina Undergraduate Bioethics Scholars, and the Departments of Anthropology, Philosophy, and Social Medicine. All of the contributors to this volume were invited speakers at this conference, although several of the original conference speakers were not able to participate in this volume due to competing demands.

3. *Qualitative research* is a method of inquiry traditionally associated with the social and behavioral sciences that relies heavily on textual and observational data collected in a naturalistic setting. Qualitative research often seeks in-depth understandings of human behavior, focusing on a small subset of a broader population to produce descriptive information. *Quantitative research,* by contrast, relies on numerical data, typically collected from a large sample, to produce generalizable knowledge about a population. Both qualitative and quantitative research are *empirical*—that is, they are forms of knowledge based on direct observations or experiences in the world. *Theoretical* research, on the other hand, investigates and constructs conceptual scaffolds through which to analyze and understand our values and ideals as well as empirical or experiential data. Some people might contrast empirical with *normative* (of or having to do with social standards or norms), but we find this contrast problematic since empirical work is also, in our view, normative. Importantly, of course, empirical work also invokes and employs theory. A related set of binary terms is *descriptive* versus *prescriptive* research. Whereas descriptive research seeks to represent things as they

are, prescriptive research implies an effort to shape events or behavior by imposing a guiding rule or set of standards.

4. The idea of procedural justice is not particular to libertarianism. Most famously, it is a core feature of John Rawls's liberal egalitarian theory.

5. Arguably, virtue-based approaches such as Plato's, which attend primarily to agent-relative questions regarding justice and its role in governing a balanced soul and polis, need take no specific stand on which distributive mechanism is to be supported.

6. Such a substantive notion is present in John Rawls's notion of "fair" equality of opportunity, which he prioritizes, and presents in conjunction with the distribution of primary goods as discussed below.

7. In her chapter, for example, Jennifer Ruger is careful to carve out a role for individual and group responsibility.

8. Many scholars have explored at length the ways historical relationships of colonialism and other forms of political and economic exploitation that continue to the present day intersect with and must be conceptualized together with cultural values concerning health, illness, and healing (e.g., Beckfield and Krieger 2009; Farmer 2001, 2006; Krieger 2001, 2008a, 2008b; Lock and Nguyen 2010; Petryna 2009, 2013; Singer and Baer 1995).

9. In particular, we see importance similarities between their approach and the concerns of the sociologist Pierre Bourdieu (1984), feminist intersectionality scholars, and, in public health, Nancy Krieger's oeuvre (e.g., Krieger 2001, 2008a, 2008b; Beckfield and Krieger 2009) on the ways political-economic and social relations of domination result in the personal embodiment of inequality.

10. Barriers to access are deeper than outright "discrimination," construed as deliberate efforts to extend unequal treatment. Access involves tacit processes of negotiating numerous kinds of barriers and layered costs, often manifest in symbolic forms of exclusion such as gestures of disdain, bureaucratic hurdles, and silent neglect.

REFERENCES

Arneson, Richard. 2013. "Egalitarianism." In *The Stanford Encyclopedia of Philosophy*, edited by Edward N. Zalta, Summer 2013. http://plato.stanford.edu/archives/sum2013/entries/egalitarianism/. Accessed 23 August 2015.

Beauchamp, Tom L., and James F. Childress. 2001. *Principles of Biomedical Ethics*. New York: Oxford University Press.

Beckfield, Jason, and Nancy Krieger. 2009. "Epi + Demos + Cracy: Linking Political Systems and Priorities to the Magnitude of Health Inequities—Evidence, Gaps, and a Research Agenda." *Epidemiologic Reviews*, January, mxp002. doi:10.1093/epirev/mxp002.

Berlant, Lauren. 2007. "On the Case." *Critical Inquiry* 33 (4): 663–72. doi:10.1086/521564.

Best, Rachel Kahn. 2012. "Disease Politics and Medical Research Funding: Three Ways Advocacy Shapes Policy." *American Sociological Review* 77 (5): 780–803. doi:10.1177/0003122412458509.

Bourdieu, Pierre. 1984. *Distinction: A Social Critique of the Judgement of Taste.* Translated by Richard Nice. Cambridge, MA: Harvard University Press.

Buchbinder, Mara, and Stefan Timmermans. 2014. "Affective Economies and the Politics of Saving Babies' Lives." *Public Culture* 26 (1): 101–26.

Cassels, Tracy. 2014. " 'Is Breast Really Best?' The Debate Doesn't End Here . . . " *Evolutionary Parenting.* February 14. http://evolutionaryparenting.com/is-breast-really-best-the-debate-doesnt-end-here/. Accessed 23 August 2015.

Colen, Cynthia G., and David M. Ramey. 2014. "Is Breast Truly Best? Estimating the Effects of Breastfeeding on Long-Term Child Health and Wellbeing in the United States Using Sibling Comparisons." *Social Science and Medicine* 109: 55–65.

Daniels, Norman, Bruce Kennedy, and Ichiro Kawachi. 1999. "Why Justice Is Good for Our Health: The Social Determinants of Health Inequalities." *Daedalus* 128 (4): 215–51.

Farmer, Paul. 2001. *Infections and Inequalities: The Modern Plagues.* Updated ed. Berkeley: University of California Press.

———. 2006. *AIDS and Accusation: Haiti and the Geography of Blame.* Updated ed. Berkeley: University of California Press.

Grob, Rachel. 2013. "The Heart of Patient-Centered Care." *Journal of Health Politics, Policy and Law* 38 (2): 457–65.

Grose, Jessica. 2014. "New Study Confirms It: Breast-Feeding Benefits Have Been Drastically Overstated." *Slate,* February 27. http://www.slate.com/blogs/xx_factor/2014/02/27/breast_feeding_study_benefits_of_breast_over_bottle_have_been_exaggerated.html. Accessed 23 August 2015.

Horton, Richard. 2014. "Offline: The Moribund Body of Medical History." *The Lancet* 384 (9940): 292.

Jain, S. Lochlann. 2013. *Malignant: How Cancer Becomes Us.* Berkeley: University of California Press.

Kaufman, Sharon R., and Lakshmi Fjord. 2011. "Medicare, Ethics, and Reflexive Longevity: Governing Time and Treatment in an Aging Society." *Medical Anthropology Quarterly* 25 (2): 209–31.

Klawiter, Maren. 2008. *The Biopolitics of Breast Cancer: Changing Cultures of Disease and Activism.* Minneapolis: University of Minnesota Press.

Krieger, Nancy. 2001. "Theories for Social Epidemiology in the 21st Century: An Ecosocial Perspective." *International Journal of Epidemiology* 30 (4): 668–77.

———. 2008a. "Ladders, Pyramids and Champagne: The Iconography of Health Inequities." *Journal of Epidemiology and Community Health* 62 (12): 1098–1104.

———. 2008b. "Proximal, Distal, and the Politics of Causation: What's Level Got to Do with It?" *American Journal of Public Health* 98 (2): 221.

Lewis, Kristen, and Sarah Burd-Sharps. 2014. "American Human Development Report: The Measure of America 2013–2014." *Measure of America.* http://www.measureofamerica.org/measure_of_america2013-2014/. Accessed 23 August 2015.

Lock, Margaret, and Vinh-Kim Nguyen. 2010. *An Anthropology of Biomedicine.* Malden, MA: John Wiley & Sons.

Martin, Melanie. 2014. "Manufactured Mommy Wars. Le Sigh." *Mammals Suck . . . Milk!* March 1. http://mammalssuck.blogspot.com/2014/03/manufactured-mommy-wars-le-sigh.html. Accessed 23 August 2015.

Moyer, Virginia A., Ned Calonge, Steven M. Teutsch, and Jeffrey R. Botkin. 2008. "Expanding Newborn Screening: Process, Policy, and Priorities." *Hastings Center Report* 38 (3): 32–39.

Moyn, Samuel. 2010. *The Last Utopia: Human Rights in History*. Cambridge, MA: Harvard University Press.

Mulligan, Jessica M. 2014. *Unmanageable Care: An Ethnography of Health Care Privatization in Puerto Rico*. New York: New York University Press.

National Commission for the Protection of Human Subjects of Biomedical and Behavioral Research. 1979. *The Belmont Report: Ethical Principles and Guidelines for the Protection of Human Subjects of Research*. April 18. http://www.hhs.gov/ohrp/humansubjects/guidance/belmont.html. Accessed 23 August 2015.

Oberlander, Jonathan. 2003. *The Political Life of Medicare*. Chicago: University of Chicago Press.

Petryna, Adriana. 2009. *When Experiments Travel: Clinical Trials and the Global Search for Human Subjects*. Princeton, NJ: Princeton University Press.

———. 2013. *Life Exposed: Biological Citizens after Chernobyl*. Reissue ed. Princeton, NJ: Princeton University Press.

Pilnick, Alison, and Robert Dingwall. 2011. "On the Remarkable Persistence of Asymmetry in Doctor/Patient Interaction: A Critical Review." *Social Science and Medicine* 72 (8): 1374–82.

Powers, Madison, and Ruth Faden. 2006. *Social Justice: The Moral Foundations of Public Health and Health Policy*. Issues in Biomedical Ethics. New York: Oxford University Press.

Quinn, Elizabeth A. 2014. "Biomarkers and Milk: Signifying Nothing: A Response to 'Is Breast Truly Best?'" *Biomarkers and Milk*. March 2. http://biomarkersandmilk.blogspot.com/2014/03/signifying-nothing-response-to-is.html. Accessed 23 August 2015.

Ragin, Charles C., and Howard Saul Becker. 1992. *What Is a Case? Exploring the Foundations of Social Inquiry*. New York: Cambridge University Press.

Rawls, John. 1958. "Justice as Fairness." *Philosophical Review* 67 (2): 164–94.

Sen, Amartya K. 1979. "Equality of What?" Paper presented at the Tanner Lectures on Human Values, Stanford University, Stanford, CA, May 22.

Storeng, Katerini T., and Dominique P. Béhague. 2014. "'Playing the Numbers Game': Evidence-Based Advocacy and the Technocratic Narrowing of the Safe Motherhood Initiative." *Medical Anthropology Quarterly* 28 (2): 260–79.

Timmermans, Carsten. 2014. "Not Moribund at All! An Historian of Medicine's Response to Richard Horton." *The Guardian*, August 4, Science section. http://www.theguardian.com/science/the-h-word/2014/aug/04/not-moribund-historian-medicine-response-richard-horton. Accessed 23 August 2015.

Watson, Michael S., Marie Y. Mann, Michele A. Lloyd-Puryear, Piero Rinaldo, and
  R. Rodney Howell. 2006. "Newborn Screening: Toward a Uniform Screening Panel
  and System: Executive Summary." *Genetics in Medicine* 8 (S5): 1S–11S.
WHO (World Health Organization). 1948. *Constitution of the World Health Organization.*
  Geneva: World Health Organization.
———. 2014. "World Health Statistics 2014." *WHO.* http://www.who.int/gho/
  publications/world_health_statistics/2014/en/. Accessed 23 August 2015.

PART I

Interrogating Normative Perspectives
on Health Inequality and Justice

1

Health Difference, Disparity, Inequality, or Inequity—What Difference Does It Make What We Call It?

An Approach to Conceptualizing and Measuring Health Inequalities and Health Equity

Paula Braveman

ABSTRACT

Over the past two and a half decades, distinct approaches have been taken to defining and measuring health inequalities or disparities and health equity. Some efforts have focused on technical issues in measurement, often without addressing the implications for the concepts themselves and how that might influence action. Others have focused on the concepts, often without addressing the implications for measurement. This chapter contrasts approaches that have been proposed, examining their conceptual bases and implications for measurement and policy. It argues for an approach to defining health inequalities and health equity that centers on notions of justice and has its basis in ethical and human rights principles as well as empirical evidence. According to this approach, health inequality or disparity is used to refer to a subset of health differences that are closely linked with—but not necessarily proven to be caused by—social disadvantage. The term "inequity," which means injustice, could also be used, but arguments are presented for using it somewhat more sparingly, for those inequalities or disparities in health or its determinants that we know are caused by social disadvantage.

BACKGROUND AND OVERVIEW

Over the past two and a half decades, distinct approaches have been taken to defining and measuring health inequalities or disparities and health equity. Some efforts have focused on technical issues in measurement, at times without addressing the implications for the concepts themselves and how that might influence action. Others have focused on the concepts, sometimes without adequately addressing the implications for measurement. This chapter contrasts a few different approaches, examining their conceptual bases and the implications for measurement and policy. It argues for an approach to defining health inequalities and health equity that centers explicitly on notions of justice and has its basis in ethical and human rights principles as well as empirical evidence.

According to this human-rights-based approach, health inequalities or disparities are potentially avoidable differences in health that adversely affect socially disadvantaged groups, and, more specifically, groups that have experienced discrimination or social exclusion.[1] The concept of "health inequalities" refers to a subset of health differences that are closely linked to, but not necessarily proven to be caused by, social disadvantage. The differences may have been caused by social disadvantage, but proof of their causation is not required to call them inequalities/disparities. These health differences are unfair because they put an already socially disadvantaged group at further disadvantage with respect to their health, and health is needed to escape social disadvantage. These differences can be measured. The term "inequity," which means injustice, could also be used for such differences, but arguments are presented here for using that term somewhat more sparingly, to refer to those inequalities or disparities in health or its determinants that we know are caused by social disadvantage. The sharpest contrast with the rights-based approach is with an approach that may be referred to as the "ungrouped" or "univariate" approach, which compares individuals based only on their health, rather than examining how health is distributed across different social groups. Another approach is to compare groups but not restrict the comparisons to those reflecting social advantage. This chapter discusses these approaches, their conceptual foundations, and their implications.

Unlike the other two approaches, the human-rights-based approach acknowledges that values inevitably play an important role in science, shaping the questions we ask and sometimes the methods we use. For example, King comments in this volume that "normative judgments about inequity are often embedded in measures of inequality" (218). And in her chapter on global health inequalities and justice, Ruger notes, "An essential first step in redressing wrongs is exposing the wrongs and making explicit the values on which proposed action is based" (70). Wrongs can be hidden in data that are not broken down by meaningful markers of social advantage and disadvantage. I believe that our values are always operating, regardless of whether we are aware of them, and should be made explicit. Scientists must constantly strive to eliminate distortion of the truth arising from any source, including consciously or unconsciously held values.

↳ how, when unconscious?

THE NEED FOR A CONCEPTUALLY SOUND DEFINITION
OF HEALTH INEQUALITIES AND EQUITY

Health disparity or inequality is hardly a household term anywhere, but over the course of the last fifteen to twenty-five years it has become increasingly familiar in public health and medical circles in the United States and elsewhere. It is, however, rarely defined. In the United States, without further explanation, health disparity is generally assumed to refer to racial or ethnic disparities in health. The term "health disparities" first came into wide use with initiatives around the year 2000, including the establishment of the Office of Minority Health within the U.S. Department of Health and Human Services. The National Institutes of Health defines health disparities as differences in health among "specific populations," without identifying the criteria that would help one decide which groups are relevant. If interpreted literally, this definition would include all differences in health among any groups of people, such as relatively worse health among the elderly than among young adults, or a higher incidence of arm or leg fractures among skiers than among nonskiers. The label is also used at times to refer to socioeconomic and other forms of disparities (e.g., gender, sexual orientation, gender identity, or disability) as well. Outside the United States, the term "health inequalities," which first came into widespread public health usage in the United Kingdom and Western Europe in the 1990s, has prevailed. There, "health inequalities" has primarily been used to refer to differences in health among different socioeconomic groups, although it also has been used at times to refer to health differences by gender, ethnic group, nativity, and other social characteristics. In this chapter, "inequality" and "disparity," whose dictionary definitions are the same, are used interchangeably, while the related terms "equity" and, by implication, "inequity" are seen as distinct.

The term "health inequity" has also been used both within and outside the United States. A succinct and eloquent definition of health inequity was coined by Margaret Whitehead in the United Kingdom almost twenty-five years ago. She defined health inequities as differences in health that are avoidable, unnecessary, unfair, and unjust (Whitehead 1992). That definition has provided inspiration and guidance globally. However, in some situations, notably those where a strong sense of social solidarity is lacking, more specificity may be needed. Notions of what is avoidable and unnecessary vary greatly. For example, many believe that "the poor will always be with us" and that the poor will tend to have worse health because they often have poor health-related behaviors for which they are to blame. Similarly, notions of what is fair and just can be strikingly different. For example, in the United States, attitudes toward progressivity in taxation vary dramatically, and in some parts of the world it is considered fair that women have few legal rights because of deeply held beliefs about women's proper roles in the society. Agencies charged with addressing health disparities may sometimes face pressures to allocate their limited resources to address health differences affecting groups that are not socially disadvantaged, such as a health difference between two affluent communities. Given the lack of clarity regarding the concepts of health inequalities/disparities and equity, over the past two decades, a series of technical and sometimes political challenges have emerged, threatening to derail efforts to achieve greater social justice in the health domain. I have attempted to produce a definition that can withstand many of the actual and potential challenges that could jeopardize efforts toward greater health equity. Key criteria for a definition are that it be both conceptually and technically sound and that it can be operationalized for the purpose of measurement; without measurement there is no accountability.

DEFINING HEALTH INEQUALITIES AND EQUITY
BASED ON HUMAN RIGHTS AND ETHICS

Based on principles from the fields of ethics and human rights (discussed below), health inequalities or disparities are defined as potentially avoidable differences in health that adversely affect socially disadvantaged groups, particularly groups that have experienced discrimination or social exclusion. The differences must be systematic, not exceptions (Starfield 2001). Avoidability does not have to be proven, but it must be at least theoretically plausible, that is, biologically plausible based on the best available scientific knowledge. It is not essential to know that the inequalities were caused by social injustice. To determine whether a potentially avoidable difference is a health inequality or not, it is only necessary to establish that the difference involves worse health (or greater health risk) among groups that are socially disadvantaged. (Differences in the factors that shape health and that adversely affect disadvantaged groups also may be thought of as health inequalities or more precisely as inequalities in opportunities to be healthy.)

Equity and equality are not the same. Equity is an ethical value. Merriam-Webster Online (2014) defines equity as "fairness or justice in the way people are treated." Health equity means fairness or justice in how people are treated, insofar as it affects their health. It means equal opportunities to be healthy. While equal rights and equal treatment under the law reflect values, equality, like parity, may refer simply to numerical equivalence. Equal treatment for all groups may be unjust when some groups, such as those who are socially disadvantaged, need more resources or services to be healthy than those who are better off. In some societies that are particularly oppressive to women, for example, women's life expectancy is equal to that of men. However, in all societies in which women are not extremely disadvantaged by their gender, women generally live longer than men. Several scholars have concluded that this is biologically based (Fukuda-Parr and Shiva Kumar 2003; Holden 1987; Sen 1992; Anand and Sen 1996; Waldron 1983) rather than reflecting inequitable treatment of males. Thus, equal life expectancy for men and women would not be equitable. Similarly, disparity or inequality could potentially refer neutrally just to any difference, without qualification, but both terms generally imply that there is something about the specified difference that does not seem right.

One might ask whether we can just use "inequality" and "disparity" in a value-neutral way, and use "inequity" to refer to differences seen as unfair. On the surface, this has strong appeal. I believe, however, that there is value in retaining the terms "health inequality" or "disparity" in the public health lexicon to refer not only to any differences or variations in health and its determinants but, more specifically, to those differences or variations that raise concerns about justice, even though definitive proof of their causation may not be available. There may be limited acceptance for calling many important health differences "health inequities" when knowledge of their causes is lacking, as is often the case. Examples of health inequity, following this perspective, would include shorter life expectancy among American Indians and African Americans than among European Americans in the United States, higher rates of child mortality in many resource-poor countries than in more affluent nations, and higher rates of lead poisoning among children in poor families than among children in more affluent families. Many would not consider the black-white disparities in birth weight, premature birth rate, and breast cancer mortality health inequities because their causes are unknown. They would, however, qualify as health inequalities/disparities, warranting inclusion in the health equity research agenda.

Not all health differences are health inequalities or disparities. Furthermore, not all health differences that warrant concerted attention are health inequalities; criteria in addition to equity, such as effectiveness and efficiency, need to be considered along with equity. Health inequalities are a particular subset of health differences that are closely linked to social advantage and disadvantage. They adversely affect groups of people who are socially disadvantaged, as reflected by their low levels of wealth, influence, prestige, or acceptance in society. Socially disadvantaged groups include, but are not limited to, people who have low incomes, low educational levels, little wealth, or low-status jobs; members of disadvantaged racial or ethnic groups; members of sexual minority groups (defined by sexual orientation or gender identity); disabled persons; in many contexts, women; and other groups that have historically experienced discrimination, exclusion, or marginalization (Braveman, Kumanyika, et al. 2011; USDHHS and ODPHP 2011). Whether a group has historically experienced discrimination or been excluded or marginalized can be documented empirically.

While distinct, health equity and health inequalities are intrinsically intertwined. Equity is the value, the principle that underlies a commitment to reduce and ultimately eliminate health inequalities. Inequalities/disparities in health and in the determinants of health, including social determinants as well as medical care, are the metric used to assess progress toward greater equity in health. Health equity means social justice in health. Pursuing health equity means striving for the highest possible standard of health for all people while giving special attention to the needs of those at greatest risk of poor health on the basis of their social conditions. A reduction in health inequalities (in absolute and relative terms) is evidence that we are moving toward greater health equity. The reference group for equity comparisons should be the most socially advantaged group in a society; their health indicates what should be possible for everyone. Moving toward greater equity is achieved by selectively improving the health of those who are socially disadvantaged, not by a decline in the health of those in advantaged groups.

THE EMPIRIC, ETHICAL, AND HUMAN RIGHTS BASIS FOR DEFINING HEALTH INEQUALITIES BASED ON SOCIAL ADVANTAGE AND DISADVANTAGE

What is the basis for singling out a particular category of health differences, namely those linked with social disadvantage, for special attention? The characteristics that define the *relevant* groups—wealth, education, occupational rank, race or ethnic group, gender, sexual orientation or gender identity, disability—are not chosen on a whim. They are chosen based on extensive evidence collected over centuries that social disadvantage is powerfully linked with ill health, and on widely held values articulated in the fields of ethics and human rights.

Empirical Evidence

A massive body of evidence strongly links social disadvantage with avoidable illness, disability, suffering, and premature death. Many, but not all, who have studied this evidence believe the links are causal (Braveman 2010; Adler and Stewart 2010; WHOCSDH 2008; Krieger 2001; Virchow 2006; Rosen 1993; Winslow 1948). King (chapter 8, this volume) claims that the evidence that social advantage affects health consists only of associations, not causal links. I disagree. The evidence base repeatedly links various forms of social advantage/disadvantage with diverse health outcomes in diverse settings and populations, and it includes far more than just observed associations. The body of knowledge on the social determinants of health comes from research with a range of designs, including longitudinal studies that establish the temporal sequence of predictors and outcomes and quasi-experimental studies using varied techniques to address potential bias. The evidence base includes some experimental evidence, although the latter is more limited largely because it is often unethical or unfeasible to randomly assign which people will receive an intervention whose health effects (which the study aims to examine) may be uncertain but whose other benefits (e.g., additional schooling or income, better housing) are known or widely believed to be substantial for reasons other than health. The extent and depth of the evidence showing that social advantage/disadvantage affects health is particularly remarkable because social factors often exert their effects over long and complex pathways that may take decades or generations to manifest, with opportunities for interaction at each step.

Criteria for causal inference include consistency and reproducibility, temporal plausibility (the hypothesized cause precedes the effect), and biological plausibility. In addition, observing a dose-response relationship between predictor and outcome greatly increases the strength of a causal inference. The evidence base on the social determinants of health meets all of these criteria. In the past two decades, science has taken enormous leaps toward elucidating the pathways and biological mechanisms through which social advantage influences health, including not only physiologic responses to stress, but also the complex phenomena leading to and sustaining obesity, the physiology of addiction, and increased knowledge of how hazardous physical exposures (e.g., to pollutants) can lead to ill health.

There is ample evidence of the biological plausibility of social disadvantage as a cause of ill health (Adler and Stewart 2010). For example, research in the basic sciences has found that chronic stress can disrupt physiological systems (e.g., neuroendocrine, immune) in ways likely to markedly increase the risk of chronic disease and premature mortality in adulthood (Seeman et al. 2010; Evans and Kim 2007). Chronic stress can lead to the shortening of telomeres, the caps on the ends of chromosomes that predict cellular aging (Puterman et al. 2015). Children aged seven to thirteen whose parents had never attended college were shown to have shorter telomeres than children of college-educated parents (Needham et al. 2012). Children from disadvantaged backgrounds have been shown to have heightened activation of stress-response systems, and altered neural development in particular areas of the brain (Center on the Developing Child 2015; Shonkoff 2011). Many studies have identified chemical mediators of inflammation triggered by stress patterned according to social class (e.g., G. Miller et al. 2014; Seeman et al. 2010). In a randomized trial, high-quality early childhood intervention programs have been shown to result in a reduced risk of cardiovascular and metabolic disease in adulthood, narrowing the socioeconomic gap in these outcomes (Campbell et al. 2014). Sleep quality is believed to be an important mediator of some adverse health effects of social disadvantage (Hale et al. 2013). Poverty may directly impede cognitive function (Mani et al. 2013), which in turn results in social disadvantage. A dose-response relationship has been documented repeatedly between measures of social disadvantage and a wide range of important health outcomes across the life span (Braveman 2010). These are just a few of many examples; they do not, of course, establish a causal relationship with complete certainty.

However, complete certainty is an illusory goal. Even though the results of randomized controlled trials were for decades considered the gold standard for causal inference in medicine and public health, one cannot infer with certainty that the relationships observed in trials are generalizable to other populations and settings. One of the main obstacles to studying health outcomes of social factors such as wealth or education is that the health effects are typically quite lagged in time and often, particularly for experiences in childhood, do not manifest themselves for decades. Studies rarely have the resources to follow participants over such long periods of time. In addition, the causal pathways from such "upstream" (i.e., fundamental) factors to health are complex, with opportunities for effect modification at every step in a long causal chain (Braveman, Egerter, et al. 2011). Considering the difficulties of studying how social factors affect health, it is in fact remarkable that they are so pervasively and repeatedly observed to do so across such a range of conditions. And it is not at all surprising that there are many exceptions. One would expect effect modification by different factors that can interact, modifying the relationship between social factors and health—for some factors, some populations, and some health outcomes—but these are exceptions to a pervasively observed rule.

Experience has shown that social disadvantage can be ameliorated by social policies such as minimum wage laws, progressive taxation, high-quality early childhood development programs, and statutes barring race-based discrimination in hospitals. The health consequences of social disadvantage also have been shown to be ameliorable at least to some extent by social policies (Almond, Chay, and Greenstone 2006; Bailey and Danziger 2013; Campbell et al. 2014; Zhao and Luman 2010; Zhao and Smith 2013).

Ethics

The proposed group approach to defining health inequalities also has a basis in principles from the field of ethics. Daniels and other ethicists have pointed out that health is needed for functioning in every sphere of life. The economist Amartya Sen advanced the notion that human development should be measured not in economic terms but in terms of the growth of human capability to freely pursue quality of life, with health among the essential capabilities. Therefore, the resources needed to be healthy—including not only medical care (Daniels 1983) but also health-promoting living and working conditions—should not be treated as commodities like designer clothing or luxury cars. Rather, they should be distributed according to need, not privilege. An aversion to health inequalities reflects widely held social values that call for everyone to have a fair chance to be healthy, given that health is crucial for well-being, longevity, and economic and other social opportunities. The philosopher John Rawls argued for the ethical obligation to maximize the welfare of those who are worse off. This notion has been influential in shaping ethical theories relevant to health equity. While not specific to the domain of health, this idea is clearly applicable to the concept of a societal obligation to make concerted efforts to improve the health of socially disadvantaged groups (Rawls 1971, 1985).

Human Rights

In addition to empirical observations and ethical notions, laws, treaties, and principles from the field of human rights also provide a basis for the proposed approach to defining health inequalities, one that is perhaps both more extensively developed and more powerful. By now, a vast majority of countries have signed, if not ratified, major human rights agreements that are of great relevance to health disparities. Signing without ratifying implies agreeing in principle without agreeing to be monitored or held accountable. These agreements are the products of discussions including representatives of virtually every country. While human rights agreements are all too often violated, they represent a global consensus on fundamental values that, hammered out over many years, greatly strengthens the basis for defining the concept of health inequalities. Under international human rights laws and agreements, countries are obligated to protect, promote, and fulfill the human rights of everyone in their populations. Recognizing that many countries lack the resources to remove all obstacles to all rights for everyone immediately, human rights agreements require that countries demonstrate "progressive realization"—in other words, that they make gradual, incremental progress toward realizing the rights of their populations. Of particular relevance for understanding health inequalities and health equity is the implicit obligation to pay particular attention to those segments of the population that experience the most social obstacles. Presumably, social obstacles are of particular concern because of their amenability to social interventions.

Think about Brazil's "right to health" & judicialization

The "right to health," defined as the right to attain the highest attainable standard of health, is the principle that generally comes to mind first when considering human rights in relation to health. The rights-based approach proposed in this chapter maintains that, for the purpose of measurement, the highest possible standard of health is indicated by the level of health enjoyed by the most socially privileged group in a society (Braveman 2006). One could argue from the perspective of a global society that this is a conservative standard because the highest level of health in one's own society—for example, in a resource-poor nation—may be quite low compared with the highest level of health in affluent nations, which arguably should be used as the standard. In practice, however, human rights agreements allow countries to design implementation measures in relation to their own populations. Thus, in practical terms, using the highest standard of health within one's nation is likely to prevail. We should not forget, however, the aspirational goal for all to reach the standard of health in the most affluent nation, which echoes Ruger's call for "a new understanding of obligations, both national and international" (81).

The right to health is not only a right to health care. This principle has an empirical basis, given that a large body of knowledge, including sources cited above, indicates that the resources needed to be healthy include not only quality medical care, but also education and health-promoting physical and social conditions in homes, neighborhoods, and workplaces. Furthermore, human rights principles call for countries to remove obstacles to health in any sector—for example, in education, housing, or transportation—and explicitly call for the right to a standard of living necessary to protect and promote health (UNGA 1966; Braveman 2010). "The right to health means that States must generate conditions in which everyone can be as healthy as possible" (OHCHR and WHO 2013); it does not mean the right to be healthy.

Equally relevant to defining health inequalities are the human rights principles of nondiscrimination and equality. According to these principles, everyone has equal rights, and nations are obligated to prohibit policies that have either the intention or the effect of discriminating against particular social groups. This is important because it is often very difficult to establish persons' or institutions' intentions. In addition, at the population level in the United States currently, greater harm to health may be done as a result of unintentional discriminatory processes and structures that persist as the legacy of slavery and Jim Crow (both of which were legal and intentionally discriminatory in their time), even when conscious intent to discriminate cannot be documented. Examples of such processes and structures include bank policies that exacerbate racial segregation, criminal justice codes that result in disproportionate incarceration of African American men, and school funding policies that rely on local property tax bases. These may no longer reflect conscious intent to discriminate; nevertheless, they persist and transmit economic and other social disadvantages with health consequence across generations (D. R. Williams and Collins 2001; D. R. Williams and Mohammed 2009).

Because human rights agreements and principles prohibit de facto (unintentional, institutional, or structural) as well as intentional discrimination, we do not have to know the causes of a given health difference to call it a health inequality. Health inequalities reflecting poorer health among a socially disadvantaged group are inequitable, even when we do not know the causes, because they put an already socially disadvantaged group at further disadvantage with respect to their health. Furthermore, health is necessary to overcome social disadvantage (Braveman 2006; Braveman, Kumanyika, et al. 2011). There will inevitably be a higher bar regarding the issue of causation when using the term "inequity" than when using "inequality" or "disparity." In theory one could argue, as I have done here, that health differences adversely affecting socially disadvantaged groups can be called inequities regardless of their causes because they have the effect of compounding the disadvantage of an already disadvantaged group. In practice, however, I believe it would be difficult to mobilize public and policy-maker opinion to take action to address an "inequity" if one could not account for the causes and make a good case that they were likely to be unjust. By contrast, labeling a difference such as the racial difference in preterm birth a "health inequality" that deserves concerted public policy attention has more chance of succeeding. The terms "inequality" or "disparity" express concern without making causal attributions. This will probably remain a contentious issue.

EQUITY ACROSS SOCIAL GROUPS OR AMONG INDIVIDUALS?

Both the Whitehead definition (implicitly) and the proposed approach (explicitly) focus on the distribution of health across different social groups, and specifically across groups with different levels of social advantage. Some have argued, however, that we should not approach health inequalities, which they define as any potentially avoidable differences or variations in health, without reference to social advantage or disadvantage from a perspective based on a priori assumptions about their nature. Contending that examining health inequalities across different predetermined social groups inevitably leads to such biased assumptions, they have proposed that we simply measure health differences among ungrouped individuals (Murray, Gakidou, and Frenk 1999). This would entail comparing the healthiest individuals to the sickest individuals and those individuals in between without grouping them according to preselected social characteristics, such as income, education, occupation, or area of residence. While the proponents of this approach have not explicitly mentioned race as a relevant characteristic, their arguments would, presumably, apply to race as well as to other individual characteristics, such as gender, disability status, and so on. Once the healthiest and the sickest are identified, according to the proponents of this ungrouped approach, we can embark on an investigative process of seeking the likely sources of the differences. This may be thought of as a univariate approach, the single variable being the level of health. By contrast, traditional approaches to measuring health inequalities typically are at least bivariate; they examine health differences by socioeconomic characteristics (e.g., education, occupation, income, wealth), by racial or ethnic group, and/or by other markers of social advantage/disadvantage (e.g., gender, disability, sexual orientation, or gender identity). The main argument for abandoning the traditional grouped approach is that it prejudges causality, potentially obscuring full inquiry into the nature of health differences. This perspective, in one form or another, has at different times won over a surprising number of advocates, principally those attracted by its novel, technical appeal.

The ungrouped or univariate approach undeniably has some attractions. At first glance, it seems simpler than the standard approach, because it removes the necessity of having data disaggregated by the dimensions of inequality of interest; the availability of meaningfully disaggregated data is a challenge globally. Using the univariate approach, one just arrays the data on health according to the degree of health (or ill health), and then embarks on a path of discovery from that point, using whatever tools one has at one's disposal, to try to determine what explains the health differences between the groups. This sounds conceptually elegant. Unfortunately, however, once one has shown the dispersion of health (without regard for its distribution), one has to undertake a complex process of inquiry to discover the causes of these differences, which requires multivariate statistical techniques that are outside the capabilities of most state and local health agencies in the United States as well as globally. Furthermore, there is nothing in the univariate approach that dictates that social disadvantage be considered in looking for the causes of health differences. The univariate approach thus runs the risk of removing questions about the role of social disadvantage in health differences from the agenda for research and action to address health inequalities.

Another stated advantage of the ungrouped or univariate approach is its potential to avoid bias. The ungrouped approach's proponents claim that when we routinely examine inequalities from the starting point of comparisons based on some predetermined social characteristic—for example, social class—we are biasing inquiry toward confirming an a priori assumption that social class is the cause of the inequalities. This seems unfounded, given that anyone with scientific training knows that associations do not prove causation. It should be acknowledged, however, that most people, including most policy makers, lack scientific training and may often assume that, for example, an association between income and a health measure necessarily implies causation. The ungrouped or univariate approach, at least in theory, lessens the potential for bias, particularly among nontechnical persons, in prejudging causality.

There is, however, a fatal flaw in the ungrouped approach when it is used to assess health inequality as implicitly understood by those who have devoted their careers to reducing health inequalities. The ungrouped approach does not consider the issues of social justice or equity that constitute the very core of any examination of health differences patterned according to social advantage and disadvantage. Furthermore, with respect to the critique of the grouped or bivariate approach that is more vulnerable to bias, it is part of basic scientific training in all disciplines to avoid the error of inferring causation from association. There is widespread awareness that if a variable used to stratify a population is found to be associated with a given outcome, one cannot infer that that variable per se is necessarily a cause of the outcome. Particularly in a nonacademic context, a statement interpreting a given set of descriptive observations may infer a causal connection, based on integrating knowledge from multiple sources and not only the observed associations that were cited. Observing the associations that were identified may be helpful in suggesting what kinds of factors should be considered in searching for causal explanations. Exploration of causes generally requires more in-depth and complex analyses. The fact that inadequately trained people may make unjustified causal attributions is an argument for more training and ongoing professional education, but it is not a good argument for abandoning the investigation of how health is distributed by markers of social advantage.

HOW DOES THE PROPOSED APPROACH ADDRESS CHALLENGES
IN DEFINING AND MEASURING HEALTH INEQUALITIES?

The proposed approach addresses a number of important challenges faced in defining and measuring health inequalities, such as the burden of proof regarding causation, how to prove causation, whether to compare groups or individuals, which groups should be compared, which group should serve as the reference group for the comparison, and whether health equity should be concerned only with equity in health care and health status itself or with the social determinants of health.

Burden of Proof Regarding Causation

Research proposed here addresses potential challenges related to the burden of proof regarding causality. It would be more succinct and intuitive to define health inequalities/disparities as health differences caused by injustice. The causes of many important health inequalities, however, may not be known or may be debatable. The proposed definition deliberately avoids the need for making inferences about the causes of health inequalities, which are defined simply on the basis of how they are patterned socially, which can be observed: a health inequality is a difference in health that adversely affects a socially disadvantaged group. This approach removes the burden of proving whether a given health difference was caused by injustice in order to consider it an inequality/disparity. This is important because it is generally difficult to establish causal connections between social indicators and health. And it is particularly difficult to do so in the case of upstream social determinants such as wealth or racial discrimination because the causal chains from such upstream determinants to health effects are generally long (often over decades, perhaps generations) and highly complex (Braveman, Egerter, et al. 2011).

It is also important to have a definition that does not require knowing the causes of the relevant health differences because the causes of many health differences that represent a tremendous burden of ill health for disadvantaged groups are unknown. This is true, for example, of racial disparities in preterm birth (PTB) and low birth weight (LBW). PTB and LBW are strong predictors not only of infant mortality, but also of child development, adult chronic diseases such as heart disease and diabetes, and premature mortality in adulthood. They are doubtless among the most important health indicators. Given the marked differences in PTB and LBW rates and their lifelong health consequences between African Americans (blacks) and European Americans (whites), addressing these differences should be an important part of an agenda to reduce racial disparities in health. Yet if we define health disparities as differences caused by injustice, these differences probably would be off the agenda because their causes are currently unknown; it will seem questionable to many to call a situation unjust if we do not know its causes. Many of us have hypotheses about the underlying causes of racial disparities in birth outcomes that, if proven true, would indeed demonstrate that injustice is a contributing cause. However, our hypotheses, while biologically plausible, are unproven. Therefore, if demonstrating that injustice is the cause of a given health difference constitutes a criterion for calling that difference a disparity/inequality, these important health differences would not meet the criteria and would not receive attention on the health inequalities agenda. This does not seem right. Similarly, large black-white differences in breast cancer mortality are seen even among women presenting at the same stage. While some researchers have concluded that these differences can be largely explained by socioeconomic factors and/or differences in care received (Mandelblatt, Sheppard, and Neugut 2013), others believe that genetic differences are also likely contributors (Danforth 2013; Dunn et al. 2010; Setiawan et al. 2009).

Regardless of the causes of a given health inequality, however, adverse health in a socially disadvantaged group deserves concerted attention because it puts an already disadvantaged social group at further disadvantage with respect to its health. Social disadvantage is further compounded because health is needed to escape it. Such compounding of disadvantage will be widely viewed as unfair. Therefore, it could be argued that all health inequalities, as defined here, are inequities because they compound the disadvantage of vulnerable groups, and that it would be better to dispense with the ambiguity of inequalities/disparities in favor of the more explicit term "inequities." It seems wise, however, to use the term "inequities" very judiciously, particularly when referring to inequalities whose causes are not known; this use of "inequities" sparingly, in favor of "inequalities" or "disparities," would avoid challenges on technical grounds, and it may be more effective in communicating to wide audiences that this strong term should be reserved for comparisons where injustice can be more easily explained. I also believe it would be a strategic error to abandon the use of "health inequalities/disparities" and treat those terms as if they are equivalent to the value-neutral "differences" or "variations." Domestically and globally, in the health sphere, they are widely understood to refer to differences that raise concerns about justice; abandoning those terms could undermine progress that has been made to date in building consensus and momentum in health policy and in social policy overall.

Relevant Groups and Comparisons

The human-rights-based approach indicates that comparisons between social groups, rather than individuals, are relevant, and it specifies the groups to be compared. These are groups with different levels of social advantage and disadvantage—that is, with different levels of resources, power, prestige, and social acceptance. Human rights agreements help to specify the relevant groups, including racial, ethnic, tribal, caste, and socioeconomic groups, as well as groups defined by gender, gender identity, sexual orientation, or physical and mental disability. Human rights treaties and other agreements name these groups (and others) as examples of vulnerable groups whose human rights deserving special efforts toward the protection, promotion, and fulfillment of their human rights. The implicit criterion for designating these groups as warranting special attention is that these groups have historically experienced discrimination, exclusion, or marginalization. The proposed approach makes it clear that the relevant measurements are across groups, not individuals, and disadvantaged groups may have individual members who do not appear to be economically disadvantaged. The fact that the United States has an African American president, thus, does not imply that African Americans are no longer a disadvantaged group.

Furthermore, the human-rights-based approach specifies that relevant comparisons are ones in which disadvantaged groups do worse than the advantaged. This stipulation is needed because challenges have been mounted that demand that resources to address health inequalities be used to address one or more of the very few situations in which a more advantaged group actually does worse on a health indicator. Example of such situations include a higher incidence of breast cancer among white women (despite the higher mortality from breast cancer among black women), a shorter life expectancy among whites than among Latinos, and a shorter life expectancy among men than among women.

Measurement Challenges: Defining Disadvantage

Ascertaining whether a group is disadvantaged can be accomplished through comparisons based on, for example, levels of wealth or income, representation in high political office or executive positions, or experience of hate crimes. Data are generally available on all of these for large racial and ethnic groups, although data are often lacking for American Indians and for groups defined by sexual orientation or gender identity. A commitment to equity would call for more studies of the health of American Indians and LGBT populations.

Particularly if inequalities by age and gender are considered, the groups considered socially disadvantaged could comprise a large proportion of the population, even in an overall affluent country like the United States, potentially rendering the notion of health equity to have little meaning in practice. Priorities must be set for an equity agenda that considers both the depth and extent of social disadvantage and of ill health experienced by potentially relevant groups. In the United States, these considerations would place disparities by race, particularly those affecting African Americans and American Indians, as well as income-based disparities very high on the equity agenda.

Measurement Challenges: The Reference Group

There has been controversy about the appropriate reference group(s) for equity comparisons. The proposed approach, drawing on ethical and human rights principles, specifies that the reference group should be one with a relatively high level of social advantage. By contrast, in the ungrouped approach, the reference group includes individuals with the highest levels of health, regardless of their nonhealth characteristics, such as wealth, racial or ethnic group, or gender. Others who do not subscribe to the ungrouped approach have often used overall population average as the reference group (Minority Health and Health Disparities Research and Education Act 2000). The justification for making the most socially advantaged group the reference for equity comparisons is based on the ethical principle of egalitarianism and the right-to-health principle, which asserts the right of all people to enjoy the highest possible standard of health. The health of the most socially privileged group (the ones with the greatest influence, wealth, or prestige, e.g., wealthy individuals, households, or neighborhoods, or, for racial/ethnic comparisons, the health of non-Latino whites) indicates what should be possible for all groups. It may be argued that those who are most socially privileged attained that status in part because they were especially healthy, rather than being healthy because of social advantage. Differences in health according to social advantage/disadvantage may reflect in part that some individuals experience declines in income because of poor health. Considerable evidence, however, suggests that reverse causation (poor health causing lower income) plays a lesser role than forward causation (low income leading to poor health), and it supports the conclusion that the primary relationship is one in which social disadvantage produces or exacerbates ill health (Kaplan, Shema, and Leite 2008; Kawachi, Adler, and Dow 2010; Marmot 2002; Muennig 2008). If, however, the comparisons were to be made solely according to levels of health, without considering how health is distributed socially, a sizable proportion of the healthiest group might consist of individuals with more favorable genotypes. This would limit the utility of comparing the sickest with the healthiest without considering social characteristics.

Average levels of health are too low a standard for equity comparisons. In a society with a large proportion of people who are disadvantaged, the level of health of many disadvantaged groups will be close to the average level because the groups' size drives the average, but this is hardly an indicator of equity.

Measurement Challenge: Absolute versus Relative Comparisons

As King notes (chapter 8, this volume), questions have often arisen regarding whether absolute or relative comparisons are appropriate for assessing health equity. Both are important to consider because, as King illustrates well, important information could be hidden by considering only relative or only absolute measures.

Conceptual Challenge: Allocation of Resources for Health according to Need versus a Minimum Basic Level (of Services and Health) for All

To some, equitable allocation of resources for health should be based on need, while others have interpreted equity to require only a basic minimum level of services for everyone. The reasoning articulated immediately above regarding the appropriate reference group for health inequality/disparity comparisons calls for the comparison to include the most socially advantaged group in a society, based on the human rights concept of "the highest attainable standard of health." This principle implies that bringing everyone only to a basic minimum level of health would be insufficient. In practical terms, however, in many societies, it would in fact be a tremendous step toward health equity to ensure a basic minimum level of health for everyone if that level were a decent one. Yamin has noted that while ensuring a minimum essential level of health care, housing, education, and other living conditions would reduce absolute deprivation, equality is a matter of relative deprivation (Yamin 2009). While there may not be a sufficient societal consensus to create the political will to commit to achieving the highest attainable standard of health for everyone, it should be kept on the agenda as an ultimate goal.

Measurement Challenges: Which Determinants of Health?

The question has arisen whether it is appropriate in striving for health equity to focus on inequalities in the social (i.e., nonmedical) determinants of health, such as income, education, and other living and working conditions repeatedly demonstrated to be tightly associated with health. The chapter by King (chapter 8, this volume) argues that the evidence base linking social factors with health outcomes is weak, consisting only of associations with inadequate bases for causal inference. In the earlier section on empirical evidence, I presented arguments to the contrary, acknowledging that absolute certainty is not an appropriate standard. In civil law, the standard for making a decision that a plaintiff is guilty is preponderance of evidence of guilt; in criminal law the standard is "beyond a reasonable doubt." The U.S. Air Force probably did not conduct randomized trials to test whether parachutes save lives before providing parachutes to paratroopers (G. Smith and Pell 2003). As King points out, knowledge of a causal link between social disadvantage and ill health does not necessarily reveal the interventions that would be most effective and efficient for either mitigating social disadvantage or buffering its deleterious effects on health; figuring that out will, in most cases, require repeated trial and error.

Striving for health equity requires striving to reduce and ultimately eliminate inequalities in the determinants of health that are under the control of policies in any realm, including both medical care and the social (i.e., nonmedical) determinants of health. It would seem irrational to exclude from consideration as targets of action toward health equity an entire group of potentially modifiable factors demonstrated to have great influence on health and health equity. In addition, human rights principles, such as the indivisibility of all rights, including all the economic, social, and cultural as well as the civil and political rights, support a broad focus on social as well as medical determinants of health (Braveman 2010).

The human rights notion of governments' obligation to progressively remove obstacles to the attainment of all rights by all their people, with particular attention to those who have experienced discrimination or exclusion, seems to provide a mandate in this respect. Some scholars have pointed out, however, that human rights instruments are not explicit about the need to address nonmedical social factors and that this limitation has reduced their usefulness in guiding national health agendas (Chapman 2010). I agree, but I believe that there is enough justification for the proposed approach based on implicit grounds. An obligation to address social factors believed to be important determinants of health also seems justified based on the human rights principle of the indivisibility of all human rights, including the economic, social, and cultural rights as well as the civil and political rights.

Challenges Not Addressed by the Proposed Approach

The proposed approach does not answer all the important questions that have arisen in discussions of the meaning of equity or justice in health. It does not answer all questions regarding what constitutes justice; it does, however, provide some guidance on this issue, notably, that the reference group should be the group with the greatest level of social advantage, which would imply a goal of greater than just a minimum level. It does not clarify whether the focus should be, as espoused by Rawls (1971, 1985), on improving the welfare of the worst-off. The proposed approach does not specify the timetable on which inequalities should be reduced; the human rights principle of progressive realization could serve as an excuse for countries to do little to reduce inequalities. Furthermore, no approach to concepts or their measurement will ever be adequate to ensure relevant action; countries may adopt rights- and ethics-based rhetoric while doing little on the ground to reduce health inequalities.

Chapman (2010) and Yamin (2009) have pointed out that human rights instruments do not adequately address health equity or the social determinants of health, in part because they do not explicitly articulate the connections among them. While many of the important concepts are implicit rather than explicit, I believe that the connections can be inferred, as illustrated by previous literature (Braveman and Gruskin 2003a, 2003b).

DIFFERENCES, DISPARITIES, INEQUALITIES, INEQUITIES?

As noted earlier, there is a level of ambiguity associated with the terms "disparity" and "inequality." On the one hand, they can be used to denote any difference or variation, which do not have ethical or human rights connotations. Without further information about their nature, differences, or variations are value-neutral. Both disparity and inequality, by contrast, carry a connotation, admittedly a subtle one, of a difference that should generate some concern. And that is undoubtedly why those who led efforts to draw attention to health disparities or inequalities wisely chose those terms when they launched health equity initiatives in the 1980s (Europe) and 1990s (United States).

Health differences in general include all of the following: worse health among the elderly than among young adults, higher rates of arm or leg fractures among people who ski, and the occurrence of a particular health problem in a particular affluent community. However, addressing such differences is unlikely to make a contribution toward greater health equity. During the 1990s in the United Kingdom, there were heated debates about whether to replace "inequalities" with the more value-neutral "variations." In the United States, the official definition of health disparities for the National Institutes of Health defines them as health differences between "specific" population groups, without specifying which groups or which criteria should be used to identify them (NIH and USDHHS 2013).

Increasingly in the United States, the term "health inequity" is being used instead of "health disparity." As discussed earlier, this is a welcome shift because it makes explicit the social justice concerns at the heart of the concept of health disparities. On the other hand, this practice may be vulnerable to challenges based on the fact that the causes of many very important health differences adversely affecting socially disadvantaged groups are unknown or debatable. An example mentioned earlier is the persistent two- to threefold disparity in birth outcomes (premature birth and low birth weight) between African Americans and European Americans in the United States, whose causes remain unknown despite many plausible hypotheses. Some of those hypotheses involve long-term race-based social disadvantage, acting through physiologic pathways involving stress; this is biologically plausible in terms of current knowledge of physiology, but unproven. Other researchers believe there is a strong genetic component, although their speculation is also unproven. If we do not know the causes of a health difference, can we call it an inequity? Inequity is a very strong word because it unambiguously invokes injustice and unfairness. Can we refer to the racial disparity in birth outcomes as an inequity without knowing the causes? According to the approach espoused here, we could do that because it is an important health difference that adversely affects a socially disadvantaged group. However, many scientists and decision makers may not be comfortable with that; the argument presented here may seem too abstract. The terms "inequality" or "disparity" convey the sense that there is reason for concern about potential inequity, without falling into a potential trap that is unlikely to produce forward movement. I think it is wise, therefore, to use the term "inequity" but to use it sparingly, for situations in which claims of injustice are more easily and strongly made. I also believe that champions of equity should be clear that it is important to make the consideration of justice explicit and that the proposed definition of health inequalities justifies considering adverse health in a socially disadvantaged group to be inequitable, regardless of the causes, because such a difference puts socially disadvantaged groups at further disadvantage on their health. While I find the wholesale substitution of health "inequity" for health "inequality" to be potentially problematic, those reservations do not apply to the use of the positive word "equity."

Whether or not "inequity" is used for any health difference adversely affecting socially disadvantaged groups, I believe it would be a strategic political error to abandon the terminology of health inequality and disparity as referring to health differences linked to social disadvantage. The limited resources that have been allocated to address inequalities/disparities would then not be reserved for that purpose; they could be used to address any health difference, including differences in health among highly advantaged individuals or communities.

IT MATTERS WHAT WE CALL IT

This discussion is not just a matter of academic interest. Concepts and how they are expressed can have major effects on policies, programs, and resources. The ideas they reflect can be used to garner or undermine support for policies among policy makers and the public. Furthermore, concepts drive measurement, and without measurement there is no accountability for the effects of policies and programs. For example, a global initiative to strengthen resource-poor countries' capacity to monitor social inequalities in health was terminated, apparently because that initiative used the grouped (bivariate) rather than the ungrouped (univariate) approach to conceptualizing and measuring health inequalities. Initiatives in many countries and subnational areas rely on the ability to follow trends in the magnitude of disparities in relation to socioeconomic status, race, ethnicity, and religion in order to assess and, if appropriate, advocate for the need for continued and/or increased resources. While these data are never sufficient to achieve action, if countries lack evidence of how health and its determinants are distributed among rich versus poor and among dominant versus marginalized groups, struggles for social justice are made far more difficult. Without evidence documenting a problem, it is much more difficult to keep an issue on the policy agenda and impossible to assess the effects of any policies on it.

There is a bidirectional relationship between concepts and measurement. It may be obvious that concepts can drive measurement, but it is also true that approaches to measurement can implicitly shape concepts because, even when not explicit, they reflect hidden concepts. For example, the "ungrouped" approach implicitly but absolutely removes questions about social justice from the agenda for public health monitoring. King (chapter 8, this volume) illustrates how measurement—for example, the choice of absolute versus relative measures of inequality—can both reflect and influence value judgments. The ungrouped approach and grouped approaches that do not consider social disadvantage are examples of measurement approaches that have the capability of removing social justice considerations from efforts labeled as "equity" initiatives, without anyone ever articulating an explicit challenge to the concept of equity.

The proponents of the univariate or ungrouped approach to measurement of health inequalities have implicitly—perhaps unintentionally—defined the concept of health inequalities in a way that would strip it of its essence, which is a concern with social justice. The ungrouped approach is a perfectly legitimate epidemiological method for studying health differences in general, which encompass much more than the study of social justice in health. Indeed, this approach comprises all of the discipline of epidemiology, which is the study of health differences (in general) and their risk factors across different populations. Health inequalities, by contrast, are a subset of health differences that are tightly associated with social advantage/disadvantage, adversely affecting groups with underlying social disadvantage. Public health assessments of health equity have traditionally and almost invariably involved comparisons of health (or health determinants) among groups with different levels of social advantage—among the rich compared with the poor, for example, or among European Americans compared with African Americans, Latinos, or American Indians. The practical and theoretical basis for these comparisons has generally not been articulated, but the approach has been taken for granted as the norm.

The ungrouped approach, like other approaches that compare groups without regard to social advantage, effectively removes explicit and systematic consideration of equity from the measurement, routine monitoring, and reporting of health inequalities. Proponents of the ungrouped (or grouped but without considering social advantage) approaches have sometimes maintained that they are not abandoning a commitment to equity because any avoidable differences in health, not only those that are patterned according to social advantage, are inequitable. This reflects a definition of equity that lacks relevance to social justice, distributive justice, and the human rights principle that those groups who face more obstacles to realizing their rights should receive more attention. Health inequalities as defined here do not comprise all differences in health, or even all differences warranting attention. Health inequalities are not the only health differences that need to be addressed by policy. As a very specific subset of health differences that reflect worse health among socially disadvantaged groups, they deserve explicit and focused attention because of ethical values and human rights principles. Many other kinds of health differences may have merit in that they improve the health of the overall population or certain not socially disadvantaged groups, but they do not address justice.

Proponents of the ungrouped approach have argued that social disadvantage can be considered at a second stage of inquiry, after individuals are grouped according to their levels of health. In theory and in academia, this is true. However, this approach neglects to consider the implications for the work of public health agencies where lack of time, analytic resources, and staff trained in health equity analysis limit their monitoring efforts to two-by-two tables. Explicit questions about how health is distributed according to social disadvantage need to be an essential, required component of the routine basic monitoring activities of health agencies. Otherwise, whether or not the issue of social disadvantage comes up in further analytic stages involving multivariate analyses will be a hit-or-miss affair, left to the discretion of individual analysts. It is unrealistic to expect that analytic processes that did not include explicit questions about equity up front would nevertheless address those considerations during subsequent stages of analysis, in part because subsequent stages generally will not occur. If the bivariate monitoring of health by indicators of disadvantage is not institutionalized in routine analysis and reporting, indicators of social advantage may or may not even be considered as possible contributors to health inequalities. And if health information disaggregated by markers of social disadvantage is not part of routine surveillance, there will not be pressure to ensure the inclusion of adequate markers of disadvantage/advantage in data sources.

The human-rights-based approach has several strengths. First and foremost, it keeps equity explicitly on the agenda for research, monitoring, and action. Furthermore, consistent with empirical knowledge as well as widely held ethical and human rights principles, it makes explicit the imperative to consider social disadvantage. Human rights principles in particular provide a firm basis for this by reflecting a global consensus about values. Another major strength of this approach is the way it addresses the burden of proof regarding causation. It defines health inequality as a health difference adversely affecting socially disadvantaged groups, not a health difference *caused by* social disadvantage. Society should be concerned with health differences that adversely affect groups at underlying social disadvantage regardless of their causes because when already socially disadvantaged groups have ill health, they are doubly disadvantaged. Furthermore, good health is needed to escape social disadvantage. This compounded disadvantage and constrained opportunity for health violates a basic sense of fairness held by many societies. In addition (and related to the removal of the burden of proof regarding causation), it avoids the need for a decision about fairness (which requires both knowing the causes and judging them to be unfair) every time one wants to assess whether a given difference is an inequality. This is important because fairness is highly subjective and may be difficult to determine based on available knowledge. Finally, the proposed definition can be operationalized for the purposes of measurement.

The major—and not inconsequential—weakness of the proposed approach is that it is somewhat awkward and technical and probably not very intuitive to nonacademic audiences. It is worth considering using the eloquent and succinct Whitehead definition in nontechnical contexts and using the proposed definition as a backup, when needed in the face of technical challenges. A limitation of the rights-based approach that should be recognized is that many scientists are uncomfortable with explicitly addressing issues of values; they equate considering values with compromising scientific rigor. The ungrouped or univariate approach to defining and measuring health inequalities was presented by its proponents as a way to avoid bias based on social values; the social values underlying and reflected by that approach—that there is no societal obligation to improve the well-being of socially disadvantaged groups—were not acknowledged by the proponents. Scientists need to recognize that their work is inevitably shaped by their own and their society's values even if they can't identify or systematically examine those values. It should also be made clear that when we study health inequalities and health equity our values shape only our research questions; they do not and should not compromise our adherence to using rigorous scientific standards in studying those questions.

However, it also needs to be made clear that potential for bias is not unique to the study of explicitly value-laden issues, such as health equity. All scientists, regardless of the nature of their research questions, inevitably face challenges to their integrity in the form of temptations to compromise their methods and reporting so that they reflect desirable findings. The best approach is to make one's values explicit and expose one's work to rigorous criticism.

The ungrouped approach to health inequalities, as well as grouped approaches that do not specify that the relevant comparisons involve social disadvantage, open the door to potential diversion of the (often meager) resources that might have been devoted to health equity for other purposes. Striving for greater equity in health is always an uphill battle because it means advocating for the poor, the powerless, the excluded, and the marginalized. Therefore, efforts to ensure equity will often be perceived as a threat by those who are advantaged. If we are not clear about where we are headed and why, we can become lost and our efforts diverted in this uphill climb over many daunting obstacles.

NOTE

1. Throughout this chapter, "social" is construed to include economic.

REFERENCES

Adler, Nancy, and Judith Stewart, eds. 2010. *The Biology of Disadvantage: Socioeconomic Status and Health*. Vol. 1186, Annals of the New York Academy of Sciences. Boston: Wiley-Blackwell.

Almond, Douglas, Kenneth Y. Chay, and Michael Greenstone. 2006. "Civil Rights, the War on Poverty, and Black-White Convergence in Infant Mortality in the Rural South and Mississippi." *MIT Department of Economics Working Paper*, no. 07-04. http:// papers.ssrn.com/sol3/Papers.cfm?abstract_id=961021. Accessed 24 July 2015.

Anand, Sudhir, and Amartya Sen. 1996. "Gender Inequality in Human Development: Theories and Measurement." In *Background Papers: Human Development Report 1995*, 1–20. New York: United Nations Development Programme.

Bailey, Martha J., and Sheldon Danziger, eds. 2013. *Legacies of the War on Poverty*. New York: Russell Sage Foundation.

Braveman, Paula A. 2006. "Health Disparities and Health Equity: Concepts and Measurement." *Annual Review of Public Health* 27: 167–94. doi:10.1146/annurev .publhealth.27.021405.102103.

———. 2010. "Social Conditions, Health Equity, and Human Rights." *Health and Human Rights* 12 (2): 31–48.

Braveman, Paula A., Susan A. Egerter, Steven H. Woolf, and James S. Marks. 2011. "When Do We Know Enough to Recommend Action on the Social Determinants of Health?" *American Journal of Preventive Medicine* 40 (suppl. 1): S58–66. doi:10.1016/j.amepre.2010.09.026.

Braveman, Paula A., and Sofia Gruskin. 2003a. "Poverty, Equity, Human Rights and Health." *Bulletin of the World Health Organization* 81 (7): 539–45.

———. 2003b. "Defining Equity in Health." *Journal of Epidemiology and Community Health* 57 (4): 254–58. doi:10.1136/jech.57.4.254.

Braveman, Paula A., Shiriki Kumanyika, Jonathan Fielding, Thomas LaVeist, Luisa N. Borrell, Ron Manderscheid, and Adewale Troutman. 2011. "Health Disparities and Health Equity: The Issue Is Justice." *American Journal of Public Health* 101 (S1): S149–55. doi:10.2105/AJPH.2010.300062.

Campbell, Frances, Gabriella Conti, James J. Heckman, Seong Hyeok Moon, Rodrigo Pinto, Elizabeth Pungello, and Yi Pan. 2014. "Early Childhood Investments Substantially Boost Adult Health." *Science* 343 (6178): 1478–85. doi:10.1126/science.1248429.

Center on the Developing Child at Harvard University. 2015. "The Foundations of Lifelong Health Are Built in Early Childhood." Working paper, 1 August 2015. http://developingchild.harvard.edu/resources/reports_and_working_papers/foundations-of-lifelong-health/.

Chapman, Audrey R. 2010. "The Social Determinants of Health, Health Equity, and Human Rights." *Health and Human Rights* 12 (2): 17–30.

Danforth, David N. 2013. "Disparities in Breast Cancer Outcomes between Caucasian and African American Women: A Model for Describing the Relationship of Biological and Nonbiological Factors." *Breast Cancer Research* 15 (3): 208. doi:10.1186/bcr3429.

Daniels, Norman. 1983. "Health Care Needs and Distributive Justice." In *In Search of Equity: Health Needs and the Health Care System*, edited by Ronald Bayer, Arthur L. Caplan, and Norman Daniels, 1–41. The Hastings Center Series in Ethics. New York: Plenum.

Dunn, Barbara K., Tanya Agurs-Collins, Doris Browne, Ronald Lubet, and Karen A. Johnson. 2010. "Health Disparities in Breast Cancer: Biology Meets Socioeconomic Status." *Breast Cancer Research and Treatment* 121 (2): 281–92. doi:10.1007/s10549-010-0827-x.

Evans, Gary W., and Pilyoung Kim. 2007. "Childhood Poverty and Health: Cumulative Risk Exposure and Stress Dysregulation." *Psychological Science* 18 (11): 953–57. doi:10.1111/j.1467-9280.2007.02008.x.

Fukuda-Parr, Sakiko, and A. K. Shiva Kumar, eds. 2003. *Readings in Human Development: Concepts, Measures, and Policies for a Development Paradigm*. New York: Oxford University Press.

Hale, Lauren, Terrence D. Hill, Elliot Friedman, F. Javier Nieto, Loren W. Galvao, Corinne D. Engelman, Kristen M. C. Malecki, and Paul E. Peppard. 2013. "Perceived Neighborhood Quality, Sleep Quality, and Health Status: Evidence from the Survey of the Health of Wisconsin." *Social Science and Medicine* 79 (February): 16–22. doi:10.1016/j.socscimed.2012.07.021.

Holden, C. 1987. "Why Do Women Live Longer than Men?" *Science* 238 (4824): 158–60.

Kaplan, George A., Sarah J. Shema, and Cláudia Maria A. Leite. 2008. "Socioeconomic Determinants of Psychological Well-Being: The Role of Income, Income Change, and Income Sources during the Course of 29 Years." *Annals of Epidemiology* 18 (7): 531–37. doi:10.1016/j.annepidem.2008.03.006.

Kawachi, Ichiro, Nancy E. Adler, and William H. Dow. 2010. "Money, Schooling, and Health: Mechanisms and Causal Evidence." *Annals of the New York Academy of Sciences* 1186 (February): 56–68. doi:10.1111/j.1749-6632.2009.05340.x.

Krieger, Nancy. 2001. "The Ostrich, the Albatross, and Public Health: An Ecosocial Perspective—or Why an Explicit Focus on Health Consequences of Discrimination and Deprivation Is Vital for Good Science and Public Health Practice." *Public Health Reports* 116 (5): 419–23.

Mandelblatt, Jeanne S., Vanessa B. Sheppard, and Alfred I. Neugut. 2013. "Black-White Differences in Breast Cancer Outcomes among Older Medicare Beneficiaries: Does Systemic Treatment Matter?" *Journal of the American Medical Association* 310 (4): 376–77. doi:10.1001/jama.2013.8273.

Mani, Anandi, Sendhil Mullainathan, Eldar Shafir, and Jiaying Zhao. 2013. "Poverty Impedes Cognitive Function." *Science* 341 (6149): 976–80. doi:10.1126/science.1238041.

Marmot, Michael. 2002. "The Influence of Income on Health: Views of an Epidemiologist." *Health Affairs* 21 (2): 31–46.

Merriam-Webster Online. 2014. S.v. "equity." http://www.merriam-webster.com/dictionary/equity. Accessed 20 January 2014.

Miller, Gregory E., Gene H. Brody, Tianyi Yu, and Edith Chen. 2014. "A Family-Oriented Psychosocial Intervention Reduces Inflammation in Low-SES African American Youth." *Proceedings of the National Academy of Sciences of the United States of America* 111 (31): 11287–92. doi:10.1073/pnas.1406578111.

Minority Health and Health Disparities Research and Education Act. 2000. Public Law No. 106-525.

Muennig, Peter. 2008. "Health Selection vs. Causation in the Income Gradient: What Can We Learn from Graphical Trends?" *Journal of Health Care for the Poor and Underserved* 19 (2): 574–79. doi:10.1353/hpu.0.0018.

Murray, Christopher J., Emmanuela E. Gakidou, and Julio Frenk. 1999. "Health Inequalities and Social Group Differences: What Should We Measure?" *Bulletin of the World Health Organization* 77 (7): 537–43.

Needham, Belinda L., Jose R. Fernandez, Jue Lin, Elissa S. Epel, and Elizabeth H. Blackburn. 2012. "Socioeconomic Status and Cell Aging in Children." *Social Science and Medicine* 74 (12): 1948–51. doi:10.1016/j.socscimed.2012.02.019.

NIH (National Institutes of Health) and USDHHS (U.S. Department of Health and Human Services). 2013. *NIH Health Disparities Strategic Plan and Budget 2009–2013.* http://www.nimhd.nih.gov/documents/NIH%20Health%20Disparities%20Strategic%20Plan%20and%20Budget%202009-2013.pdf. Accessed 9 August 2013.

OHCHR (Office of the United Nations High Commissioner for Human Rights) and WHO (World Health Organization). 2013. "The Right to Health." *World Health*

Organization. November. http://www.who.int/mediacentre/factsheets/fs323/en/. Accessed 20 January 2014.

Puterman, Eli, Jue Lin, Jeffrey Krauss, Elizabeth H. Blackburn, and Elissa S. Epel. 2015. "Determinants of Telomere Attrition over 1 Year in Healthy Older Women: Stress and Health Behaviors Matter." *Molecular Psychiatry* 20 (4): 529–35. doi:10.1038/mp.2014.70.

Rawls, John. 1971. *A Theory of Justice.* Cambridge, MA: Belknap Press of Harvard University Press.

———. 1985. "Justice as Fairness: Political Not Metaphysical." *Philosophy and Public Affairs* 14 (3): 223–51.

Rosen, George. 1993. *A History of Public Health.* Expanded ed. Baltimore: Johns Hopkins University Press.

Seeman, Teresa, Elissa Epel, Tara Gruenewald, Arun Karlamangla, and Bruce S. McEwen. 2010. "Socio-Economic Differentials in Peripheral Biology: Cumulative Allostatic Load." *Annals of the New York Academy of Sciences* 1186 (February): 223–39. doi:10.1111/j.1749-6632.2009.05341.x.

Sen, Amartya K. 1992. *Inequality Reexamined.* Cambridge, MA: Harvard University Press.

Setiawan, Veronica Wendy, Kristine R. Monroe, Lynne R. Wilkens, Laurence N. Kolonel, Malcolm C. Pike, and Brian E. Henderson. 2009. "Breast Cancer Risk Factors Defined by Estrogen and Progesterone Receptor Status: The Multiethnic Cohort Study." *American Journal of Epidemiology* 169 (10): 1251–59. doi:10.1093/aje/kwp036.

Shonkoff, Jack P. 2011. "Protecting Brains, Not Simply Stimulating Minds." *Science* 333 (6045): 982–83. doi:10.1126/science.1206014.

Smith, Gordon C. S., and Jill P. Pell. 2003. "Parachute Use to Prevent Death and Major Trauma Related to Gravitational Challenge: Systematic Review of Randomised Controlled Trials." *British Medical Journal* 327 (7429): 1459–61. doi:10.1136/bmj.327.7429.1459.

Starfield, Barbara. 2001. "Improving Equity in Health: A Research Agenda." *International Journal of Health Services* 31 (3): 545–66.

UNGA (United Nations General Assembly). 1966. *International Covenant on Economic, Social and Cultural Rights.* December 16. http://www.ohchr.org/EN/ProfessionalInterest/Pages/CESCR.aspx. Accessed 23 August 2015.

USDHHS (U.S. Department of Health and Human Services) and ODPHP (Office of Disease Prevention and Health Promotion). 2011. *Healthy People 2020.* http://www.healthypeople.gov/2020/about/disparitiesAbout.aspx. Accessed 8 April 2014.

Virchow, Rudolf Carl. 2006. "Report on the Typhus Epidemic in Upper Silesia." *American Journal of Public Health* 96 (12): 2102–5.

Waldron, Ingrid. 1983. "Sex Differences in Human Mortality: The Role of Genetic Factors." *Social Science and Medicine* 17 (6): 321–33.

Whitehead, Margaret. 1992. "The Concepts and Principles of Equity and Health." *International Journal of Health Services* 22 (3): 429–45.

WHOCSDH (World Health Organization Commission on the Social Determinants of Health). 2008. *Closing the Gap in a Generation: Health Equity through Action on the Social Determinants of Health.* Geneva: World Health Organization.

Williams, David R., and Chiquita Collins. 2001. "Racial Residential Segregation: A Fundamental Cause of Racial Disparities in Health." *Public Health Reports* 116 (5): 404–16.

Williams, David R., and Selina A. Mohammed. 2009. "Discrimination and Racial Disparities in Health: Evidence and Needed Research." *Journal of Behavioral Medicine* 32 (1): 20–47. doi:10.1007/s10865-008-9185-0.

Winslow, C. E. A. 1948. "Poverty and Disease." *American Journal of Public Health and the Nation's Health* 38 (1, part 2): 173–84.

Yamin, Alicia Ely. 2009. "Shades of Dignity: Exploring the Demands of Equality in Applying Human Rights Frameworks to Health." *Health and Human Rights* 11 (2): 1–18.

Zhao, Zhen, and Elizabeth T. Luman. 2010. "Progress toward Eliminating Disparities in Vaccination Coverage among U.S. Children, 2000–2008." *American Journal of Preventive Medicine* 38 (2): 127–37. doi:10.1016/j.amepre.2009.10.035.

Zhao, Zhen, and Philip J. Smith. 2013. "Trends in Vaccination Coverage Disparities among Children, United States, 2001–2010." *Vaccine* 31 (19): 2324–27. doi:10.1016/j.vaccine.2013.03.018.

2

Global Health Inequalities and Justice

Jennifer Prah Ruger

ABSTRACT

Moral philosophers have for some time been arguing that global poverty and associated human suffering are universal concerns and that there is a moral obligation, not just a matter of charity, for wealthier countries to do more. If we are serious about addressing the problem of global health inequalities, we need to develop a conception of global health justice. Moreover, addressing global health inequalities requires a reexamination of the norms and principles underlying global institutions in order to offer proposals for a better global health policy. This chapter sketches some analytical components of provincial globalism, a framework that takes individuals to be the moral unit in both domestic and global contexts and that improves the prospects of alleviating global health inequalities. Provincial globalism takes the realization of individuals' health capabilities as basic, since health capabilities are both an intrinsically and instrumentally valuable dimension of individuals' overall capability set. Provincial globalism supports a shared health governance that enables institutions to reexamine the objectives, policy goals, and decision-making procedures of the global health architecture. Shared health governance provides standards for regulating global and domestic institutions and practices to create the conditions for realizing individuals' health capabilities. In this chapter I will first discuss some of the challenges of global health inequalities and the current global health policy system. I will then turn to some of the components of the provincial globalism and shared health governance frameworks. Paula Braveman's argument for defining and measuring health inequalities and health equity in terms of justice (this volume) supports the arguments made in this chapter that new forms of global health governance can achieve global health justice.

INTRODUCTION

Moral philosophers have for some time been arguing that global poverty and associated human suffering are universal concerns, and that there is a moral obligation, not just a matter of charity, for wealthier countries to do more to alleviate global poverty. The scope of this moral concern is the topic of considerable debate, and it is unclear to many that this obligation is grounded in justice, rather than in humanitarian duties to foreigners. In this chapter I suggest that if we are serious about addressing the problem of global health inequalities, we need to develop a better conception of global health justice. Moreover, addressing global health inequalities requires a reexamination of the global basic structure, global institutions, and norms and principles that underlie it in order to offer proposals for better global health policies. One approach to addressing these issues would be to take the moral status of states as the primary unit of analysis (a nationalist perspective), but if one is concerned about the health and well-being of individuals, then the individualist focus of the capabilities approach, an alternative to welfare and normative economics in political and moral philosophy, can better assist us in determining the goods and resources to be distributed both within and among countries. Because equality among individuals does not necessarily follow directly from equality between states, the norms and principles underlying domestic social arrangements and distribution must align with the norms and principles that underlie the global basic structure.

It is in this context that this chapter briefly sketches some, although not all, analytical components of provincial globalism, an alternative framework to a states-based approach that takes individuals to be the moral unit of analysis in both domestic and global contexts and that improves the prospects for ensuring the alleviation of global health inequalities. Provincial globalism takes the realization of individuals' health capabilities as basic, since health capabilities are both an intrinsically and instrumentally valuable dimension of individuals' overall capability set. Shared health governance offers an institutional approach to reexamining the objectives, policy goals, and decision-making procedures of the global health architecture (the global basic structure). Shared health governance provides standards by which to regulate both the global and domestic basic structure so that global and domestic institutions and practices create the conditions for the realization of individuals' health capabilities. In this chapter I will first discuss some of the challenges of global health inequalities and the current global health policy system. I will then turn to some of the components of the provincial globalism and shared health governance frameworks.

GLOBAL HEALTH INEQUALITIES AND GLOBAL HEALTH POLICY

Parents in Mali, where approximately one in five children dies of the disease before age five, live in dread of malaria. Indeed, every man, woman, and child in this western African nation of about 16 million is at risk of contracting malaria and its debilitating fevers and, if severe, its attendant neurological and respiratory complications. The national health information system reported 2.1 million clinical cases in 2012, a quarter of them severe. A critical shortage of public health staff undermines the nation's best efforts to combat malaria, as does a lack of laboratory capacity, since only 10 percent of reported cases are actually confirmed by lab tests (USAID 2014). Mali's climate, so congenial to the *Anopheles* mosquitoes that carry malaria, is partly to blame, but in Ecuador, a country whose climate is also conducive to malaria, the rate of infection is vanishingly low, and the disease no longer regularly claims lives (WHO 2009a, Annex 2). These and countless other examples illustrate the grim reality: the burden of disease and ill health is distributed with harsh inequality. That this reality is well-known, widely covered in the press, and thoroughly studied by scholars makes it no less unjust.

Interest in global health inequality has grown over the past several decades. The World Health Organization (Jong-Wook 2003; WHO 1999, 2000), the World Bank (Gwatkin 2000; World Bank 1997), UNICEF (UNICEF 1997, 1999), the Pan American Health Organization, the United Nations Development Programme (Anand and Sen 1996; UNDP 1996, 2003), the UK Department of International Development (UKDFID 2000), and the broader global health community (Evans et al. 2001; Foege 1998; Howson, Fineberg, and Bloom 1998) have made the issue of global health inequalities a priority. More recently, as Paula Braveman's chapter in this volume points out, discussion has focused on the different conceptualizations and measures of health inequalities and health inequities. In Braveman's chapter, an argument is made for defining and measuring health inequalities and health equity in terms of justice (chapter 1, this volume). These points support the arguments made in this chapter regarding global health justice and governance, as both chapters emphasize the significance of incorporating concepts of justice into considerations of health inequalities. The lack of a sound knowledge base, grounded in ethical reasoning, regarding global health justice hampers global policy formulation aimed at closing the gap in health attainment between industrialized and developing countries, and within countries as well.

Global health inequalities have potential resolutions in global health policy through the institutions and behavior of global and domestic actors. While the nation-state remains the most important actor in both domestic politics and international relations, global institutions and actors, public and private, play an increasingly important role. The UN system itself, including the World Bank and the World Health Organization (WHO), is responsible for a number of global arrangements that impact global health inequalities.

Acceleration of globalization, increasing economic interdependence, and vast international movements of people and products ushered in an era of global health governance. Recognizing that infectious diseases emerging or reemerging anywhere can have repercussions everywhere gave new urgency to addressing health on a global scale. Global health governance is dramatically complex, with a plethora of new actors, a lack of clear structure, a deluge of uncoordinated activities, and operational chaos.

The bulk of global health policy literature affirms the continuing primacy and ultimate responsibility of nation-states in health governance, national and global (Buchanan and DeCamp 2006; Gruskin 2004; Helfer 2004; Kickbusch and Buse 2000; Lee and Dodgson 2000; Ruger 2006a; Taylor 2004; Walt 1998; WHO 2000). Bilateral funding still constitutes the greatest single source of global health assistance (IHME 2009; *The Lancet* 2009), and national resources (public and private), even in low- and middle-income countries, still fund most national health spending (WHO 2009b, 108–17).[1] Disease surveillance and control, despite their global implications, depend on the capacity and decisions of national governments. Rich and powerful states further contribute to global health inequality by promoting intellectual property rights and protecting their pharmaceutical, tobacco, and food industry interests. States are also relevant in other ways. Domestically, public sector or mixed public-private health systems tend to outperform strictly private sector ones in achieving equity (Roemer and Roemer 1990; WHO 2000), supporting a major role for the nation-state. Public health success stories—the trachoma control campaign in Morocco, and the HIV/AIDS programs in Brazil and Thailand (Levine, WWWG, and Kinder 2004; Okie 2006), for example— have also demonstrated state efforts' effectiveness.

The rise of nonstate actors and major global health initiatives driven by public-private partnerships, foundations, G8, and other non-UN entities has diminished the importance of WHO and health-related UN organizations in global health governance (Godlee 1994; *The Lancet* 2009; Lee 2004; Szlezák et al. 2010; Whyte, McCoy, and Rowson 2005). As an example, disillusionment with WHO inefficiency and ineffectiveness has arguably spurred engagement of nonstate actors (Buse and Walt 2000, 2002a, 2002b). Initiatives such as the Global Fund and the Joint United Nations Programme on HIV/AIDS (UNAIDS) have taken away WHO's purview over major diseases (Godlee 1994; Hein and Kohlmorgen 2008). Other multilateral organizations, not traditionally health-related, have gained importance in global health governance. The World Bank, the G8, and the G20 are all increasingly involved in global health.

The UN and WHO are beset with criticisms regarding their role and efficacy in promoting global health goals. The UN lacks a "master plan" for health, leading to competition and duplication among UN agencies (Lee et al. 1996). WHO is vulnerable to bilateral influence and political pressure and has no enforcement powers. Critics charge that it is too focused on technical matters and vertical programs, too bureaucratic, and insufficiently engaged with civil society (Al-Mazrou et al. 1997; GHW 2005; Godlee 1994; Walt 1993; Whyte, McCoy, and Rowson 2005). Its conflicting roles as advocate, adviser, and evaluator further limit its effectiveness (Murray, Lopez, and Wibulpolprasert 2004). In the past, it has been unable—and it continues to be reluctant—to use the power of international law (Gostin 2007a, 2007b). For all of WHO's flaws, however, the global health community continues to look to it as the leading global health governor and the institution best situated to address global health inequalities, in the absence of a real alternative.

Despite global health policy's profusion of new actors and the absence of clear governance structure, striking examples of global health successes show that these operational difficulties can be overcome. National governments, international organizations, nongovernmental organizations (NGOs), the private sector, and individuals have managed fruitful collaborations. The African Programme for Onchocerciasis, polio and guinea worm eradication, lymphatic filariasis and measles elimination campaigns, and the PARTNERS project on multi-drug-resistant tuberculosis exemplify successful global health efforts involving many national, international, nonprofit, and corporate actors. Still, widely acknowledged global health successes are notable partly because they remain relatively rare. The main global policy approaches to health challenges today are either vertical or horizontal, trending into calls for a diagonal third way, which combines the two. Vertical programs or selective primary health-care targets are disease-specific, while horizontal programs or comprehensive primary health-care programs entail broad-based health systems development and strengthening.

Increasingly, global health is understood as a multisectoral issue that does not exist in isolation from other sectors, especially in a globalizing world (Drager and Sunderland 2007; Drager and Beaglehole 2001; Nishtar 2007; Piot and Coll Seck 2001; Plotkin and Kimball 1997; WHO 2006). Greater intersectoral coordination (Ruger 2005) to better integrate health concerns into broader policy making is essential to ensure coherent policies that protect health interests (Ruger 2004). Economic globalization and trade liberalization have the potential to lead to a globalized health crisis. But these policy trends also link to economic growth, which is necessary for health systems development and sustainability.

Greater local ownership of businesses and institutions and participation in global health initiatives are important for development and sustainability of health initiatives (De Renzio and Maxwell 2005) and have contributed to the recent successes against malaria, onchocerciasis, and guinea worm, for example (Keusch et al. 2010; Levine, WWWG, and Kinder 2004). Local ownership better represents and addresses local needs (Trubek and Das 2004) and offers hope for closing global health inequalities gaps. However, the ability of countries and localities to undertake projects is a concern. These efforts must take human resources and financial capacities into account (Caines et al. 2004) and include key stakeholders. Many governments might lack competence and integrity (Easterly 2006; Gostin 2007b), which require strengthening. Ownership may also be difficult to wrest from donors reluctant to give up pet initiatives (Maxwell 2007).

The current global health policy and system is inadequate. And the global health governance literature is essentially untethered to a theorized framework able to illuminate and evaluate global health governance in accordance with moral values, values that aid in constructing an approach to addressing global health inequalities. Effective governance demands new solutions. A key component to any such solution is a theory of justice and governance in global health. Why are global health inequalities a matter of justice—or are they? What globally shared values and priorities are central? We need answers to these questions to understand our obligations and effectively promote global health justice. The provincial globalism / shared health governance line of reasoning, grounded in capability theory, offers a new approach. The ethical principles on which this approach rests include the intrinsic value of health to well-being; the importance of health for individual and collective agency; the concept of shortfall inequality, measuring the gaps between different groups' health achievement; and the need for a disproportionate effort to help disadvantaged groups. Shared health governance is a theory of global health governance that is based on a commitment to the principles inherent in a theory of global health justice, namely provincial globalism.

International and national responses to global health problems must derive from shared ethical values about health: widely held ethical claims have the power to motivate; to delineate principles, duties, and responsibilities; and to hold global and national actors morally responsible for achieving common goals.

An essential first step in redressing wrongs is exposing the wrongs and "mak[ing] explicit the values on which proposed action is based" (Whitehead, Dahlgren, and Gilson 2001). In the provincial globalism view, a global community that allows individuals to die prematurely and suffer unnecessary morbidity when it could create the social and economic conditions necessary to support health is behaving unjustly. Alternatively, in supporting universal health attainment, provincial globalism would address conditions that reduce individuals' capability to function, including those particularly prevalent among disadvantaged groups, such as tuberculosis, malaria, and AIDS. Global health justice also raises issues about the allocation of moral responsibility in global health. The provincial globalism perspective parcels out respective roles and responsibilities at the global, national, local, and individual levels based on functional requirements and needs, identifying actors and institutions, their obligations, and how they are held accountable.

The world needs a new way forward, and shared health governance (Ruger 2012, in press; Wachira and Ruger 2011) provides a framework (Ruger 2012). Shared health governance calls for melding values among different global, national, and local actors—a shared vision of health and health provision. Shared health governance advances health agency for all; involving affected and marginalized groups in national and global health initiatives is critical for addressing aid recipients' needs effectively and reining in powerful industry and national interests. Under shared health governance, the global community recognizes health as a meaningful and operational right, the realization of which requires voluntary resource redistribution from rich to poor to narrow the vast and unjust gaps in health and health services. Actors internalize shared moral norms for equity in health and commit to meeting the health needs of others. The provincial globalism account, under development for several years (Ruger 1998, 2009a, 2009b, 2012), illustrates the various components, theoretical and empirical, needed to build a morally grounded global health justice theory that provides guidance for implementation and the specific obligations and requirements of shared health governance. Provincial globalism argues for the application of the health capability paradigm as a theoretical foundation for the right to health and for rethinking the right to health as an ethical demand for health equity.

PROVINCIAL GLOBALISM

The provincial globalism view starts with a universal ethical norm—the general duty to promote human flourishing and human capabilities, or, more specifically, central health capabilities; then it assesses moral responsibility with respect to that duty. Provincial globalism builds on the health capability paradigm, which argues from an Aristotelian/capability perspective that health capabilities are the central focal variable for evaluating justness and efficiency in health policy. The Aristotelian/capability view asserts that humans' capability to flourish is the proper end of social and political activity. Given this shared goal, an obligation to promote the potential for human flourishing is universal. Health capabilities are part of a broader set of human capabilities such as moral, intellectual, and non-health-related physical abilities, and this pluralistic view of the dimensions and goals of human life provides the foundation for understanding health capabilities as the specific focal variable for global health policy.

Human flourishing is a morally central aim shared by all persons by virtue of their humanity. Human flourishing captures and incorporates the idea of human capability, what humans are able to do and be and what possibilities they have. Capability includes human agency, an essential human good to be protected and promoted. The ability to direct one's own life, to make one's own choices, is an essential human interest: people flourish by making their own decisions and shaping their own circumstances. Agency includes health agency, the ability to make decisions and choices about one's health.

The distinction between achievement and the freedom to achieve is important in this capabilities-based view. Functionings are a person's achievements, what they do and are—their activities and states of being, for example. Capability is a person's freedom to achieve the functionings that she values. Examining individuals' potential to function, even if they are not functioning at that level at a given time, reveals the deprivation and suffering many individuals experience throughout the world. The difference between the actual and potential functioning of the world's population is a key indicator in assessing injustices. Health capabilities enable individuals to achieve certain health-related functionings. The difference between health capabilities and health functionings is the difference between the freedom to achieve and achievement itself. Health capabilities encompass both health functionings and health agency.

The goal of planning in provincial globalism is a global and domestic distribution of the conditions enabling people to function in ways that are significant for human flourishing. Accounting for the heterogeneity existing between individuals in the world is important to assessing justice from this perspective. Individuals have various internal and external characteristics that can inform assessments of a just equality: justice requires our global community to aid people in proportion to their degree of disadvantage relative to their capabilities, in line with Aristotle's principle of proportionality. Individuals are entitled to different allocations, depending on what they need to lead a flourishing life.

In duty apportionment, provincial globalism outlines a continuity or series of gradations—rather than a sharp break—between the global and domestic realms. Domestic commitments, through national and subnational governments, must comport with global, universal commitments. Provincial globalism elaborates a multilevel governance, which for ethical and practical reasons is the best approach for achieving universal global health objectives. General and specific duties associated with this collective responsibility are discussed further below.

In focusing on the capability to achieve valuable functionings, provincial globalism entitles individuals to differential allotments of goods and circumstances needed to produce capabilities, for example for different disease severity levels, while simultaneously respecting freedom and reason in enabling all humans to make choices regarding their preferred attainments. Meeting these needs is essential for human flourishing. From this perspective, the state of being human itself, our common humanity, confers moral status. Because they undermine human flourishing, global health deficits require remedy. This obligation is not open-ended, however, as efficiency is also an important concern for justice and global health. Indeed, the measure of global success lies in the extent to which our global and domestic arrangements succeed in or fall short of enabling individuals to function at their best, given their natural circumstances and using the fewest resources possible.

Health capability sustains other facets of human flourishing, because without life itself, no other human functionings are possible. The provincial globalism approach emphasizes the importance of health for individual agency—the ability to live a life we value. Deprivations in people's health capability are unjust because they unnecessarily reduce the capability for functioning and the exercise of agency, and they undermine human flourishing. Policies to deny treatment to malaria patients, for example, or to deny antiretroviral drugs to HIV/AIDS patients, as happens in sub-Saharan Africa and other parts of the world—especially if resource allocation or rationing schemes are adopted or recommended by a global health regime that places cost-effectiveness above all else—are morally troubling not only because they constitute subliminal health care, reduce individuals' opportunity for employment, and cause suffering (as important as these problems are), but also, most fundamentally, because they reduce capabilities for physical and mental functioning, even for survival (Sen 1985, 1992). Empirical evidence from the natural and social sciences shows the effects of disease on cognition, the ability to make decisions and engage in physical activities (Dymek et al. 2000; Mitchell et al. 2005; Soto et al. 2008). Schizophrenia and Alzheimer's disease prevent sufferers from exercising free speech and agency and forming conceptions of their own good (Dymek et al. 2000; Kelly 2006; Soto et al. 2008). Some health states, like AIDS and physical disabilities, make it prohibitive to participate in the life of some faith communities (Cerhan and Wallace 1993).

The provincial globalism view implies that society should create the conditions for individuals to achieve a certain threshold level of health capability, health functioning, and health agency (Ruger 2006b). Global inequalities in, and threats to, health capabilities are morally troubling because they are morally arbitrary, so often just an accident of birth in an impoverished or remote place. Arbitrary factors should not determine one's health or survival. Thus, global health inequalities require rectification.

Once health capabilities are specified, one must determine how to measure them and at what levels to provide them. Capability, because it is the freedom to achieve functionings rather than the functionings themselves, is not directly observable; to evaluate global health policy, therefore, one must assess realized health functionings and health agency. However, this approach also offers a framework for assessing a person's potential health achievement because it is a freedom to achieve functionings rather than the functionings themselves, which is especially relevant when considering preexisting illness and disability.

Provincial globalism takes a global view of health capabilities, under which the global health community strives for coherent goals to enhance health justice. This approach does not require agreement on all goals, but on a minimal set around which global consensus might form. Determining the scope and content of health capabilities is a step toward delineating obligations of global, national, local, and individual actors.

Achieving global health justice means finding a shared standard of health on which to make interpersonal comparisons of health functionings as a proxy for health capabilities and to establish a coherent framework for setting global health goals. The challenge is to construct a conception of health that reflects the "view from nowhere" (Nagel 1986; Sen 1993). This quest for universality in health morality is highly contentious and open to criticism on both philosophical and political grounds. Provincial globalism seeks not to justify, theoretically, a universal view of health but, rather, to determine a minimalist account of health, to identify certain health aspects critical to human functionings that can form a global consensus, and to ground this shared vision in a transpositionally objective worldview.

In 1948, the WHO defined health as "a state of complete physical, mental and social well-being, and not merely the absence of disease or infirmity." An incompletely theorized agreement seems to be emerging on core dimensions of health, moving toward a shared view. This emerging global view is clear, grounded, and agreed-upon, and thus useful in understanding how to assess health policies and interventions.

Health capabilities represent individuals' ability to achieve certain health-related functionings and the freedom to achieve those functionings. Because health functionings and achievements map directly onto health capabilities, they are effective as indicators of health functionings and proxies for health capabilities. Health agency is another component of health capability; it can also serve as a proxy for, and can be causally linked to, both health functioning and health capability.

Why should we be concerned with health capabilities? Why not make the ethical perspective attend to health or health functionings alone? Taking health capabilities as central allows us to distinguish between achieving a given health outcome through coercion versus voluntary action. Just looking at health outcomes alone (e.g., fertility rates), while a key component of this theory and helpful for practical policy purposes, will not show how these outcomes came about—through coercive sterilization, pregnancy termination, or one-child policy laws, for instance. This approach includes health agency, an individual's or group's ability to pursue valuable health goals and to effectively bring about health. Also, health capabilities, through health agency, incorporate a role for individual responsibility, a crucial element in any theory of health and global justice. This approach demonstrates the role of individual responsibility in health outcomes, as lifestyle and behavior are fundamental health determinants. At the same time, health capabilities are socially dependent. Socially dependent capabilities are intended to directly incorporate at the individual level the extent to which group-level factors influence individual health capabilities.

Health agency is a core value in provincial globalism. Individual choices do not occur in a vacuum: there are personal and societal consequences from individual choices. Individuals are owed assistance in meeting health agency needs, and individuals owe the global, and their domestic, communities responsible exercise of health agency. The privilege of individual health agency entails the obligation to make wise choices that do not harm others. Health agency requires self-governance, management skills, and the ability to link behavior and outcomes. Under provincial globalism, for example, public policy regarding vaccinations would place a greater emphasis on enhancing the public's health agency around vaccine risks and benefits than on coercion. In this way full and effective internalization of a public moral norm would result in widespread voluntary compliance with recommended vaccination schemes, thus promoting individual health agency as well as public health.

The case of Andrew Speaker also illustrates this point (Ruger 2010). In 2007, Speaker allegedly disobeyed health officials by traveling internationally between the United States, Europe, and Canada while suspected to have extensively drug-resistant TB. The regulatory instruments currently operating in public health and governance did not combine voluntary and ethical considerations with legal enforcement. The system did not adequately promote Speaker's health agency by informing him of risks to himself and others or of the possibility for legal action if he chose to travel. Under provincial globalism, there would be an international standard of rules and procedures for communication, education, and deliberation among patients and health workers or officials.

Promoting central health capabilities depends on health agency development. For example, efforts to reduce the spread of HIV and AIDS depend critically on the ability to acquire and effectively employ knowledge of HIV/AIDS transmission, of preventive measures, and of the costs and benefits of health behaviors. Living successfully with AIDS requires individuals' health agency in adhering to treatment. Because much ill health derives from individual behaviors, individuals must use their health agency to improve their own health.

At the collective level, groups must have the agency to demand conditions enabling good health, especially through the public health and health-care systems. Agency to demand systems that provide medically necessary and appropriate care on a cost-effective basis and to create and reform institutional arrangements through political engagement is necessary under provincial globalism. For example, under provincial globalism nations would enshrine a positive universal entitlement to adequate health care. The U.S. Constitution does not presently include such a right. Legislators have attempted to fill this void through the passage of the Affordable Care Act and other statutory laws that created programs such as Medicare and Medicaid, though these laws are challenged in the courts. Additionally, individual claims for health care in the United States are often viewed as secondary to a judicial doctrine that favors negative liberties (Hamel et al. 2015). Until there is a positive comprehensive entitlement to health internalized as a public moral norm of health equity in the United States, legal precedent will continue to undermine attempts by American lawmakers and citizens to exercise their collective agency and democratically demand the legal and institutional arrangements necessary for good health under provincial globalism.

Both collective and individual health agency depend in turn on health values, goals, and norms—hence the importance of internalizing norms about the value of both health-related goals and behaviors, such as those related to vaccination policy, the control of infectious disease, efforts to reduce the spread of HIV/AIDS, and the pursuit of a positive entitlement to health.

For a global pledge to improve individuals' health capabilities and reduce inequalities in them, understanding health needs is key. Health needs map directly onto health functionings, which in turn map directly onto health capabilities. Health needs, through their relation to functioning, define what is required to improve individuals' health capabilities. For example, a person might suffer from malnutrition or diabetes or a broken leg. Improving her health capabilities requires preventing, curing, and compensating for conditions that curtail her capabilities for health functioning, because only then will she have the improved capability of health agency that will allow her to make future choices about her health functionings. Thus, how well we meet health needs is an objective measure of our success in improving health capabilities. The concepts of medical necessity and medical appropriateness are essential considerations and help to clarify the account of health needs under the health capability paradigm.

While the universal ethical norm of health equity—a reduction in shortfall inequalities in central health capabilities—rests on a normative framework of human flourishing, the health capabilities approach applies a functionalist perspective on allocating responsibility for achieving health equity. In this approach, health functioning and health agency are both the ends and the means of a global enterprise comprising national health systems and global norms, actors, and institutions. This approach begins with the health capability—health functioning and health agency—of every individual person worldwide as morally significant. The approach then works outward toward the enveloping necessary conditions, starting with the local and national environment.

It is essential, then, to analyze health needs and health agency needs and the extent to which structures at the individual, local, national, and global levels can meet those needs. The immediate and local nature of meeting needs (think of a nurse and doctor providing prenatal care and delivery services in a clinic with necessary equipment and medicines, for instance) requires beginning the systematic study of global health at the individual level and expanding outward from there. Even with all the varied promises of telemedicine, foreign aid, management, and global governance, ultimately, a local provider in a local hospital or facility with drugs and medical devices on hand will provide medical attention to the person in need of health services. The near-eradication of malaria in Eritrea illustrates the effectiveness of local design and implementation, as compared to the WHO global Malaria Eradication Program, which failed largely because of its insistence on a single top-down strategy and failure to draw on local expertise or adapt to diverse local conditions (Packard 2007, 168–69). Indeed, under provincial globalism there can be no optimally functioning global health system without national and local health systems to meet the needs of local populations. The Speaker case also demonstrates the critical importance of more oversight and standardized procedures early in infectious disease control and at the local level (Ruger 2010). The public health officials operating in this case enjoyed too much latitude. Local and national regulations are more easily enforced than global regulations and closer to the ground-level origins of health problems.

The provincial globalism approach to global distributive justice starts with a set of principles to be applied, progressively as needed, so that all individuals worldwide have the opportunity to be healthy. Provincial globalism, while recognizing the importance of all aspects of quality of life, acknowledges that at this juncture there is no way to guarantee a minimum income to all. Thus in provincial globalism the focal variable for global health justice is central health capabilities. Still, it aims to bring all individuals' health to the level of the highest international average (life expectancy in Japan), and to do so as efficiently as possible, even if this goal is progressive in its realization. Provincialism globalism thus offers a robust concept of global distributive justice. It is impossible to guarantee equal health outcomes or equal amounts of health care. We can, however, strive for shortfall equality, integrating three core concepts—equality, priority, and threshold. Shortfall equality takes into account a norm or threshold against which to assess health equity; it also considers concerns for the worse-off and the need for proportional allocation. Finally, it considers equality, but from a different perspective than full equality of health outcomes or access to health care. The shortfall equality concept can assess health capabilities, especially where equalizing achievements for different people is difficult.

At the global or country level, shortfall equality can be used to assess quantitatively how much a given society has realized its health potential and how much remains unrealized, by comparing the actual achievement with the possible maximum. The typical unit of analysis for comparison is the country, though the method can also compare groups within countries.

For global health, these formulations generally imply that public policy should try to bring each individual's health functioning up to a specified level (within the limits of that person's circumstances), by focusing on the gap between functioning and freedom for achieving functioning, provided such efforts do not lower the health functioning of the general population beneath the norm. Priority thus goes to individuals who exhibit a gap between their health status and the status they could achieve, and those with the greatest deficit in health status should receive the highest priority. Priority goes to deprivations below the shortfall equality norm; those above are secondary until the scope of justice can expand with greater resources.

The health capability paradigm theoretically justifies a right to health as a meaningful and operational right. Critically, it recognizes that realizing a right to health requires individual and societal commitments to public moral norms. On this view, the right to health constitutes an ethical demand for health equity. This ethical demand will probably involve legal instruments for enforcement; more importantly, it will require individuals, states, and nonstate actors to internalize public ethical norms to implement and achieve compliance with a right to health in international human rights policy and law. Actualizing a right to health involves both legal and nonlegal instruments. This commitment sees the right to health as the basis and inspiration for new legislation. It also sees it as an ethical claim, in this case on all individuals, especially the wealthier, to redistribute some of their resources to help meet the health needs of others, those who are unable to afford care.

Under the health capability paradigm, individuals internalize the public moral norm of health equity, to understand the obligations each of us has to help realize the right to health for everyone in the global community. For the right to health, this internalization process must entail a commitment to financial claims (e.g., tax contribution) to fulfill the right (e.g., through universal health insurance coverage). As individuals internalize this norm, a growing consensus will ultimately lead to public policies, legislation, and agreed-upon laws guaranteeing a right to health.

Because fulfillment of a right to health requires social organization for resource redistribution and related legislation and regulation, provincial globalism rests on an ethical commitment among the global community for health capability for all people. Without this ethical commitment, redistributing resources from the wealthy to those less fortunate and from the well to the sick will not be possible, because redistribution must be voluntary in the sense that such acts are formed under fair conditions in which there is no duress or coercion. The ethical significance of the right to health provides strong grounding for individual and state action to respect, protect, and fulfill this right through institutional change. Obligations and duties fall on all individuals, but the allocation of specific responsibility for respecting, protecting, and fulfilling the right to health depends on the roles of institutions and individuals at different levels of society—global, national, and subnational.

Borders and states (nations) do have moral significance. The world's system of state sovereignty, with its principle of self-determination, requires respect for the collective agency of peoples and mutual respect among states. Citizens' ability to cooperate to achieve collective goals is an important element of human agency. People must be able—indeed, encouraged—to participate politically, and their actions should result in meaningful collective achievements. On the other hand, countries and cultures often embrace destructive public norms and engage in morally repugnant, even evil practices like slavery, widow burning, or genocide (Gewirth 1994). The debate in global justice has been one of seemingly irreconcilable tension between nationalism and state sovereignty on the one hand and cosmopolitanism on the other.

Provincial globalism, a middle-ground view, offers a gradualist approach of collective responsibility, whereby duty allocation illuminates mutual accountability, legitimacy, and potential recourse when actors fail to meet their responsibilities. Provincial globalism does not deny the close connections between personal identity and cultural community that evolve from nationalism (Tamir 1993) or even subnational units of analysis, as would some utilitarian cosmopolitanism schemes for resource redistribution (Singer 2015). But there is more to social identity than just national identity. Group affiliations—gender, race, ethnicity, class, caste, occupation, religion, sport, and other avocations—define persons as well, and there seems to be no limit to social ties that can constitute identity for individuals. There is also no reason why political identities cannot be established to support global health justice. Who, then, is responsible for realizing health equity at the global level? What duties and responsibilities do global and state actors and institutions have? Provincial globalism acknowledges the relevance of causality, remediation, and partiality in determining obligations, but argues that the allocation of responsibilities derives particularly from the roles, abilities, and effectiveness of actors and institutions.

Allocation begins with a universal ethical principle of health equity and a general obligation, through shared health governance, for global and national actors to address global health inequalities and threats. Its principles encompass voluntary commitments and functional requirements and needs: voluntary commitments among individuals and groups at the global, national, and local levels to share resources and relinquish some autonomy through collective action to address health problems, and functional requirements assigning institutions and agents roles in addressing health issues.

Reducing global health disparities and addressing externalities require social organization and collective action around four key functions: (1) redistribution of resources; (2) related legislation and policy; (3) public regulation and oversight; and (4) creation and distribution of public goods. Redistribution of resources occurs within and among societies. Policy measures enable transfers and include progressive taxation, equitable and efficient risk pooling, redistributive expenditure patterns, subsidies, and cash transfers. National health systems exist as structures for self-determination and collective action. The postmodern state is certainly open to critique on its evolution and legitimacy. Nonetheless, it is the contemporary unit of international relations. Provincial globalism asserts a strong duty for states to reduce shortfall inequalities in their populations' central health capabilities. Global actors also have responsibilities under this general duty, but these essential global health functions reach beyond what individual states can accomplish.

The sovereign state has primary responsibility, given its central function in raising and redistributing revenue and creating and implementing policies and laws. We have no global government. The policies and laws required to promote central health capabilities gain legitimacy at the state level through the joint political project of democratic self-governance and the authority of the state as the functional structure through which individuals give up their autonomy and resources to pursue common goals. The need for public action and especially voluntary resource redistribution makes public moral norms indispensable. Individuals must sacrifice some of their resources and autonomy to be regulated and redistribute those resources to others. Once individuals internalize these ethical commitments, they freely enter into them and create obligations to obey them.

In many respects, the current makeup of global and national institutions and programs is dysfunctional, failing to close global health inequality gaps. We need a new understanding of obligations, both national and international. Further needed are institutions through which state and international players, NGOs, communities, businesses, foundations, families, and individuals can collaborate in shared health governance to correct and prevent global health injustice. Ultimately, individuals themselves, through their individual and collective health agency, must control much of what it takes to prevent and treat disease, to maintain and improve health.

Global health functions are measures that are beyond the reach of individual governments and independent groups but that benefit all countries, developing and disseminating public goods, for example. International health actors have different roles in these global functions. Global institutions and actors, whether they act bilaterally or multilaterally, have a duty to remedy global inequities in affluence, power, and opportunities. Though global actors serve a secondary role in addressing global health injustices, they nonetheless represent the international community's will to rectify global market failures, create public goods, and address equity concerns on a global scale.

The sovereign nation-state is well placed to meet health needs and health agency needs. It raises and redistributes revenues and passes and implements legislation. No global structures exist to perform these functions. The state is a functional structure through which individuals cede some resources and autonomy to pursue common goals. Of course existing state (national) boundaries are neither undisputed nor immutable. Multiple examples today demonstrate the yearnings of peoples for their own states (nations). But these yearnings themselves underscore the state's moral and political significance in contemporary international relations.

State actors assume primary responsibility for fostering individuals' capability to be healthy; states are in the best position to reduce the shortfall between potential and actual health and to develop health agency. This responsibility includes efforts to deal with the social, economic, and political determinants of health. States also assume primary responsibility for creating equitable and affordable health care and public health structures. This obligation includes creating equal access to quality health-related goods and services, including public health and health literacy goods, and to proximal and controllable determinants, including nutritious and safe food, potable water, sanitation, and adequate living conditions. Stewardship obligations include public health surveillance systems, similar to the U.S. Centers for Disease Control and Prevention (CDC), that feed into the WHO's global surveillance system. Overall, national systems must ensure that their populations are able to seek and obtain goods and services when health needs arise.

Providing medically necessary and medically appropriate health care and public health services for all is part of the job of justice. And when national governments are unjust, regardless of their level of development, the global community has the responsibility to work for health equity within the confines of those societies' self-determination and self-governance. Even democratic societies can be unjust: the United States, with all its wealth, has not fulfilled the requirements of health justice.

CONCLUSION

The provincial globalism approach sets high standards: it aspires to self-actualized societies in which governments and peoples internalize a commitment to the central health capabilities of their fellow men and women. Where incompetent states fail to deliver effective public health and healthcare systems, the global community must provide assistance and oversight. An important area for further exploration is the study of social movements and their influence in changing norms and governance through the norm internalization and value formation process.

National (state) and subnational entities best fulfill health system functions due to the local nature of health service provision, disease prevention, and health promotion programs. National government efforts have achieved notable health successes, such as Thailand's "100 percent condom program" for HIV prevention, Sri Lanka's reduction in maternal mortality, and Chile's Hib immunization program (Levine, WWWG, and Kinder 2004). States are

thus still the normatively and empirically most appealing primary locus for so-
cial cooperation on health. Finally, provincial globalism specifies *global health citizenship,* by which any individual on the planet knows that wherever she is, and wherever she travels, the conditions are in place to protect and promote her health and prevent disease and injury. While this goal is not currently within reach, it is an important aspiration for this global health theory.

NOTE

1. In WHO 2009b, see Table 7, "Health Expenditures."

REFERENCES

Al-Mazrou, Yagob, Seth Berkley, Barry Bloom, S. K. Chandiwana, Lincoln Chen, Moses
Chimbari, Julio Frenk, et al. 1997. "A Vital Opportunity for Global Health: Supporting
the World Health Organization at a Critical Juncture." *The Lancet* 350 (9080): 750–51.
doi:10.1016/S0140-6736(05)62559-7.

Anand, Sudhir, and Amartya Sen. 1996. "Gender Inequality in Human Development:
Theories and Measurement." In *Background Papers: Human Development Report 1995,*
1–20. New York: United Nations Development Programme.

Buchanan, Allen, and Matthew DeCamp. 2006. "Responsibility for Global Health."
Theoretical Medicine and Bioethics 27 (1): 95–114.

Buse, Kent, and Gill Walt. 2000. "Global Public-Private Partnerships: Part I: A New
Development in Health?" *Bulletin of the World Health Organization* 78 (4): 549–61.

———. 2002a. "Globalisation and Multilateral Public-Private Health Partnerships: Issues
for Health Policy." In *Health Policy in a Globalising World,* edited by Kelley Lee, Ken
Buse, and Suzanne Fustukian, 41–62. Cambridge: Cambridge University Press.

———. 2002b. "The World Health Organization and Global Public-Private Health
Partnerships: In Search of 'Good' Global Health Governance." In *Public-Private Partnerships
for Health,* edited by Michael Reich, 170–95. Cambridge, MA: Harvard University Press.

Caines, Karen, Kent Buse, Cindy Carlson, Rose-marie de Loor, Nel Druce, Cheri Grace,
Mark Pearson, Jennifer Sancho, and Rajeev Sadanandan. 2004. *Assessing the Impact of
Global Health Partnerships.* London: DFID Health Resource Centre.

Cerhan, James R., and Robert B. Wallace. 1993. "Predictors of Decline in Social
Relationships in the Rural Elderly." *American Journal of Epidemiology* 137 (8): 870–80.

De Renzio, Paolo, and Simon Maxwell. 2005. *Financing the Response to HIV/AIDS: Future
Options and Innovations.* London: Overseas Development Institute.

Drager, Nick, and Robert Beaglehole. 2001. "Globalization: Changing the Public Health
Landscape." *Bulletin of the World Health Organization* 79 (9): 803.

Drager, Nick, and Laura Sunderland. 2007. "Public Health in a Globalising World:
The Perspective from the World Health Organization." In *Governing Global Health:*

Challenge, Response, Innovation, edited by Andrew Cooper, John Korton, and Ted Schrecker, 67–78. Aldershot, UK: Ashgate.

Dymek, Maureen P., Paul Atchison, Lindy Harrell, and Daniel C. Marson. 2000. "Competency to Consent to Medical Treatment in Cognitively Impaired Patients with Parkinson's Disease." *Neurology* 56 (1): 17–24.

Easterly, William Russell. 2006. *The White Man's Burden: Why the West's Efforts to Aid the Rest Have Done So Much Ill and So Little Good*. New York: Penguin Press.

Evans, Timothy, Margaret Whitehead, Finn Diderichsen, Abbas Bhuiya, and Meg Wirth, eds. 2001. *Challenging Inequities in Health: From Ethics to Action: Summary*. New York: Oxford University Press.

Foege, William H. 1998. "Global Public Health: Targeting Inequities." *Journal of the American Medical Association* 279 (24): 1931–32.

Gewirth, Alan. 1994. "Is Cultural Pluralism Relevant to Moral Knowledge?" *Social Philosophy and Policy* 11 (1): 22–43.

GHW (Global Health Watch). 2005. *Global Health Watch 2005–2006: An Alternative World Health Report*. London: Zed Books.

Godlee, Fiona. 1994. "WHO in Retreat: Is It Losing Its Influence?" *British Medical Journal* 309 (6967): 1491–95.

Gostin, Lawrence O. 2007a. "A Proposal for a Framework Convention on Global Health." *Journal of International Economic Law* 10 (4): 989–1008.

———. 2007b. "Meeting the Survival Needs of the World's Least Healthy People: A Proposed Model for Global Health Governance." *Journal of the American Medical Association* 298 (2): 225–28.

Gruskin, Sofia. 2004. "Is There a Government in the Cockpit: A Passenger's Perspective on Global Public Health: The Role of Human Rights." *Temple Law Review* 77: 313–33.

Gwatkin, Davidson R. 2000. "Health Inequalities and the Health of the Poor: What Do We Know? What Can We Do?" *Bulletin of the World Health Organization* 78 (1): 3–18.

Hamel, Mary Beth, Jennifer Prah Ruger, Theodore W. Ruger, and George J. Annas. 2015. "The Elusive Right to Health Care under U.S. Law." *New England Journal of Medicine* 372 (26): 2558–63.

Hein, Wolfgang, and Lars Kohlmorgen. 2008. "Global Health Governance Conflicts on Global Social Rights." *Global Social Policy* 8 (1): 80–108.

Helfer, Laurence R. 2004. "Politics, Power, and Public Health: A Comment on Public Health's New World Order." *Temple Law Review* 77: 291–95.

Howson, Christopher P., Harvey V. Fineberg, and Barry R. Bloom. 1998. "The Pursuit of Global Health: The Relevance of Engagement for Developed Countries." *The Lancet* 351 (9102): 586–90.

IHME (Institute for Health Metrics and Evaluation). 2009. *Financing Global Health 2009: Tracking Development Assistance for Health*. Seattle: University of Washington.

Jong-Wook, Lee. 2003. "Global Health Improvement and WHO: Shaping the Future." *The Lancet* 362 (9401): 2083–88.

Kelly, Brendan D. 2006. "The Power Gap: Freedom, Power and Mental Illness." *Social Science and Medicine* 63 (8): 2118–28.

Keusch, Gerald T., Wen L. Kilama, Suerie Moon, Nicole A. Szlezak, and Catherine M. Michaud. 2010. "The Global Health System: Linking Knowledge with Action: Learning from Malaria." *PLoS Medicine* 7 (1): 28.

Kickbusch, Ilona, and Kent Buse. 2000. "Global Influence and Global Responses: International Health at the Turn of the 21st Century." In *International Public Health*, edited by Michael Merson, Robert Black, and Anne Mills, 701–37. Gaithersburg, MD: Aspen.

Lee, Kelley. 2004. "The Pit and the Pendulum: Can Globalization Take Health Governance Forward?" *Development* 47 (2): 11–17.

Lee, Kelley, Sue Collinson, Gill Walt, and Lucy Gilson. 1996. "Who Should Be Doing What in the International Health: A Confusion of Mandates in the United Nations?" *British Medical Journal* 312 (7026): 302.

Lee, Kelley, and Richard Dodgson. 2000. "Globalization and Cholera: Implications for Global Governance." *Global Governance*, 213–36.

Levine, Ruth, WWWG (What Works Working Group), and Molly Kinder. 2004. *Millions Saved: Proven Successes in Global Health*. Vol. 3. Washington, DC: Center for Global Development.

Maxwell, Simon. 2007. "Can the International Health Partnership Deliver a New Way of Funding Health Spending?" *Overseas Development Institute*. http://www.odi.org/comment/4151-can-international-health-partnership-deliver-new-way-funding-health-spending. Accessed 12 March 2014.

Mitchell, Alex J., Julián Benito-León, José-Manuel Morales González, and Jesús Rivera-Navarro. 2005. "Quality of Life and Its Assessment in Multiple Sclerosis: Integrating Physical and Psychological Components of Wellbeing." *Lancet Neurology* 4 (9): 556–66.

Murray, Christopher J. L., Alan D. Lopez, and Suwit Wibulpolprasert. 2004. "Monitoring Global Health: Time for New Solutions." *British Medical Journal* 329 (7474): 1096.

Nagel, Thomas. 1986. *The View from Nowhere*. Oxford: Clarendon.

Nishtar, Sania. 2007. "Politics of Health Systems: WHO's New Frontier." *The Lancet* 370 (9591): 935–36.

Okie, Susan. 2006. "Fighting HIV: Lessons from Brazil." *New England Journal of Medicine* 354 (19): 1977–81.

Packard, Randall M. 2007. *The Making of a Tropical Disease: A Short History of Malaria*. Baltimore: Johns Hopkins University Press.

Piot, Peter, and Awa Marie Coll Seck. 2001. "International Response to the HIV/AIDS Epidemic: Planning for Success." *Bulletin of the World Health Organization* 79 (12): 1106–12.

Plotkin, Bruce Jay, and Ann Marie Kimball. 1997. "Designing an International Policy and Legal Framework for the Control of Emerging Infectious Diseases: First Steps." *Emerging Infectious Diseases* 3 (1): 1.

Roemer, Milton I., and Ruth Roemer. 1990. "Global Health, National Development, and the Role of Government." *American Journal of Public Health* 80 (10): 1188–92.

Ruger, Jennifer P. 1998. "Aristotelian Justice and Health Policy: Capability and Incompletely Theorized Agreements." PhD diss., Harvard University.

Ruger, Jennifer Prah. 2004. "Ethics of the Social Determinants of Health." *The Lancet* 364 (9439): 1092–97.

———. 2005. "Global Tobacco Control: An Integrated Approach to Global Health Policy." *Development* 48 (2): 65–69.

———. 2006a. "Ethics and Governance of Global Health Inequalities." *Journal of Epidemiology and Community Health* 60 (11): 998–1002.

———. 2006b. "Toward a Theory of a Right to Health: Capability and Incompletely Theorized Agreements." *Yale Journal of Law and the Humanities* 18 (2): 3.

———. 2009a. "Global Health Justice." *Public Health Ethics* 2:261–75.

———. 2009b. *Health and Social Justice*. Oxford: Oxford University Press.

———. 2010. "Control of Extensively Drug-Resistant Tuberculosis (XDR-TB): A Root Cause Analysis." *Global Health Governance* 3 (2): 1–20.

———. 2012. "Global Health Governance as Shared Health Governance." *Journal of Epidemiology and Community Health* 66 (7): 653–61. doi:10.1136/jech.2009.101097.

———. In press. *Global Health Justice and Governance*. Oxford: Clarendon.

Sen, Amartya K. 1985. *Commodities and Capabilities*. Amsterdam: North-Holland.

———. 1992. *Inequality Reexamined*. Cambridge, MA: Harvard University Press.

———. 1993. "Positional Objectivity." *Philosophy and Public Affairs* 2 (2): 126–45.

Singer, Peter. 2015. *The Most Good You Can Do: How Effective Altruism Is Changing Ideas about Living Ethically*. New Haven, CT: Yale University Press.

Soto, Maria E., Sandrine Andrieu, Christopher Arbus, Matthieu Ceccaldi, Philippe Couratier, Thierry Dantoine, J.-F. Dartigues, et al. 2008. "Rapid Cognitive Decline in Alzheimer's Disease: Consensus Paper." *Journal of Nutrition, Health and Aging* 12 (10): 703–13.

Szlezák, Nicole A., Barry R. Bloom, Dean T. Jamison, Gerald T. Keusch, Catherine M. Michaud, Suerie Moon, and William C. Clark. 2010. "The Global Health System: Actors, Norms, and Expectations in Transition." *PLoS Medicine* 7 (1): 1–4.

Tamir, Yael. 1993. *Liberal Nationalism*. Princeton, NJ: Princeton University Press.

Taylor, Allyn L. 2004. "Governing the Globalization of Public Health." *Journal of Law, Medicine and Ethics* 32 (3): 500–508.

Trubek, Louise G., and Maya Das. 2004. "Achieving Equality: Healthcare Governance in Transition." *DePaul Journal of Health Care Law* 7: 245–79.

UKDFID (United Kingdom Department for International Development). 2000. *Better Health for Poor People: Strategies for Achieving the International Development Targets*. London: Department for International Development.

UNDP (United Nations Development Programme). 1996. *Human Development Report 1996: Economic Growth and Human Development*. New York: Oxford University Press.

———. 2003. *Human Development Report 2003: Millennium Development Goals: A Compact among Nations to End Human Poverty.* New York: Oxford University Press.

———. 2014. *Human Development Report 2014: Sustaining Human Progress: Reducing Vulnerabilities and Building Resilience.* http://hdr.undp.org/en/2014-report. Accessed 29 August 2015.

UNICEF (United Nations Children's Fund). 1997. *UNICEF Annual Report 1997.* New York: United Nations Children's Fund.

———. 1999. *The Progress of Nations 1999.* New York: United Nations Children's Fund.

USAID (U.S. Agency for International Development). 2014. *President's Malaria Initiative: Malaria Operational Plan: Mali Fiscal Year 2012.* http://www.pmi.gov/docs/default-source/default-document-library/malaria-operational-plans/fy12/mali_mop_fy12 .pdf. Accessed 20 June 2014.

Wachira, Catherine, and Jennifer Prah Ruger. 2011. "National Poverty Reduction Strategies and HIV/AIDS Governance in Malawi: A Preliminary Study of Shared Health Governance." *Social Science and Medicine* 72 (12): 1956–64.

Walt, Gill. 1993. "WHO under Stress: Implications for Health Policy." *Health Policy* 24 (2): 125–44.

———. 1998. "Globalisation of International Health." *The Lancet* 351 (9100): 434–37.

Whitehead, Margaret, Göran Dahlgren, and Lucy Gilson. 2001. "Developing the Policy Response to Inequities in Health: A Global Perspective." In *Challenging Inequities in Health: From Ethics to Action,* edited by Timothy Evans, Margaret Whitehead, Finn Diderichsen, Abbas Bhuiya, and Meg Wirth, 308–24. New York: Oxford University Press.

WHO (World Health Organization). 1999. *The World Health Report 1999: Making the Difference.* Geneva: World Health Organization Press. http://www.who.int/whr/1999/ en/. Accessed 20 March 2014.

———. 2000. *The World Health Report 2000: Health Systems: Improving Performance.* Geneva: World Health Organization Press. http://www.who.int/whr/2000/en/. Accessed 20 March 2014.

———. 2006. *International Trade and Health: WHA59.26.* Geneva: World Health Organization Press. http://www.who.int/trade/trade_and_health/en/. Accessed 20 March 2014.

———. 2009a. *World Malaria Report 2009.* Geneva: World Health Organization Press. http:// www.who.int/malaria/world_malaria_report_2009/en/. Accessed 20 March 2014.

———. 2009b. *World Statistics 2009.* Geneva: World Health Organization Press. http:// www.who.int/whosis/whostat/2009/en/. Accessed 20 March 2014.

"Who Runs Global Health?" 2009. *The Lancet* 373 (9681): 2083.

Whyte, Alison, David McCoy, and Mike Rowson, eds. 2005. *Global Health Action: Global Health Watch Campaign Agenda.* Nottingham, United Kingdom: Russell Press. http:// www.ghwatch.org/sites/www.ghwatch.org/files/GlobalHealthAction0506.pdf. Accessed 21 March 2014.

World Bank. 1997. *Health, Nutrition, Population Sector Strategy.* Washington, DC: World Bank.

3

Health Inequalities and Relational Egalitarianism

J. Paul Kelleher

ABSTRACT

Much of the philosophical literature on health inequalities seeks to establish the superiority of one or another conception of luck egalitarianism. In recent years, however, an increasing number of self-avowed egalitarian philosophers have proposed replacing luck egalitarianism with alternatives that stress the moral relevance of distinct relationships, rather than the moral relevance of good or bad luck. After briefly explaining why I am not attracted to luck egalitarianism, I distinguish and clarify three views that have been characterized in the philosophical literature as forms of relational egalitarianism. I call these three relational views equality of treatment, equality of concern, and social egalitarianism. I argue that each deserves the title "egalitarianism" and (more importantly) that these three views are not competitors; rather, each brand of relational egalitarianism describes a plausible plank of distributive justice that bears on the evaluation of health inequalities and on the political institutions that create, sustain, or exacerbate them. To illustrate this pluralistic relational egalitarian approach, I draw on a case study by Horton and Barker (this volume) to discuss how each of the three planks might be brought to bear on the evaluation of oral health disparities among the children of migrant Latino farmworkers in California.

INTRODUCTION

If one wishes to evaluate inequalities in health from the perspective of justice, it is natural to turn to philosophical conceptions of egalitarianism. Such views aim to explain why inequalities (or at least certain inequalities) are morally problematic, and why social and political institutions that engender inequalities are unjust and need repair. There is, however, a vigorous debate within political philosophy as to how egalitarianism should be conceived. In recent years, a broad division has emerged between so-called luck egalitarians, on the one hand, and "relational" egalitarians, on the other. The main aim of this chapter is to explain this debate and to distinguish further between three types of relational egalitarianism. Although I will not offer a comprehensive critique of it, I will explain why I am not attracted to luck egalitarianism. Then, after distinguishing between the three types of relational egalitarianism, I will suggest that these should not be viewed as competitors; rather, each describes a plausible plank of distributive justice that bears on the evaluation of health inequalities and the political institutions that create, sustain, or exacerbate them. To illustrate this pluralistic egalitarian approach, I will draw on a case study by Horton and Barker (this volume) to discuss how each of the three planks might be brought to bear on the evaluation of oral health disparities among the children of migrant Latino farmworkers in California.

LUCK EGALITARIANISM AND RELATIONAL EGALITARIANISM

There are many versions of luck egalitarianism, but they all endorse the claim that inequalities are *pro tanto* unjust, unless they can be shown to result from the responsible choices of individuals. ("*Pro tanto*" indicates that the injustice can be outweighed by other moral factors; for example, a policy that widens unchosen inequalities may nevertheless be just, all things considered, if the increase in inequality is morally outweighed by significant improvements in the well-being of the worst-off.) Luck egalitarians believe that (*pro tanto*) injustice attaches to inequalities that result from bad brute luck, but not to inequalities traceable to individuals' responsible choices or gambles.[1] Different versions of luck egalitarianism focus on different kinds of inequality—some focus on inequalities in health as such, whereas others care about health only insofar as health bears on the wider category of well-being. Again, though, all versions tie judgments of justice and injustice to facts about chance and choice.

For the moment, let us assume that all relevant inequalities (whether inequalities in health or inequalities in well-being) arise from bad brute luck (and thus not from gambles and choices for which individuals can be held responsible). Luck egalitarianism would thus condemn the inequalities. But

Figure 3.1. Social Position and Mortality Rate: Two Versions

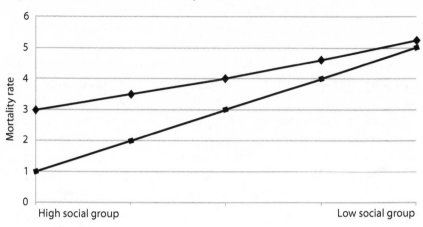

Source: Marmot 2004.

why? Consider the diagram (figure 3.1), which replicates a diagram first drawn
by Michael Marmot and discussed in his book *The Status Syndrome* (Marmot
2004, 246).

The diagram shows the mortality effects of two different policies on
five social groups arranged from left to right in descending order of social advantage. Call the two policies Square (indicated by the bottom graph) and
Diamond (indicated by top graph). Suppose Diamond reflects current policy
and we are considering a move to Square. Should we make the move? Square
would obviously lead to greater health inequalities than Diamond, but Square
also offers Pareto improvements with respect to life expectancy, since each
social group in Square has lower mortality than the corresponding social
group in Diamond. (Assume that changing policies would not change who
is in which group.) Marmot drew the diagram during a conversation with
the health economist Angus Deaton. Deaton then asked Marmot whether
he cared more about reducing distributive inequalities than he did about reducing poor health. Here's how Marmot responded: "I demurred. [Deaton]
was in no doubt that all economists would choose the bottom graph because
everyone is better off. . . . [He] suspected that I went for the one with less
inequality where everyone suffered more. . . . It is my view that we should
reject both alternatives and aim for a society where health for everyone has
improved and inequality is less" (Marmot 2004, 245–46).

This answer of Marmot's probably did not satisfy Deaton. For Deaton
was trying to call attention to the downside of claiming that equality itself

is intrinsically important. Marmot's response suggests that he endorses (or would endorse) a philosophical position that very often underlies luck egalitarian views. This position is known as *telic egalitarianism*, and it says simply that equality is intrinsically good, and inequality intrinsically bad. Larry Temkin is a leading proponent of telic egalitarianism, and he has elsewhere offered a Marmot-like response to scenarios similar to Square-vs.-Diamond that force one to choose between greater equality and less sickness and death. As Temkin puts it: "The essence of the egalitarian's view is that comparative unfairness is bad, and that if we could do something about life's unfairness, we have some reason to. . . . But, the anti-egalitarian will incredulously ask, do I *really* think that there is some respect in which only some being blind is worse than all being blind? Yes. Does this mean that I think it would be better if everyone else was blind? No. As noted previously, equality is not all that matters. But it does matter *some*" (Temkin 2003, 775, 780).[2]

Temkin here associates unchosen inequalities with what he calls "comparative unfairness." In Temkin's view, it is simply unfair when some have better health than others through no fault of their own. It is a short step from here to the conclusion that unchosen inequalities are unjust, as many people believe in a tight connection between fairness and justice. Temkin admits, however, that this unfairness generates only a pro tanto reason to eliminate the inequality. Thus, in a scenario like Square-vs.-Diamond, Temkin's view leaves open the possibility that it is ultimately more important to avoid Diamond's costs in health and well-being than it is to secure its more equal distribution. Nevertheless, telic egalitarianism, or something quite like it, is at the heart of most luck egalitarian approaches to distributive justice.

Now, in the very large literature on telic egalitarianism there are two objections to it that are worth noting here. The first objection maintains that telic egalitarianism has little right (and certainly no exclusive right) to the name "egalitarianism." Elizabeth Anderson was among the first to lodge this objection. She writes: "There must be a better way to conceive of the point of equality. To do so, it is helpful to recall how egalitarian political movements have historically conceived of their aims. . . . Inequality referred not so much to distributions of goods as to relations between superior and inferior persons" (Anderson 1999, 312). More recently, Daniel Hausman and Matt Waldren argue that six discrete objectives—none of which resembles telic egalitarianism—"have been prominent among the objectives of those who have fought under the banner of equality" (Hausman and Waldren 2011, 578). I will return to Anderson's and Hausman and Waldren's views below.

A second objection to telic egalitarianism would apply even if telic egalitarians agreed that other views also merit the label "egalitarian." This second objection claims that distributive equality has *no* moral importance because it is not connected in the right way to the interests of individuals. Roger Crisp puts it like this: "The worry arises from the idea that what matters morally could be something that was independent from the welfare of individuals" (Crisp 2003, 747). Since pursuing equality in Square-vs.-Diamond (and in other examples Temkin himself constructs) would harm *everyone's* interests in absolute terms, Crisp finds it hard to see why one should care intrinsically about distributive equality at all. Where does its value come from? As Martin O'Neill writes, "On the Telic view . . . the ideal of equality can seem merely *arithmetic,* instead of being a properly intelligible political value" (O'Neill 2008, 139). For this reason, Hausman and Waldren refer to telic egalitarianism as "fundamentalist egalitarianism," since "it relies on what it regards as a fundamental intuition" about the injustice of unchosen inequalities (Hausman and Waldren 2011, 569). In a scenario like Square-vs.-Diamond, telic/fundamentalist egalitarians "can only thump their guts. . . . The problem is that . . . their argument for equality does not share anything with arguments for competing moral concerns" (Hausman and Waldren 2011, 574).

I am very sympathetic to Crisp's, O'Neill's, and Hausman and Waldren's doubts about the intrinsic value of distributive equality, and thus I am sympathetic to this second objection to the telic luck egalitarian principle. Many philosophers who lack the fundamentalist intuition about the intrinsic value of distributive equality will suggest that equality only *appears* to be valuable because the pursuit of equality so often overlaps with the pursuit of arrangements that benefit the worst-off. But these philosophers are quick to note that a commitment to improving the prospects of the worst-off is not the same as a commitment to distributive equality. After all, sometimes improving the situation of the worst-off will require *increasing* inequalities (as it would in a move from Diamond to Square). In order to give voice to these non-telic-egalitarian concerns, Derek Parfit introduced *prioritarianism,* the view that "benefitting people matters more the worse off these people are" (Parfit 1997, 213). Thus on a prioritarian view, there might be *nothing at all* wrong with a policy that maximally benefits the worst-off while also increasing distributive inequality. Temkin, by contrast, wants to say that although such a policy might be all-things-considered morally permissible (or even morally required), it is nevertheless morally regrettable because it clashes with telic luck egalitarianism. But if Crisp and O'Neill and Hausman and Waldren are all correct to doubt or reject the fundamentalist intuition that underlies luck egalitarianism, then prioritarianism will be attractive because it is an ideal that is quite clearly connected to the interests of persons. For *whenever* prioritarianism recommends a policy, that is because the policy will at least make *someone* better off. Telic egalitarianism cannot say the same.

While I believe that prioritarianism is an improvement over telic egalitarianism (and thus over luck egalitarianism), I do not believe it provides the basis for a plausible conception of distributive justice. To see why, note that as Parfit paints the view, prioritarianism requires a prioritarian response to all the needs one is in a position to address. As he puts it: "[The Priority View] naturally has universal scope. If it is more important to benefit one of two people, because this person is worse off, it is irrelevant whether these people are in the same community, or are aware of each other's existence. The greater urgency of benefitting this person does not depend on her relation to the other person, but only on her lower absolute level" (Parfit 1997, 214).

Drawing on a similar interpretation of prioritarianism, Richard Norman argues that the prioritarian perspective derives from "the standpoint of benevolent and sympathetic concern." Norman goes on to distinguish "the ethics of benevolence" from the ideal of social justice, thereby implying that prioritarian concern is what we are obligated to display to others regardless of our particular relationship to them (Norman 1999, 184, 185). Given this, I fear that *both* telic egalitarianism *and* prioritarianism run afoul of an important objection that W. D. Ross made long ago against utilitarianism. Ross writes:

> In fact the theory of "ideal utilitarianism" . . . seems to simplify unduly our relations to our fellows. It says, in effect, that the only morally significant relation in which my neighbours stand to me is that of being possible beneficiaries by my action. They do stand in this relation to me, and this relation is morally significant. But they may also stand to me in the relation of promisee to promiser, of creditor to debtor, of wife to husband, of child to parent, of friend to friend, of fellow countryman to fellow countryman, and the like; and each of these relations is the foundation of a *prima facie* duty, which is more or less incumbent on me according to the circumstances of the case. (W. D. Ross 1930, 19)[3]

Ross agreed with utilitarianism that there is always an important moral reason to promote others' well-being, regardless of their relationship to us. And he might well have agreed with prioritarianism—if he had known about it—that the well-being of the worst-off deserves some special priority. But Ross starkly departs from utilitarianism, prioritarianism, *and* telic egalitarianism in stressing the distinct moral importance of certain special relationships. It is, of course, not news that utilitarianism sees nothing intrinsically morally important about special relationships; and Parfit observes that prioritarianism is similar to utilitarianism in this regard. And though Parfit is correct when he says that telic egalitarianism is intrinsically concerned with *relativities*, the relativities at issue here involve brute comparisons between certain *features* of people's circumstances—for instance, their health or well-being—rather than on any distinctive social, familial, political, or otherwise interpersonal relationship that people themselves might stand in with others. What would happen, then, if instead of embracing telic egalitarianism or the equally nonrelational alternative of prioritarianism, we follow a more Rossian path and seek a *relational* egalitarianism? What would a decidedly relational egalitarianism look like?

THREE KINDS OF RELATIONAL EGALITARIANISM

Although they are not always characterized as such, I believe there are at least three types of relational egalitarianism on offer in the philosophical literature. These views highlight different kinds of morally important relationships we can stand in with others, rather than simply highlighting the bare fact that one person (or group of persons) has better health or greater well-being than another. Each of these relational views has its own distinctive reasons for calling itself "egalitarian," as I will explain. What they share is the conviction that if an ideal of equality is morally important for distributive justice, it must be reinterpreted as something other than mere similarity of condition between individuals who bear no further distinctive relation to one another. Moreover, while all three relational egalitarianisms are competitors to telic luck egalitarianism, they are not necessarily competitors with each other. Indeed, after sketching each of the three in this section (with a focus on their implications for health), I will then explain more fully how these three views can be combined into a single framework that can guide the formation of health policy.

First Type of Relational Egalitarianism: Equal Treatment

The first type of relational egalitarianism comes separately from Thomas Pogge and Thomas Nagel. In a paper titled "Relational Conceptions of

Justice: Responsibilities for Health Outcomes," Pogge writes: "My view on justice in regard to health is distinctive in two ways. First, I hold that the strength of our moral reasons to prevent or to mitigate particular medical conditions depends not only on what one might call *distributional* factors, such as how badly off the people affected by these conditions are in absolute and relative terms, how costly prevention or treatment would be, and how much patients would benefit from given treatment. Rather, it depends also on *relational* factors, that is, on how we are related to the medical conditions they suffer" (Pogge 2006, 135).

To illustrate, suppose you negligently hit a child while driving, injuring her badly. On rushing her to the hospital, you learn that she is in critical condition and requires a blood transfusion. Her blood type is rare and, as it happens, matches yours. She needs a lot of blood, and you are prepared to donate. However, the doctor also informs you that two other children were also recently admitted in need of that same rare blood type. Each needs half the amount you need to give to the girl to save her life, and you cannot safely donate enough to save all three. The doctor asks you whether you'd like to donate your blood and what you want done with it. It is Pogge's view that you have a stronger obligation to the girl than to the two other children, and that this traces to the way in which you are related to her current condition. In particular, *you* caused it. So although you can save more lives by letting the girl die and giving your blood to the other two children, Pogge believes you are morally required to choose the option that fails to maximize the number of lives saved. Call this kind of relational view *causal relationism*, since it says that our causal connections with others are relevant for assigning moral responsibility.

So construed, only a strict consequentialist will reject causal relationism wholesale. But Pogge takes this nonconsequentialist line quite a bit further, arguing that a duty to redress another's neediness is a duty *of justice* only if it flows from causal relationism. Consider another of his health-related examples:

> There are . . . extremely harsh natural environments where a man
> with a higher metabolic rate cannot meet his extra food needs simply
> by moderating his discretionary spending a bit or by working a little
> overtime. In such a context, decent people will make every effort to
> ensure that the man will have enough to eat. They will do so as a mat-
> ter of basic human solidarity, realizing that, given his constitution, he
> simply cannot survive on the fruits of his own labor. But does he have
> a justice claim to such support, can he demand it as a matter of right?

Listen to what such justice claim would sound like: "I have a higher
metabolic rate than you all. As a consequence, I need 50 percent more
food each day to be equally well nourished. Six hours of labor are
needed to produce this additional food. You five therefore owe it to
me as a matter of justice to work an extra hour each day along with
me to produce the extra food I need." If this is not a plausible claim,
then we should recognize, I think, that there are moral requirements
that, however stringent and categorical, are not demands of justice.
(Pogge 2010, 53)

Pogge elsewhere admits that this approach to justice "seems committed
to the callous (if not cruel) view that we, as a society, need do no more for
persons whose health is poor through no fault of ours than for persons in
good health" (Pogge 2002, 76). Yet as is indicated in the final line of the long
quotation above, Pogge prefers instead to draw a distinction between *moral*
obligations (which might be heavily needs-based) and obligations of *justice*
(which, he says, are not). It is then open to partisans of causal relationism to
"speak of duties of humanity or solidarity" that are "quite stringent" but "do
not correlate with rights" (Pogge 2010, 53).

So how can the idea of causal relationism be used to construct a brand of
relational *egalitarianism*? Pogge's answer is that causal relationism entails that
"the core of egalitarian liberalism" consists in "the idea that a liberal society,
or state, ought to treat all its citizens equally in terms of helps and hindrances.
Such equal treatment need not be equality-promoting treatment. Preexisting
inequalities in, for example, genetic potentials and liabilities . . . are not
society's responsibility" (Pogge 2002, 75). Thus while telic egalitarianism *is*
equality-promoting—that is, it sees intrinsic value in equal outcomes—Pogge's
equality of treatment view ignores outcomes and focuses solely on equalizing
the benefits that society bestows and the burdens it imposes. For many of the
same reasons as Pogge, Thomas Nagel has also defended "the deontological
theory of justice" that "centres on equal treatment rather than the avoidance
of inequality in the broadest terms" (Nagel 1997, 305–6). Like Pogge's, Nagel's
view restricts "injustice to certain specifically social causes of inequality, whose
avoidance takes precedence over the general welfare and other goals," including
the purely distributive goals of telic egalitarianism (Nagel 1997, 313).

To see why this might be called an egalitarian view, it will help to have a
more concrete example of what Pogge and Nagel mean by equal treatment.
Consider then the reasonable complaint that a blind person might lodge in a

society that caters more to the needs of the sighted than to the blind. The telic egalitarian would highlight the unchosen, unequal, and thus unfair outcomes that result when only the sighted can easily navigate their social world. By contrast, Pogge prefers to say:

> I understand that the present organization of our society is less appropriate to your mental and[/or] physical constitution than to those of most of your fellow citizens. In this sense, our shared institutional order is not affording you genuinely equal treatment. To make up for the ways in which we are treating you worse than most others, we propose to treat you better than them in other respects. For example, to make up for the fact that traffic instructions are communicated through visible but inaudible signals, we will provide free guide dogs to the blind. In doing so, our objective is that our institutional order as a whole should afford you genuinely equal treatment. (Pogge 2010, 31)

Here, equal treatment involves equalizing the overall balance of benefits and burdens *that flow from active social policy choices*. It does not involve equalizing resulting health or well-being. Thus, if there are further disadvantages in well-being that attend blindness but are not redressed by policies affording equal treatment, Pogge and Nagel do not believe that justice requires further redress.

Equality of treatment, so construed, is a form of relational egalitarianism because its understanding of what must be equalized stems from a prior commitment to causal relationism. Causal relationism, in turn, holds that the strength of one's reason to address neediness depends largely on one's causal relation to the needs in question. On this view, once the needs that one has caused (or helped to cause) have been redressed, one has strong reason to address residual needs *only if* doing so is required to ensure that social policies distribute *socially created* benefits and burdens equally among members of society.

Second Type of Relational Egalitarianism: Equality of Concern

The distinction between moral duties and duties of justice seems clearly important, but one might doubt that Pogge and Nagel have drawn the line in the right place. For while Pogge and Nagel are surely correct to highlight justice-based duties to redress *needs* to which one is causally related, Pogge and Nagel do not take pains to argue against justice-based duties that arise out of the way one is related to *the people* who suffer the needs. Yet as Ross stresses, these latter sorts of duties arise all the time and can be quite stringent. They are present, for example, when a parent has a duty to respond to the needs of a sick child, or perhaps when a citizen has a duty to help provide health care to a soldier whose health need is not traceable to his or her military service. In each of these cases, what we owe others has to do with the special interpersonal relationship we bear *to them*, not the special causal relationship we might bear to their need. So here we have a second kind of relational view. Call it *interpersonal relationism*. Interpersonal relationism is a component of lots of distributive justice frameworks, and it is the form of relationism discussed in Samuel Scheffler's influential paper "Relationships and Responsibilities." Scheffler's discussion focuses on responsibilities that arise out of noninstrumentally valuable relationships, but it is not obvious that interpersonal relational responsibilities cannot also arise in the context of purely instrumentally valuable relationships. Nevertheless, I shall follow Scheffler in viewing interpersonal relational responsibilities as requiring a "dispos[ition] . . . to see that [other] person's needs, interests, and desires as, in themselves, providing me with presumptively decisive reasons for action, reasons that I would not have had in the absence of the relationship" (Scheffler 2001, 100). In other words, they require a certain degree of concern for another's well-being.

Just as Pogge and Nagel built a version of relational egalitarianism (i.e., equality of treatment) around the more general idea of causal relationism, so too can a distinct version of relational egalitarianism be built around the general idea of interpersonal relationism. Such a view would hold that distributive justice generates duties of *equal concern* for those to whom one stands in especially morally relevant political relationships. Views along these lines have been defended separately by Ronald Dworkin and Richard W. Miller. According to Dworkin, "equal concern is the sovereign virtue of political community," for "no government is legitimate that does not show equal concern for the fate of all those citizens over whom it claims dominion and from whom it claims allegiance" (Dworkin 2002, 1). Likewise, Miller claims that "equal concern is the more appropriate standard [of social justice] because it better reflects the moral significance of democratic citizenship. For equal concern . . . expresses the proper valuing of the institutional loyalties on which a well-ordered democracy depends" (Miller 2002, 298). According to Miller, the proper way to value others' institutional loyalties—that is, loyalty to a shared political project—is "by showing special loyalty to them, displayed in special concern for their needs" (Miller 2010, 43).

The requirements of equal concern embodies what I have elsewhere called a "supply-side" requirement (Kelleher 2013). That is, it does not in the first instance enjoin a specific pattern or level of benefits that individuals are to possess or enjoy; rather, it enjoins a degree of other-regarding concern that is to flow *from* the provider of justice (here most plausibly the political community as a corporate entity) *to* the recipients of justice (the members conceived as individuals). Thus, unlike both telic egalitarianism and Parfit's prioritarianism, which focus on the "demand-side" issue of individuals differ in the amount of health or well-being they enjoy, equality of concern stresses the supply-side factor of displaying the proper attitudes toward, and dispositions to help, those in need.

Drawing in part on both Dworkin and Miller, I have argued elsewhere that equality of concern is indeed a genuine requirement of distributive justice (Kelleher 2014). But my goal here is only to explain how that view can be seen as a distinct brand of relational egalitarianism. It is egalitarian because the concern displayed to each of a given set of individuals is to be *equal*. And it is relational insofar as the duty to show special concern is grounded in facts about interpersonal relationships that tie certain individuals to one another. Dworkin suggests how these two elements can be combined to yield a distinctive view (or at least a distinctive plank of justice). He writes, "As individuals we owe all other human beings a *measure* of concern, but we do not owe them concern equal to that we have for ourselves, our families, and others close to us" (Dworkin 2008, 95).[4] He continues, "A legitimate government must treat all those over whom it claims dominion not just with a measure of concern but with *equal* concern. I mean that it must act as if the impact of its policies on the life of any citizen is equally important" (Dworkin 2008, 97). I interpret Dworkin as claiming that certain features of the domestic political relationship justify governments (I prefer to speak of political communities) in showing *strong and equal* concern for each member of society. This is what makes it a form of relational egalitarianism.

A famous example of Thomas Nagel's is, I think, useful in beginning to tease out more practical implications of the equal concern view. (For our purposes, it is best to ignore the interpretive question of what Nagel would say is the connection between this example from 1979 and his later endorsement of causal relationism and the equal treatment view.) The example begins by asking us to imagine that Nagel has one healthy child and one suffering from a painful disability. Suppose now that he must make a choice between moving to a city where the second child could receive medical treatment but which would be unpleasant for the first child, or moving to a semirural suburb where the first child alone would benefit. Nagel stipulates that "the gain to the first child of moving to the suburb is substantially greater than the gain to the second child of moving to the city." He then claims, "If one chose to move to the city, it would be an egalitarian decision. It is more urgent to benefit the second child, even though the benefit we can give him is less than the benefit we can give the first child" (Nagel 1979, 124). In response to these claims, Parfit argued that Nagel had confused the ideas of equality and priority. For Nagel's discussion clearly suggests that he really does not care about equality *at all*; instead, his focus is on making the worst-off child as well off as possible (Parfit 1997, 215–16). But Parfit's diagnosis ignores the fact that Nagel's example seems intended to illustrate the supply-side phenomenon of equal concern. Thus Parfit can be right that if one fundamentally cares about improving the situation of the worst-off, then one should not fundamentally care about *distributive* equality in the way the telic luck egalitarian does. That is, one should not care about brute arithmetic equality between people's health or well-being, for it is (as we have seen) conceivable that the only way to improve the lot of the worst-off is via a policy that improves the better-off even more, thereby widening the gap. But—and here's the key point—even if one does not fundamentally care about distributive equality between people's health or well-being, one *can* maintain that each is entitled to robust and equal concern. And according to Nagel, equal concern for the worst-off is precisely what justifies being especially attentive to their needs. That is the very point of the example: while he loves his two children equally and is therefore equally concerned for them, he also rightly views the needs of the worst-off child "as being ahead in the queue, so to speak" (Nagel 1995, 68). Nagel's example, therefore, demonstrates how something *like* a prioritarian response to differing needs can be consistent with showing each of many different individuals the same robust degree of concern. It is therefore worth asking (as I will below) whether members of modern liberal democracies owe one another duties of equal concern that in turn justify health-promoting policies and institutions that tilt in favor of aiding the worst-off.

Third Type of Relational Egalitarianism: Social Egalitarianism

The third kind of relational egalitarianism I want to identify is a brand of what I will call *social relationism*. This sort of view is found in Elizabeth Anderson's work, in which she argues that distributive justice is not about producing a certain pattern of health or well-being between persons, but rather about fostering mutually respectful interactions between them. According to Anderson, the ideal of equality is best conceived as "a social relationship.... Two people [are] equal when each accepts the obligation to justify their actions by principles acceptable to the other, and in which they take mutual consultation, reciprocation, and recognition for granted" (Anderson 1999, 313). In this sort of view, "equality" once again does not characterize a relationship between two (or more) *quantities*, nor does it betoken similarity in the degree of other-regarding *concern*; rather, it suggests a character that the interactions between two (or more) individuals should display. Along these same lines, Samuel Scheffler has also argued that individuals are equal in the morally relevant sense when they can or do interact with one another "as equals," or "on a footing of equality" (Scheffler 2003, 26, 23). And as already noted, Hausman and Waldren claim that there are six different objectives that social egalitarians (which Hausman and Waldren call "non-fundamentalist egalitarians") will emphasize as important to a society of equals. For the social egalitarian, distributive inequalities are objectionable when they frustrate the realization of distinct social relational ideals. Hausman and Waldren's six ideals are procedural fairness, impartiality, the display of equal respect, the cultivation of fraternity, the prevention of domination, and everyone's possessing a firm basis for self-respect (Hausman and Waldren 2011, 578). Thus like the other two kinds of relational egalitarianism I have described, but unlike telic luck egalitarianism, social egalitarianism gives explicit primacy to palpable social evils that connect up in obvious ways to central human interests.

One worry about social egalitarianism is that its driving values and ideals may be too vague to explain what we owe to each other with respect to things like health. For example, Scheffler claims that "human relations must be conducted on the basis of an assumption that everyone's life is equally important." Yet it is not yet clear whether this requires individuals to share a stranger's fate by making sacrifices to help improve his health. Does one owe this to all strangers, or just certain ones? Scheffler leaves such questions unanswered. Further, while it is clearly true that the disabled should be presented with a social world that treats them as equals and is not hostile to their differences, it may seem in principle possible to eliminate the *stigma* associated with certain disabilities without requiring expensive, publicly funded measures to *prevent* or *eliminate* those disabilities in the first place. Is a single-minded focus on reducing stigma all that is required by social egalitarianism?

I raise these issues not to dismiss social egalitarianism. It is, after all, hard to deny that justice requires institutional arrangements that treat citizens "as equals" and situate them "on a footing of equality." The same goes for Anderson's claim that justice militates against hierarchy and marginalization. However, these attractive claims do not yet tell us all that we need to know when we seek to evaluate inequalities in health.

In this section I have described three kinds of relational egalitarianism. Unlike telic luck egalitarianism or prioritarianism, each follows Ross in stressing the moral importance of specific, real-world relationships. Moreover, the first two—equality of treatment and equality of concern—join telic egalitarianism in requiring equality *of something*: equality of treatment requires "equal social helps and hindrances," whereas equality of concern requires the display of equal degrees of concern for each member of a morally significant group (such as a political community). By contrast, the third form of relational egalitarianism, social egalitarianism, interprets equality not as a relationship between *quantities* (of benefits) or *degrees* (of concern), but rather as a morally attractive *type* of relationship, one involving mutually respectful interaction and discourse conducted "on a footing of equality."

COMBINING THE THREADS

As I have indicated, my own view is that the distinct relational egalitarian views are not competitors and that each describes a plausible plank of distributive justice. Whether and how each bears on the evaluation of health inequalities is a harder question. In this section I want to say a bit more about how the three relational egalitarian views might be brought together to form the core of a pluralistic approach to distributive justice. In the next section I will attempt to connect the pluralistic approach to the case study provided in this volume by Sarah Horton and Judith C. Barker concerning the oral health of Latino children.

To begin combining the theoretical threads, note that the basis of the equal treatment view, causal relationism, is endorsed by virtually all conceptions of distributive justice, including libertarianism. Causal relationism, again, is the view that the strength of one's moral reason to redress disadvantages depends greatly on one's past causal relation to that disadvantage. And libertarians tend to agree that if one causes harm to another, or if a government policy causes harm to members of society, then redress and restitution are owed. But it is of course true that libertarians will reject the aspect of the equality-of-treatment view that enjoins the provision of equal helps and hindrances to each member. So where does this demand come from? Pogge is quiet on this, but in my view this demand must also derive from the nature of the cooperative relationships that members of a society stand in with one another. For example, on the assumption that governments legitimately engage in broad macroeconomic management and steering—an assumption shared by Pogge and Nagel—many social laws and policies will conspire to yield a hierarchy of jobs and roles. Yet it is implausible to say that the relative size of a given worker's contribution to economic prosperity is proportional to the size of the salary or wage he or she earns. Jobs and roles "at the bottom" have to be taken up by someone, and those of us who do not have to take them are typically relieved that this is so. Each occupant of a useful role therefore accepts a bundle of burdens and benefits that *arguably* renders each occupant's net social contribution more or less equal. (I put the stress on *arguably* because I admit that more must be said to defend this conclusion.) If members' net social contributions are indeed roughly equal, then this would support the view that in addition to avoiding and redressing socially caused *harm*, social policies must further ensure that each member of society receive roughly equal benefits from social cooperation.

Suppose for the sake of argument that Pogge and Nagel can in fact build these additional theses into their equal treatment view. Even so, their view would not require the redress of (to use Pogge's words) "preexisting inequalities in, for example, genetic potentials and liabilities." After all, on Pogge's and Nagel's equal treatment view, if society doesn't cause the health problems, then they "are not society's responsibility and are not to be corrected or compensated at the expense of those favored by these [purely natural] inequalities" (Pogge 2002, 75–76). It is at this point that Dworkin's and Miller's relational "equality of concern" view can be brought in to supplement the equal treatment view. For according to Dworkin and Miller, the very forms of social cooperation that Pogge and Nagel can cite to require equality in social "helps and hindrances" can also be cited to defend the requirement that fellow citizens display robust and equal concern for one another. Miller is particularly helpful here, as his view highlights the ways in which actually existing democratic capitalism differs from laissez-faire libertarianism. While many self-avowed libertarians have no problem with state-protected private property, national defense, public schools, and public police forces, modern capitalism evidently requires even more in the name of stability and prosperity. Examples here include the central bank's role in setting the key price in the entire economy (the interest rate), a tool that has been used in the United States to deliberately put and keep working people out of work in the name of price stability; the central bank's role as lender of last resort; the state's bestowal of limited liability to corporate entities; and government-granted monopolies in the form of patents. After highlighting these and other functions of modern governments, Miller (in effect) argues that a focus on providing equal helps and hindrances is misguided:

> Equal concern is the more appropriate standard because it better reflects the moral significance of democratic citizenship. For equal concern, not concern for equal benefit, expresses the proper valuing of the institutional loyalties on which a well-ordered democracy depends. Morally responsible citizens of a just polity want its functioning to depend on willing civic commitments—for example, a preference for principled persuasion and empathic consideration of others' conflicting interests even when one could be part of a dominant coalition; a willingness to conform to laws with which one disagrees, even if they are somewhat unjust or quite foolish; and, if need be, a willingness to risk one's life for one's country. A proper appreciation of these shared institutional loyalties is displayed in equal concern for one's loyal coparticipants. (Miller 2002, 298)

I believe the general thought here is that when you continue to cooperate with me even though I help to coerce you through support for laws that you may not fully agree with, I owe you something significant in return (and vice versa). We might say (although Miller does not) that what we give to one another in the course of normal political cooperation is the sort of thing sports commentators refer to as an "intangible": it doesn't necessarily show up in a breakdown of yearly economic statistics, but it deserves special recognition nonetheless. This recognition, Miller suggests, should take the form of special concern for those whose lives one helps to coerce and whose civic cooperation one relies on.

This account of how a duty of equal concern arises does, I admit, suggest that equality of concern and equality of treatment are competitors. Indeed, Miller explicitly says that equality of concern is a "more appropriate standard" of social justice than equal benefit is. But I do not agree that they are competitors. Consider a more personal analogy. Suppose a parent and his adult child agree to go into business together, agreeing to split profits in half. I assume it is uncontroversial that such an arrangement generates a pro tanto duty on behalf of each to share the profits equally with the other. But the presence of such a duty is perfectly consistent with the presence of distinct duties of parental and filial love and concern. Thus, even if their business contract gives each a *pro tanto* equal claim on the business's profits, it can still be all-things-considered wrong for (say) the parent to insist on an equal share. If the child is experiencing a financial rough patch while the parent is already financially comfortable, a parental duty of love and concern may well carry the day and count against equal shares. If this is plausible, I think something similar can be said about the political case. That is, the equal treatment view can be correct that roughly equal contributions generate *pro tanto* claims to roughly equal shares of the social output. And yet the circumstances of social cooperation that Miller highlights can *also* generate *further pro tanto* obligations of concern for one's fellow cooperators. Of course, merely drawing attention to this potential blend of *pro tanto* duties does not yet make it clear what this means in practice. But I do think it shows that we needn't view "equality of helps and hindrances" and "equality of concern" as competitors.

What about the third relational egalitarian view, social egalitarianism? Does that somehow conflict with the other relational views? I noted in the third section that while social egalitarianism does embody certain important values, these values are highly abstract. This has not prevented some social egalitarians from making bold claims about the view's implications for health justice. For example, Elizabeth Anderson holds that social egalitarianism gives each citizen "a claim to a capability set sufficient to enable them to function as equals in society. . . . Democratically relevant functionings include adequate safety, health and nutrition, education, mobility and communication, the ability to interact with others without stigma, and to participate in the system of cooperation" (Anderson 2010, 83). But Anderson does not offer a substantive defense of this conclusion, and until she does so it will continue to be reasonable to question her move from the fairly abstract ideal of social equality to the conclusion that citizens have "claims to health."[5]

In elaborating his own social egalitarian view, Daniel Hausman says, "The strongest egalitarian criticisms of domestic inequalities in health rest, I think, on the values of solidarity and reciprocity, which, as I argued above, I take to be themselves [relational] egalitarian values" (Hausman 2013, 40). He continues: "To permit some to suffer, to die or to be disabled needlessly is to fail to embrace them as partners in the human enterprise. . . . But the extent to which solidarity is possible across national borders is limited, and this argument has less application to international inequalities" (Hausman 2013). This view, however, raises the following worry: if the "application" (to use Hausman's term) of solidarity at the domestic level depends on the contingent fact that the sentiment of solidary just happens to be felt at that level, doesn't the ideal of solidarity lose its normative force? Unless more is said, it is hard to see why failing to feel solidarity across borders should be thought a permissible failing, whereas failing to feel it within borders is to be viewed as a moral flaw that can be corrected with (or at least counterbalanced by) coercively enforced health-promoting institutions. Unfortunately, Hausman does not say more. But this gap may in fact be an opportunity. For if Hausman embraced something like the argument for equality of concern, he could cite that as the basis of why robust solidarity is owed at the domestic level, but not across borders. This would leave the broad contours of Hausman's view intact, and his view would be defensible for precisely the reason he indicates: participants in a domestic political project *are* partners in a morally relevant human enterprise, and the nature of their partnership *does* impose objective moral requirements to display solidarity and reciprocal concern for one another. This, as we have seen, is basically Miller's thesis, and I think this in turn shows how equality of concern and social egalitarianism can be mutually supporting (if not entirely overlapping).

RELATIONAL EGALITARIANISM AND
ORAL HEALTH DISPARITIES

Sarah Horton and Judith C. Barker's discussion in this volume of oral health in Latino farmworker children in California provides a case study that I believe implicates all three relational egalitarian threads I have highlighted. I want to end with an all-too-brief discussion of how the pluralistic framework I've developed can potentially inform our discussion of whether and how inequalities in oral health raise issues of distributive justice.

As it happens, the first step is the same for both the epidemiologist and the causal relationist, and that is to ask about causes. At first blush, however, it is not clear that oral ill health among the studied population is the result of third-party harm that can directly ground duties of compensation and restitution. At one point in their discussion of causes, Horton and Barker refer to Nancy Krieger's work showing "how the excess risk of hypertension among African Americans is the physical embodiment of myriad social and material factors—including residential and occupational segregation, exposure to toxic substances, interpersonal discrimination" (140). Here, identifiable and independently unjust social practices contribute to instances of poor health that thereby inherit the unfairness of their causes. But it is not clear that the oral health issues that Horton and Barker focus on are like that. According to Horton and Barker, the proximate causes of oral ill health are the diet and feeding practices of the children's parents. Extensive bottle feeding in early childhood, combined later with sodas, candies, and processed foods, do predictably lead to tooth decay. But here the proximate causative agents are the parents who have migrated to California to give themselves and their children a better life and who must permit others to bottle-feed their children while breast-feeding mothers are out working in the field. It is hard to treat *these* causes as morally on a par with the social causes of African American ill health that Krieger outlines.

Proximate causes are, however, just one morally relevant factor. As we have seen, even causal relationists like Pogge and Nagel hold that equal treatment requires a fair distribution of the benefits and burdens of social cooperation, and it would therefore be open to them to argue that oral ill health can be unjust *either* if its proximate causes are inherently unjust *or* if it is the indirect result of an unjust distribution of economic resources. And it is quite clear that one upstream (though not *that* far upstream) factor relevant here is the very poor access to pediatric dental care available to the children of migrant farmworkers. Horton and Barker report that California's dental program under Medicaid, Denti-Cal, has such low provider reimbursement rates that "within a fifty-mile radius of Mendota—a catchment of roughly eight hundred thousand—only five dentists accepted children under five insured by Denti-Cal" (146). And even when children do manage to see a dentist, Denti-Cal's "high standards for proof of service" (147) can mean that (as one dentist put it) "You keep sending in your Xrays and get your reimbursements denied, you get frustrated. As a result, there are very few dentists who do pulpotomies on Denti-Cal patients in the area" (147). This encourages underreimbursed and overworked Denti-Cal providers to simply extract diseased teeth, rather than restore them. While the argument cannot be fleshed out fully here, one can easily imagine Pogge or Nagel arguing that this arrangement fails to give these families and their children their fair share of social resources. Thus, even if justice does not require a dedicated concern with this population's oral *health*, it can require a dedicated concern with the fair distribution of background resources, which individuals would then predictably use to promote their *own* health. This is how an unjust distribution of resources can turn into an unjust cause by the lights of a principle of equal treatment.

A principle of equal concern can take this indictment one step further, by offering to take an active concern in Latino children's oral health itself, and not just in their access to all-purpose resources.[6] For as Horton and Barker explain, a great many (perhaps the vast majority) of these children are U.S. citizens. (Although I cannot take up the issue here, it is arguable that those who are not citizens now would be eligible to become citizens under a more just immigration system.) If Miller and Dworkin are correct that responsible citizenship carries with it a claim to the concern of the political community, then the demands of justice might not run out once resources had been distributed as a principle of equal treatment alone would require. Further adjustments may be needed to ensure that proper concern is being shown to those whose needs are especially pressing. Everyone knows that rotting teeth can be physically painful, and as Horton and Barker demonstrate, the lifelong social stigma associated with bad or missing teeth can be piercing and traumatic. So if a principle of equal concern should be combined with a principle of equal treatment, that would add further support to policies aimed at redressing the poor health of the worst-off—*not* as a way of evening out the distribution of health-related resources but, rather, as the expression of active concern for the well-being of those to whom one is specially politically related and whose needs are especially pressing.

At some point, wanting nicer teeth ceases to be a desire for improved health and becomes a desire merely for improved social status. And it is here where relational egalitarian concerns may appear especially relevant. But just how they are relevant is not immediately clear, since a main aim of relational egalitarianism is to combat and eliminate unjustified bases of stigma and status differences. Indeed, a good case can be made that the social status conferred by *beautiful* teeth—as opposed to merely healthy teeth—is unjust and should not be further entrenched by public policy. Consider, for example, a potential letter that Elizabeth Anderson imagines people receiving along with "compensation checks" from the (fictional) State Equality Board: "To the ugly and socially awkward: How sad that you are so repulsive to people around you that no one wants to be your friend or lifetime companion. We won't make it up to you by being your friend or your marriage partner—we have our own freedom of association to exercise—but you can console yourself in your miserable loneliness by consuming these material goods that we, the beautiful and charming ones, will provide. And who knows? Maybe you won't be such a loser in love once potential dates see how rich you are."

Anderson herself concludes: "Could a self-respecting citizen fail to be insulted by such messages? How dare the state pass judgment on its citizens' worth as workers and lovers!" (Anderson 1999, 305). Does this mean, then, that a relational egalitarian cannot justify tax-financed dental care for those whose are stigmatized or ostracized because their teeth aren't straight enough or attractive enough? In later work Anderson concedes that the social roots of stigma can be so difficult to extirpate that tax-financed beautification may well be the only feasible way deliver justice to stigmatized individuals. She now imagines a different, more defensible letter: "Dear Citizen, Your critique of the ways society stigmatizes you and fails to accommodate your differences exposes an injustice in society, which we are working to correct. Unfortunately, we have found that it is difficult to change unjust habits of stigmatization held by the populace against people with your physical appearance. Hence, we are offering you the alternative of plastic surgery, so that you can escape this unjust stigma" (Anderson 2010, 96).

I have no doubt that most social egalitarians would claim that their central concerns can also justify policies aimed at individuals' oral health, not just at their oral beauty. But if health-promoting policies can already be grounded in the relational planks of equal treatment and equal concern, it may be best to draw most heavily on social egalitarianism when responding to the unjust stigma that attends missing, cracked, or stained teeth. Anderson's discussion shows us how to do this.

CONCLUSION

In this essay I have explained the difference between telic egalitarianism (which is at the heart of many luck egalitarian views) and relational egalitarianism, and I have described three different types of relational egalitarianism. In the end, I think that each of the three has an important role to play in our thinking about distributive justice and in our subsequent evaluation of health inequalities. I began my discussion of relational egalitarianism by expressing sympathy with Ross's relational critique of utilitarianism. As is well-known, Ross's positive view has been very influential within bioethics, and his is by far the most famous version of moral pluralism. But Ross's view, and many of the discussions of it that exist in the bioethics literature, suggest that there is some single principle of distributive justice, which in turn is just one principle in a fuller moral view. I have argued here that there is in fact more than one principle of distributive justice, and indeed more than one principle of relational egalitarian distributive justice. I hope my discussion helps to clarify the normative and conceptual landscape against which debates about justice and health inequalities should take place.

NOTES

1. It is, of course, not easy—and perhaps it is impossible—to distinguish choices and outcomes for which people are responsible from those that result from bad brute luck. For further discussion, see Voigt 2013.

2. Emphasis in original.

3. Ross uses *"prima facie"* to make the qualification I have been making with *"pro tanto."*

4. Emphasis in original.

5. For an in-depth exploration of these and related issues, see Voigt and Wester 2015. Regrettably, Voigt and Wester's very nice article appeared too late for me to engage adequately with it here.

6. I assume, along with Ross, that there is always a reason to help those who need help, even in the absence of a special relationship to them. Since I am now trying to explain how the three relational views might work in practice, I'm choosing not to stress the relevance of nonrelational benevolence. But in the end, such benevolence might be among the strongest reasons to help the children at issue. I thank Dan Hausman for pressing me on this point.

REFERENCES

Anderson, Elizabeth S. 1999. "What Is the Point of Equality?" *Ethics* 109 (2): 287–337.

———. 2010. "Justifying the Capabilities Approach to Justice." In *Measuring Justice: Primary Goods and Capabilities*, edited by Harry Brighouse and Ingrid Robeyns, 81–100. Cambridge: Cambridge University Press.

Crisp, Roger. 2003. "Equality, Priority, and Compassion." *Ethics* 113 (4): 745–63.

Dworkin, Ronald. 2002. *Sovereign Virtue: The Theory and Practice of Equality*. Cambridge, MA: Harvard University Press.

———. 2008. *Is Democracy Possible Here? Principles for a New Political Debate*. Princeton, NJ: Princeton University Press.

Hausman, Daniel M. 2013. "Injustice and Inequality in Health and Health Care." In *Justice, Luck and Responsibility in Health Care*, edited by Yvonne Denier, Chris Gastmans, and Antoon Vandevelde, 29–42. Dordrecht: Springer Science and Business Media.

Hausman, Daniel M., and Matthew Sensat Waldren. 2011. "Egalitarianism Reconsidered." *Journal of Moral Philosophy* 8 (4): 567–86.

Kelleher, J. Paul. 2013. "Capabilities versus Resources." *Journal of Moral Philosophy*, no. 12: 2–21.

———. 2014. "Beneficence, Justice, and Health Care." *Kennedy Institute of Ethics Journal* 24 (1): 27–49.

Marmot, Michael. 2004. *The Status Syndrome: How Social Standing Affects Our Health and Longevity*. New York: Henry Holt and Company.

Miller, Richard W. 2002. "Too Much Inequality." *Social Philosophy and Policy* 19 (1): 275–313.

———. 2010. *Globalizing Justice: The Ethics of Poverty and Power*. Oxford: Oxford University Press.

Nagel, Thomas. 1986. *The View from Nowhere*. Oxford: Clarendon.

———. 1995. *Equality and Partiality*. Oxford: Oxford University Press.

———. 1997. "Justice and Nature." *Oxford Journal of Legal Studies* 17: 303–21.

Norman, Richard. 1999. "Equality, Priority and Social Justice." *Ratio* 12 (2): 178–94.

O'Neill, Martin. 2008. "What Should Egalitarians Believe?" *Philosophy and Public Affairs* 36 (2): 119–56.

Pogge, Thomas W. 2002. "Responsibilities for Poverty-Related Ill Health." *Ethics and International Affairs* 16 (2): 71–81.

———. 2006. "Relational Conceptions of Justice: Responsibilities for Health Outcomes." In *Public Health, Ethics and Equity*, edited by Sudhir Anand, Fabienne Peter, and Amartya Sen, 135–61. Oxford: Oxford University Press.

———. 2010. "A Critique of the Capability Approach." In *Measuring Justice: Primary Goods and Capabilities*, edited by Harry Brighouse and Ingrid Robeyns, 17–60. Cambridge: Cambridge University Press.

Ross, W. David. 1930. *The Right and the Good*. Indianapolis: Hackett.

Scheffler, Samuel. 2001. *Boundaries and Allegiances: Problems of Justice and Responsibility in Liberal Thought*. Oxford: Oxford University Press.

———. 2003. "What Is Egalitarianism?" *Philosophy and Public Affairs* 31 (1): 5–39.

Temkin, Larry S. 2003. "Egalitarianism Defended." *Ethics* 113 (4): 764–82.

Voigt, Kristin. 2013. "Appeals to Individual Responsibility for Health." *Cambridge Quarterly of Healthcare Ethics* 22 (2): 146–58. Erratum: 2013. *Cambridge Quarterly of Healthcare Ethics* 22 (3): 328–29.

Voigt, Kristin, and Gry Wester. 2015. "Relational Equality and Health." *Social Philosophy and Policy* 31 (2): 204–29.

4

The Liberal Autonomous Subject and the Question of Health Inequalities

Eva Feder Kittay

ABSTRACT

The bioethical principle of respect for the autonomy of the patient represents an advance over the paternalism that earlier pervaded medical practice. Yet the normative set of assumptions that accompany the principle of autonomy has its own difficulties. The notion of autonomy, derived primarily from liberal moral and political theories, makes assumptions about capability and capacity that are often belied just when patients are in need of medical care. Patients who can compensate for their diminished agency and autonomy tend to have more material and social resources at their disposal. They are those who Shim et al. (this volume) characterize as having greater social capital. Those who are presumed autonomous but lack these resources are, in Onora O'Neill's (2002) words, "abandoned to their autonomy." Others still are deemed incompetent, in which case their agency gets scarce acknowledgment. I argue that the assumption that the recipient of health care is an autonomous subject effectively skews the distribution of health resources in favor of those who are most likely to fit that norm and who, when they have diminished capacities, have the wherewithal to have their autonomy "supported" through periods of medical need. The assumption of patient autonomy thus illuminates one way in which socioeconomic inequalities result in health disparities. I utilize a study of three heart attack victims belonging to three different socioeconomic classes to illustrate how the assumptions of the autonomous patient contribute to their different health outcomes. I conclude that a better model of medical care should aim to anticipate the needs of a patient or the patient's home caregiver, identify what this patient needs to meet her medical needs, and promote ways for patients to make life choices most conducive to health.

INTRODUCTION

A *New York Times* article by Janny Scott, tellingly entitled "Life at the Top in America Isn't Just Better, It's Longer," features three New York residents of different socioeconomic classes, each of whom suffered from heart disease (Scott 2005). The article chronicles their different health outcomes following a heart attack. Scott points out that "heart attack is a window on the effects of class on health. The risk factors—smoking, poor diet, inactivity, obesity, hypertension, high cholesterol and stress—are all more common among the less educated and less affluent, the same group that research has shown is less likely to receive cardiopulmonary resuscitation, to get emergency room care or to adhere to lifestyle changes after heart attack."

The article highlights the sort of fact that is widely discussed in the health disparities literature, namely that health disparities track a number of predictable indicators: not only health insurance (or some form of reliable health-care access), but also income and wealth, education, race or ethnicity, age, disability, and sometimes gender. While this is unsurprising, more surprising is that even in nations with a good health-care system with wide coverage, those occupying each successively lower portion of the socioeconomic pyramid do worse in terms of longevity and morbidity than those above.[1] Scott's three-tiered study provides us with rich material for investigating how socioeconomic differences translate into disparities in health outcomes.

Richard Wilkerson and his colleagues have produced impressive evidence showing that the steepness of the inequality pyramid—in other words, relative rather than absolute wealth—is itself a potent factor in health disparities (see, e.g., Wilkinson 1992; Corruccini 1984; Wilkinson 1996; Mullahy and Robert 2004). As Norman Daniels et al. remark, it is "not just the size of the economic pie but how the pie is shared that matters for population health. It is not the absolute deprivation associated with low economic development... but the degree of relative deprivation within them" (Daniels, Kennedy, and Kawachi 1999, 221).

Although these conclusions, taken largely from the work of Wilkinson and colleagues, are sometimes disputed, I will not take issue with them here.[2] A critical underlying question in the literature has been: What is the pathway linking social inequality to health inequality? This complex question can be answered in part by examining the circuitous route that Shim et al. (this volume) call cultural health capital.[3] Lying at the foundation of those resources that can be called cultural capital is the capacity for autonomous actions and choices.

In this chapter, I write as a philosopher who is concerned with issues of justice and care. Considering questions of justice from the perspective of someone interested in questions of how we care for people in states of vulnerability, I have become suspicious of a notion that plays a key role in political and moral philosophy, bioethics, and medical practice: the concept of autonomy. In bioethics and health-care practices, an autonomous person is understood to be a person who is capable of making his or her own decisions regarding medical care and capable of giving informed consent to procedures that are suggested by health professionals.[4] The antithesis of the autonomous individual is the "incompetent" patient. The dichotomous classification of patients as autonomous or incompetent serves neither group well. When a person is ill, they are often not in a position to make well-considered decisions about their medical care. The less education and resources they possess, the less they are able to understand medical explanations and instructions, and the less control they have over their lives such that their desire for a healthy outcome is congruent with the ability to do what such an outcome requires. The higher a person sits on the socioeconomic pyramid, the more advantageous is the valuing of autonomy. Those who are presumed to be autonomous but lack the means to realize their justifiable desires for health and well-being are more likely to suffer than to benefit from the emphasis on autonomy, or so I shall attempt to show using Scott's example. Further, when patients are deemed "incompetent" to make decisions an autonomous person can make, medical personnel have license to run roughshod over their particular desires, aims, or concerns in favor of a general "best interest" standard.

In this essay, I put forward a hypothesis that is undoubtedly provocative: that many medical practices that crystallize around the concept of autonomy serve as one pathway by which inequalities in socioeconomic status result in unequal health outcomes. The idealization of the citizen in an affluent liberal society as an autonomous agent has infiltrated the contemporary concept of the patient. This idealization has uptake insofar as the physician accepts himself and his fellow citizens as autonomous agents. As the value of autonomy takes hold, medicine becomes an institution that is fitted to a certain sort of patient and works best when the patient best fits the model—when practice and patient are matched as lock and key.

The idealization of the patient as an autonomous individual who should have his autonomy respected is tied to a number of other values, many of which are hard to impute: self-determination, equal respect for all, individual choice. But others are more questionable: self-sufficiency, the high value placed on rationality, and individualism, among others. The different values arise out of a conception of society and a conception of the person (or the person as citizen). In Shim et al.'s (chapter 9, this volume) terms, adapted from Bourdieu, the cultural health capital, which is broadly recognized and which we can identify as the repertoire of skills that come under the heading of autonomy, arises out of the cultural capital needed to achieve social status and economic success.

That the two, cultural health capital and cultural capital, are closely aligned should on the one hand not be surprising. On the other hand, one might think health care should stand apart from the wider ideal, since medicine often deals with human beings in a vulnerable state, when they are most fragile and dependent on others. Medicine is practiced on someone in need of care—and so on someone who fails to satisfy the ideal of the autonomous agent. The two ideas—that the patient is autonomous and independent, and that the patient is a vulnerable and dependent—are reconciled through a vision of medicine as enacted on a fully capable and fully functioning person who is only temporarily in need of some fixing. The concept of autonomy that finds its way into our cultural consciousness and into bioethical ideals is one that is developed in philosophical writings on justice. Before moving on to examples and the role autonomy plays in bioethics and medical practice, we will first look at how the concept functions in the political ideal from which it is drawn.

THEORY: THE CITIZEN AS AUTONOMOUS

The theory that will help us fix our concepts is that of John Rawls, whose conception of "justice as fairness" is widely thought to best formulate the ideal of justice for a liberal and egalitarian democracy. Although Rawls's "realistic utopia," as he calls his theory, is a long way from the deeply imperfect democracy we are familiar with in the United States, its ideals are meant to serve as a measure by which we judge our society. Rawls argues that were we to know nothing of who we are and how we are situated in our society,[5] we would choose two principles (out of a list of traditional principles of justice) to govern the basic structure of society. The first principle affirms equal basic rights and liberties for all, while the second principle determines just distributions of opportunities, income, and wealth. Within the constraints of the just regulation of the basic structure, everyone is entitled to pursue their own conception of the good, and at the same time must respect others' rights to do the same. It is insofar as they are rational that participants can formulate, revise, and pursue a conception of their good. It is insofar as they are reasonable that they can come to understand the equal right of others to do so as well.

The persons in Rawls's well-ordered society are idealized as rational, reasonable, free and equal, independent, normal and fully functioning (or fully cooperating) over a complete life. The entire theory is fashioned for autonomous citizens to be able to live their lives by their own lights, while respecting the rights of others to do likewise. For this, they need what Rawls identifies as "primary goods." The two principles of justice together, chosen under fair conditions, assure a society in which everyone has the primary goods of basic liberties and freedoms, fair equality of opportunity, positions and offices open to all, wealth and income, and, most importantly, the social bases of self-respect. The importance that Rawls puts on the social bases of self-respect and autonomy go hand in hand, as one needs self-respect to form, revise, and pursue a vision of one's own conception of the good.

Although in his earlier articulations Rawls never mentions health care, Norman Daniels expanded Rawlsian theory to include it. Daniels maintains that health is needed if we are to have fair equality of opportunity. Rather than take health care as necessary for overall well-being—as the World Health Organization and many others do—Daniels believes health care belongs to a theory of justice because it returns persons to a "normal" state of full functioning,[6] which, as I pointed out earlier, thus reconciles the vulnerability and dependency of illness with the independence of the autonomous citizen.[7]

On this view, health care restores people to full functioning, allowing them to be part of the cooperative scheme in which resources are distributed and rights and liberties are respected. Daniels, taking his cue from the idealization of Rawlsian contractors as "fully functional over a normal life span—i.e., that no one would become ill or die prematurely," believes that the goal of public health and medicine should be to return people to that ideal (Daniels, Kennedy, and Kawachi 1999, 228). This view of health care does little for those who cannot be so restored or those who do not function as autonomous agents in the first place.

Only in his final restatement of the theory of justice as fairness did Rawls consider health care. Taking up Daniels's suggestion, Rawls supports this principled response to health-care needs as a way to decide what health disparities are unjust and to determine the urgency of a medical procedure. As an example, he notes that subsuming health care under equality of opportunity shows that attending to disease should have priority over cosmetic surgery. Only the former returns a person to the normal and full functioning state needed to be a fully cooperating member of society. Unfortunately, Rawls says little else about what the theory of justice as fairness can offer.

Surely we do not need the elegant and elaborate apparatus of Rawls's theory to come to the conclusion that cosmetic surgery should not be a high priority. But many conditions requiring medical care and associated hands-on daily care will not restore a person to normal and full functioning. Do these cases, then, also fall at the bottom of the list of priorities?

To see how poorly such a theory treats those who fall outside the idealized conception of the citizen, consider the situation of a caregiver who tends to her mother with Alzheimer's and as a consequence faces great financial, physical, and health costs to herself. One such daughter asked: "What can I do? Throw her [her mother] away? I can't do that, she's my mother." Neither the mother—who cannot be restored to a full cooperator—nor the daughter—who, while not ill, can enter the cooperative social arrangement only by disregarding her connection with her mother—are included in social cooperative arrangements outlined in Rawls's theory. The costs of the mother's care, and the toll taken on the caring daughter's own resources and health, fall outside the system of social bargaining among equals.

To be fair to Rawls, his principles must always be taken in the context of the whole theory, and it is hard to believe that Rawls would seriously countenance an ordering of health priorities that would place all medical needs of a person too disabled to be employed at the end of any list. Rawls's ideal is a society with inequalities in income and wealth, but inequalities in primary goods are always to be minimized and to favor those who are least advantaged (particularly along the measure of income and wealth).

On Rawls's view, any society with steep inequalities cannot be a society that complies with his two principles of justice. And if inequality itself is a critical factor in health inequalities, then the closer a society realizes Rawlsian principles, the less steep the health inequalities will be. Daniels seizes on this feature of the theory to distinguish health inequalities from health inequities. If the conditions of background justice reduce inequalities to the extent that reducing them further would disadvantage the least well-off, then any remaining inequalities will not be intolerable inequities. They would be justifiable within the framework of justice as fairness. The upstream attention to social justice would come as close as possible to eliminating health inequities—at least for those who are fully functioning, with "normal" medical needs.[8]

Daniels responds to a possible criticism that his Rawlsian approach does not fare well with ailments of old age, as these individuals would not be likely to be restored to full functioning. Daniels replies that functioning and opportunity are relative to age, so we would want to restore functions that are open to individuals of advanced age. But that still implies that care for the Alzheimer's sufferer will probably be low on the list of priorities for care given to the elderly.[9]

Although Daniels removes the idealizing condition that members of Rawls's well-ordered society are full cooperators, the idealization guides his recommendation in ways that are unlikely to be beneficial to those who, medically speaking, are "the worst off." The modified Rawlsian just society would doubtless have fewer health inequalities than our present situation, but would retain many of the same gross inequalities we now see, where people with significant illnesses and severe disabilities, together with their families, are both poorer and less well served by the medical community than the rest of the population.

The idealization that guides the Rawlsian project is not helpful. There are times when we are not fully functioning and cannot be restored to full functioning. There are individuals who are not "normal" in any fixed sense of normalcy. We often lack the skills, resources, or wherewithal to pursue our rational interests even when we have successfully identified them. We are vitally connected to others for whom we are willing sacrifice our own advantage. The fact that we get ill and have disabilities and need the care and assistance of others is not just a step down from the ideal: it is a feature of any human society, no matter how well ordered. These conditions need not necessarily make a life go badly if social structures are organized with these aspects of human life as an integral part of how we order a just society.

Bioethics translates the purely philosophical conceptions of morality and justice into principles that ought to govern our actual medical practices. The bioethics in a liberal society models its conception of the ideal patient on the idealized citizen of a liberal state. What we find is that those who cannot be restored to full functioning are not the only ones who fare poorly. Many who may be returned to full functioning fail to be—when, and to the degree that, they fall short of the expectations of the ideal patient. Like the idealized citizen, the ideal patient is an autonomous, rational, independent agent. If a theory of justice for a society populated with idealized persons does a poor job in helping determine which health inequalities are inequities, then a bioethics based on the same presumptions will be similarly flawed.

AUTONOMY, BIOETHICS, AND HEALTH-CARE PRACTICES

Beauchamp and Childress provide the by now very familiar principles meant to guide medical practitioners: respect for autonomy, beneficence, nonmaleficence, and justice. Autonomy has become the principle that has received the most attention. The emphasis on autonomy is not surprising, although it is fairly new. The "respect for autonomy" principle, often to the exclusion of principles such as beneficence and nonmaleficence, reflects the norm of the person as free, rational, independent, and autonomous.

What is autonomy and why do we value it? On a Kantian model, autonomy is the capacity to direct our actions by reference to the categorical imperative (moral law) and take responsibility for those choices; on a model derived from John Stuart Mill's theory, it is the capacity to direct the course of our lives; on a Rawlsian model, it is the capacity to formulate and revise one's own conception of the good. Many contemporary authors characterize autonomy as a self-reflective capacity that permits an individual to be self-determining, to make choices for which one can take responsibility and choices with which one identifies—that is, an expression of who one is and what one authentically desires.

On all these conceptions, the value of autonomy is seen to be a feature of persons (or, on the Kantian model, of the will) that both reflects and confers dignity on persons (see, e.g., O'Neill 2002). Some views are purely procedural and require only a self-reflexivity that identifies some desire as a desire that I desire to have. Others such as the Kantian view are not merely procedural but have content, a choice to act according to a maxim that we could not but will to become a universal law. Mixed views define a procedure for autonomous action but also place constraints on the content of that action. Desiring a job that involves degrading oneself, for example, could be ruled out as an autonomous desire even if, on reflection, it is what we desire to desire. Such a mixed view may invoke a set of competences, a "repertoire of coordinated skills that makes self-discovery, self-definition and self-direction possible" and that contain some vision of what an autonomous life looks like.[10]

Autonomy in the philosophical sense is demanding in the competences and cognitive capabilities it must engage—often too demanding, especially when we are feeling ill, are facing overwhelming and confusing medical options, or are anticipating frightening medical outcomes. Even though the bioethical and medical conceptions are far thinner and less demanding, they value, and to some extent expect or presume, these same capacities in the patient whose autonomous decisions are to be respected. But the demanding competences required for autonomy may be beyond us when, in our older years, we experience diminishment or impairment of the sensory and cognitive capacities required to take in and process information. Without a good education (a major determinant of health outcomes), we may feel unprepared to make decisions. We may fail to give the physician any confidence that we can comply with the demands of aftercare. We may not come across as sufficiently rational to be viewed as deserving of the respect due to the autonomous person. Furthermore, sensing such condescension, we may feel that we cannot fully trust the medical personnel.

Even a simple, terse definition of autonomy such as Sarah Buss's—"To be autonomous is to be a law to oneself; autonomous agents are self-governing agents" (Buss 2002)—requires more than most of us can muster at the best of times. To be self-governing, a law to oneself, one must be capable of high cognitive functioning: one must understand the concept of law, know how to apply it to one's own actions, and be able to engage in self-scrutiny. In a medical context, we need to be able to convey our capacity to be self-determining if we are to have medical personnel take our needs and desires seriously.

Although the notion of autonomy has historically been tied to a conception of the self as "an inner citadel"—a self that can stand up to outside forces that hope to influence it—feminist theorists who expound a more relational conception of the self speak instead of "relational autonomy" (see, e.g., Mackenzie and Stoljar 2000; Friedman 2003; Nedelsky 2011). A relational understanding of the self understands the development of autonomy as itself emerging from social interactions that provide us with competencies we need for autonomy. Furthermore, proponents of the relational self argue that maintaining autonomy requires a network of relationships on which we can rely to help us formulate, revise, and enact what we genuinely desire (or desire to desire). Although this is not the notion of autonomy that prevails in the medical context, it is in fact operative for those whose autonomy is respected in a medical crisis. When we are ill and unable to make decisions for ourselves, we need to have decisions made for us that reflect our wishes and desires and that call attention to our needs to an otherwise busy medical staff. We need people around us who care about us and for us. When we are in need of medical attention, we need advocates: advocates who understand how the system works, who can demand respect and attention, and who can understand our needs and translate these to the medical staff and interpret the medical staff's questions and instructions. Without education and social connections we cannot maintain our "autonomy" in the face of illness. We will see how critical such connections are as we examine some illustrations of how class, social connectedness, and autonomy are determinative of medical outcomes.

Until relatively recently, the medical field has been exempted from assumptions about persons as autonomous because of the seemingly irremediable asymmetry of knowledge and skill between patient and medical provider. Instead the medical profession relied on a paternalistic model of care. The asymmetry once thought to be an obstacle to the autonomous decision-making of a patient has become instead the basis for the requirement that the patient be provided with information adequate to making an informed decision, thereby acknowledging the importance of respecting the patient's autonomy even in the medical context. Those who cannot consent to their medical care are deemed "incompetent."

In the bad old days of paternalistic medicine, we were all treated as incompetents—at least with respect to having a voice in our medical care. As late as the 1970s in the United States, physicians would not think of burdening patients with the details of the treatments they were to undergo or even the names of the medications they were prescribing.[11] Physicians thought patients who were dying ought not be informed of their ill fate (Oken 1961, 1120).[12] We do not wish to return to that model of medicine, one that may well not have a better record of equity than the autonomy model I am criticizing. While I am attempting to show how the emphasis on autonomy may contribute to health inequalities and inequities, I want to be clear that I do not think the paternalistic medical model was free of such inequities. Paternalistic medicine is authoritarian, and how the good of medicine is dispensed will depend on how physicians choose to dispense that good. Instead I want to point the reader to a view of health care as first and foremost care, which, at its best, is not paternalistic but requires respect for the agency of the cared-for. Care requires not only attention to the needs of the other as the caregiver sees them, but as the cared-for understands her higher-order needs—what it is that she really wants and cares about. It requires neither paternalistic treatment nor the unreflective assumption of the patient's autonomy.

CLASS, AUTONOMY, AND HEALTH OUTCOMES

Each of the three subjects portrayed by Janny Scott in her *New York Times* essay is assumed to be competent and so is treated as an autonomous patient. The more fully these subjects are able to meet the expectations of an autonomous individual, the better their health outcome. But their ability to meet such expectations depends on how well that "autonomy" is supported by the circumstances of their lives.

The difference in health care begins with the circumstances of the heart attack and the choice of hospital. When he suffered a heart attack, Mr. Miele, an architect, was in midtown Manhattan with business colleagues, returning from an expensive lunch. When he collapsed on the sidewalk, his companions ignored his request for a taxi and immediately called for an ambulance. He was given the choice of hospitals, each equipped and capable of responding to cardiac problems with the latest technology. Miele chose the private research hospital over Bellevue, a large public hospital with a notoriously crowded emergency room. He was immediately met by his doctor, received excellent care, including a surgical procedure, and was out of the hospital in two days, and back on his feet within weeks.

Note how the forms of advantage conformed to the model of the patient and citizen as autonomous. Miele worked as a professional in a job in which he had significant control over his hours and workload. The architect was given a choice and was sufficiently well informed to understand that the hospital in which you are treated makes a difference. Being in Manhattan meant that he *actually did have a choice* between two hospitals, each of which was equipped to handle his emergency care. (Note another important socioeconomic fact smuggled in here: that the quality of medical services is uneven across neighborhoods.) His social network included others who were equally well situated and informed. They were in a position to support his autonomy, even as his own was compromised by his medical condition. Because they understood the gravity of the situation, they were able to override Miele's own ill-considered desire to minimize the situation, and immediately called for an ambulance. (Were Miele himself fully apprised of the gravity of his situation and fully competent at the time he would also have chosen the ambulance—thus, even though they overrode his choice, they were respecting what a fully rational consideration on his part would be.)[13] Miele's social network extended to his brother-in-law, a surgeon, and to his brother, the chairman of the board of another hospital, both of whom checked in to be assured that the hospital was doing all that it needed to do. Again, these individuals could be said to support the autonomy and the status of Mr. Miele as an autonomous individual who had the wherewithal to rationally pursue his own good, at a time when Mr. Miele himself was less able to do so.

Describing the treatment that followed, Scott writes: "Within minutes, Mr. Miele was on a table in the cardiac catheterization laboratory, awaiting an angioplasty to unclog his artery—a procedure that many cardiologists say has become the gold standard in heart attack treatment. When he developed ventricular fibrillation, a heart rhythm abnormality that can be fatal within minutes, the problem was quickly fixed" (Janny Scott 2005). The heart damage was minimal. At home, Miele had the support needed to enable him to make the rational decisions to alter his diet and take up exercise. He was not only returned to full functioning; he was in better condition than he had previously been.

Mr. Wilson, an African American office worker, had his heart attack after a substantial meal with his fiancée. He first assumed his symptoms were indigestion, but his fiancée insisted on calling an ambulance. In this, she, like Miele's companions, supported his autonomy, but did so much more hesitantly, allowing some time to pass before putting in a call. Mr. Wilson was given a choice between Brooklyn Hospital Center and a city-run hospital that serves Brooklyn's poorest neighborhoods. He chose the former. Unlike Mr. Miele, who was immediately given the gold standard of care, Mr. Wilson was given a drug to break up a clot blocking an artery to his heart. Brooklyn Hospital was not able to perform the needed surgery, and Wilson was transferred to a Manhattan hospital that could provide the needed angioplasty. His hospital stay was longer, and he returned home with the same instructions given to Miele: to change his diet, start exercising, and stay on prescription medication that was costly. Wilson stayed on course until he felt better, but then returned to the lifestyle that damaged his heart the first time and stopped taking the medication. It was Wilson himself who made his choices when he resumed his diet of red meat, let up on his exercise regime, and stopped his medication. Wilson, unlike Miele, as we will see, had a less supportive network to help him change the damaging habits. Perhaps here we ought to say that Wilson was "abandoned to his autonomy" (O'Neill 2002).

The third person, Ms. Gora, a recent Polish immigrant from a working-class background, was employed as a cleaning lady and lived in one of the boroughs of New York. She was not feeling well while at home with her husband. She hoped her symptoms would go away, but eventually allowed her husband to call an ambulance. Even when the ambulance arrived she resisted going. She was given no choice in hospitals and was simply taken to the same public hospital that Mr. Wilson had rejected. She had to wait two hours before she was seen by a nurse practitioner, and it was several hours before tests confirmed that she was experiencing a heart attack. (One can be quite certain that had Miele been taken to this hospital instead, his insistent colleagues and his network of well-connected relatives would not have tolerated a two-hour wait in the face of a probable cardiac incident.) Her treatment was drugs for the clotting and blood pressure, and only on the following day was she transferred to Bellevue (the hospital that Miele turned down) for an angiogram. By that time the heart attack was over, but she was to have an angiogram to assess the likelihood of a second attack. She came down with a fever, so the angiogram was canceled. She was sent home without any further procedures being performed. The suboptimal treatment comports with a Baylor report that "the health care safety and quality problems exist because of limited infrastructure and outmoded care systems, which result in a cycle of suboptimal care being repeated throughout the many levels of care" (Mayberry et al. 2006). Such care is found largely where the poor who lack the means to demand better treatment are located (ibid.).

Gora's condition was never fully explained, and she was not send home with admonitions to change her habits. When she arrived at Bellevue for her first follow-up exam, she asked her doctor: "Doctor, I don't know what I have, why I was in hospital. What is this heart attack? I don't know why I have this. What I have to do to not repeat this?" (Scott 2005). Either she had not fully understood what she was told in the hospital because of her poor English or no one had explained her situation fully. Gora's competency in being able to understand and direct what happening to her fell far short of that of either Mr. Miele or Mr. Wilson. In addition to the outmoded care she received, she had very few supports available to her and numerous obstacles to overcome. But the medical professionals—well meaning though they might have been—and the system of medical care had few tools at their disposable to deal with a patient who didn't fully understand and didn't have the cultural health capital to know what questions to ask. Scott chronicles a daunting cascade of difficulties that followed Gora's heart attack.

There are also gender elements that one can point to. Miele and Wilson both had women who looked after them. Miele's wife became fully informed of what he required, helped him shop for the foods that would reduce his chance of having another attack, reminded him of appointments and medications, and urged him on as he undertook his exercise regime. Where he fell short, she stepped in. Wilson's fiancée was helpful to a lesser degree as she was less well informed and things such as shopping for the right foods was more daunting in the neighborhood they lived in. Gora's husband did little to adjust or to support her. He insisted on her preparing the same foods he had been used to and that she had been warned off. He did not stop smoking and did not accompany her to appointments. The contrasts are not only heavily class laden, but gender laden as well.

It seems reasonable to say that no rational person would willingly make the choices that lead to their own demise. Knowing that some of her heart muscle was irreparably damaged was a source of great distress to Gora. She made many efforts to stop smoking and change her eating habits, but as she stopped smoking, her weight increased considerably. In her increasingly distressing and lonely life, food was an irresistible way of comforting herself. To act in such a way that you can endorse your decision requires more than a strong will. It requires an environment that helps, or allows one to act as a fully rational self-determining person would. In speaking of his heart attack, Wilson said: "I don't think I'll survive another one." For Wilson, abandoning the regime that could help assure that he would not suffer another attack could not in fact be an autonomous choice in the sense that self-reflective theories define autonomy. His first-order choice to resume his old diet and lifestyle are not ones he would endorse or choose to choose. Medical practice is built on the assumption that follow-up care and changes in behavior can be left to the autonomous choices people make, even though we are well aware of the fact that many are not able to abide by these resolutions, not because they don't value their health but because they do not have the wherewithal to follow through.

Miele was able to change his work schedule, had the means to buy the right foods and join the gym, and had the support of others who helped him maintain his altered ways. His wife accompanied him to doctor's visits and took notes on what he was required to do. She learned to prepare the heart-healthy foods in an appealing way and helped him maintain his exercise regime. She had both the knowledge and authority to help steer him to choices that he could autonomously endorse. Clearly one cannot and ought not to coerce people into making such life changes, but one can certainly ask whether there is not a responsibility on the part of a health-care system, in conjunction with social policy, to assist in providing supports that will help people act on what they know to be in their own best interest.

Miele had supports sufficient for the more fully autonomous choices that he made or that others made in his stead. Although it is almost oxymoronic to speak of others making autonomous choices for him, insisting on the autonomy of the patient forces such language. What I mean by it is simply that others made the choices for him that he himself would have made had he been making those choices when he was able to function autonomously. But this way of speaking underscores the idea that I am trying to press in this chapter—namely, that during periods of illness we are rarely in a position to be autonomous agents. Recognizing how we might choose were we able to act autonomously requires others who can support our autonomy. But the need to have one's autonomy supported requires more than a singular advocate. It requires advocates who have the wherewithal to feel secure in their choices, the material resources to actualize their decisions, and authority in the eyes of others and in the eyes of the patient. Furthermore, among the options one has, choices that approximate what an autonomous chooser would choose need to be available. Miele had those choices: choices among well-equipped hospitals, foods that were heart-healthy, the ability to join a gym and to cut down on hours when necessary.

These choices are increasingly less available as one descends the socio-economic ladder. Thus, while Wilson had wanted to change his diet, finding healthy foods in his neighborhood was difficult. His fiancée didn't have the knowledge to prepare these foods for him so that they had the appeal of his standard diet, and his friends were not sufficiently informed to help him keep to his new regime. It is hardly surprising that he lapsed, that he failed to make the more fully autonomous choices—the choices that he would have desired to choose.

Gora was in a still worse situation. She had as little choice in the other aspects of her life as she had in the hospital to which she was taken. While she prepared the food, her husband did little to encourage a diet that would have been helpful. She had little understanding of her own situation, and no one to help her comprehend it. She lacked the rapport with medical personnel to insist on explanations that were adequate to her understanding. She had no autonomous choices with respect to her work schedule. She could not take time off and so eventually had to leave her job. She ate her way through the boredom, gaining weight and becoming diabetic. The heart attack was the beginning of the unraveling of her health and her life.

Despite the degree of control or lack of it that the three individuals portrayed had, the medical profession assumed that all of them had the ability to control their situation in the same way. Those with the ability and presumption that they were entitled to a certain level of care could make demands on the system: consider Miele's brother and brother-in-law checking in and making certain the hospital was doing what was needed. Those without the knowledge or authority or presumption were left to wait two hours before being seen for a cardiac condition. Not only Miele but also his wife attended medical consultations, thus assuring that they got the necessary information, while Gora, without sufficient language skills, was lost amid the information dispensed, information meant to bridge the knowledge gap between physician and patient that would allow for patient autonomy.

When we make the assumption that autonomy is merely a matter of individuals choosing for themselves—and our health-care system works on the assumption that all but the incompetent would make autonomous choices—we fail to see the many ways in which such choices depend on a cultural and social forms of capital that provide networks to support autonomy. As such supported autonomy is made available to those who are socially and economically privileged, the presumption of the autonomous patient thus becomes one pathway by which social inequality results in unjust medical inequalities.

THE "INCOMPETENT" PATIENT

The dichotomy between the autonomous and the incompetent patient leaves little room for understanding that people who are functional in their daily lives are less capable of autonomous decision making when faced with health crises. The view that persons who are competent should be able to make, and should not be prevented from making, decisions for themselves (and so should take responsibility for making those decisions) is questioned only in case an otherwise competent person is not in a position to make a rationally warranted decision because he or she is not fully informed or because he or she is temporarily incapacitated. Those who are not otherwise capable of making such decisions are viewed as permanently incompetent.

The failure to be able to make autonomous decisions is captured in the inability to give "informed consent." Informed consent is the operationalized, if attenuated, version of the philosophical concept of autonomy. However, in practice the ritualized and routinized consent (as patients in the United States regularly experience it) is often obtained by having a consent form shoved across the desk to a patient by an administrator who waits impatiently for the patient's signature; or a form handed to a patient with a perfunctory explanation as the individual is about to go in for a major procedure. For many patients, especially when their education is limited, the informed consent form is intimidating. When the patient is not of the same socioeconomic class as the physician, they are less likely to insist on the clarification of obscure language or other obfuscations. When patients sense condescension from the physician, they may respond by pretending to know what they do not. And those who do not speak the dominant language are deeply disadvantaged unless they have an advocate/translator. Even the person who usually functions fully as an autonomous agent may be flummoxed when confronted by the consent form when ill and mentally in a fog.

But the idea of informed consent also sets the bar for those who appear to be utterly incapable of consent. Patients may be unconscious, or conscious but too overcome with illness or too medicated to consent to their treatment. They may appear not to be rational, or to have mental deficits that affect their ability to understand or consent to what is happening to them. In these cases, they have to either resort to someone who is legally approved or legally delegated to make medical decisions and sign the mandatory consent forms for that individual; or if no such person is reasonably available, medical staff may make decisions that they take to be in the best interest of their patient.

The relatively sharp dichotomy between the autonomous individual and the incompetent patient creates a medical and legal imperative to strip a patient who is considered to be incompetent of the authority to intervene on her own behalf. Only if the family member deciding on her care is sufficiently sensitive to her desires does the patient have any agency on her part recognized. Jonathan Glover adopted the question "Do they take sugar?" to capture this view of patients who are no longer addressed directly and are no longer consulted to determine what their own view of their good may be. The presumption of incompetence is too often made in the case of someone who is disabled even when they can in fact speak for themselves. But in the case of those who cannot speak for themselves because they are cognitively impaired, the presumption of incompetence allows for abuse and treatment that many of us would deem a violation of our dignity. Not infrequently the infantilizing, negligent, or abusive behavior is made on the assumption that these folks "won't know the difference anyway."

In bioethics and in medical practice, focusing on questions of autonomy and creating a sharp divide between the "incompetent" and the "autonomous" contributes to health-care disparities in a number of different ways. One is illustrated by the questions that emerged when, in 1955, developers of a hepatitis virus vaccine wanted to experiment on child inmates of Willowbrook State School for Children with Mental Retardation. The proponents of the experiment argued that the children were already susceptible to the virus, since it was rampant in Willowbrook. The study would subject them to a mild form of the virus but in a clean and well-kept facility where they would not be subject to the other illnesses found in Willowbrook. Opponents objected to experimenting on a population that could not give consent, and even if experimentation was done only on those children who had parents able to consent, the children had no way to object to their parent's decision. Opponents questioned whether such consent on the part of the parents could really be free and well informed. They also pointed out that there were alternate ways to control hepatitis (for example, through gamma globulin injections) and that experimenting with a vaccine was not the only way to get desired results.

But while the focus of the historical debate, and of subsequent bioethical scrutiny (Beauchamp and Childress 2001), was on whether the children and their parents were being treated paternalistically or would have their autonomy respected, what remained unquestioned were the conditions at Willowbrook that gave rise to the certain spread of hepatitis: overcrowding, understaffing, inadequate hygiene—in short, the moral scandal that was Willowbrook. Asking whether the experiment was justified on the grounds of autonomy entirely missed the most crucial moral question, which was why such institutions were allowed to exist at all. Judging that the medical system was dealing with patients who were incompetent allowed the bioethicists to take as a given the unequal health conditions that pervaded such institutions. Less charitably, we can read into the neglect the question: Why waste precious resources on these individuals who didn't know the difference anyway?

We might ask: Do the medical researchers believe that the disadvantage and abuse of a population unable to fend for themselves is unavoidable, and that their health inequalities are therefore inevitable? Unfortunately, such a false presumption might be at the heart of the health inequalities disabled people (and their families) repeatedly encounter, even when their reasoning ability is not impaired. People with disabilities find themselves treated as incompetent when they are perfectly able to handle medical decisions.

Although a patient may be able to speak for herself and be legally competent, being put in a wheelchair is often sufficient to trigger the "Do they take sugar?" response by medical providers—that is, the response of turning to the caregiver, neglecting the person in the wheelchair, to ask about what the preferences of the wheelchair user might be. Disabled people encounter numerous obstacles in their efforts to obtain the services that they require. The problems begin with obtaining the medical insurance and equipment and finding medical services that are fully accessible. They extend to the ill-informed attitudes of medical providers that result in inadequate care. I have heard and read anecdotes repeatedly from disabled women whose physicians supposed that because they were disabled they would not want to have children and proceeded to treat them as if their reproductive health was of no consequence. The National Council on Disability writes: "Lack of disability competency and knowledge [on the part of physicians] is a leading barrier to care, according to women with disabilities and those with diverse disabilities, including people who are deaf or hard of hearing, people who are blind or have vision impairments, and people with intellectual and developmental disabilities. Without appropriate training and awareness, health-care providers hold incorrect assumptions and stereotypes about people with disabilities, which can affect every aspect of care and can result in inadequate and inappropriate care" (NCD 2009).

The disabled individual, the pregnant woman (see DeBruin et al., chapter 6, this volume), the racial minority, the immigrant, and those who are poor are more likely to be judged incompetent and when judged to be autonomous, left to their own devices. When people are poor in cultural health capital, as members of these groups often are, being treated as autonomous might in theory be dignifying. But when the resources needed to realize that autonomy are lacking, when the advocacy and support that can help realize autonomy is lacking, they cannot gain from a system not developed to serve them. Like a key attempting to fit into a mismatched lock, these patients cannot unlock the wonders of modern medicine.

Rather than create a dichotomy between an incompetent and an autonomous patient, we need a medical system that is not only committed to identifying medical needs, but equally committed to understanding patients as persons who are in need of caring. Health care is first and foremost care, and when the burden of all care, except what a narrow focus on medical needs demands, is left to the individual and whatever family support they have, health care can only be as effective as the resources an individual can muster. And individuals are not equally well positioned to muster the resources they need. A health-care system needs to be more closely attentive to the lapses and inadequacies of the larger cultural and socioeconomic factors that prevent good care. It needs to be constructed to meet the demands of care in a society that itself is fashioned not for hypothetical equal and autonomous cooperators but for vulnerable, dependent, and interdependent persons.

NOTES

1. This point was documented by the Whitehall Studies conducted by Michael Marmot in Britain in the mid-1980s, and later in 1997, which studied the highly stratified civil service in Britain. Despite the universal coverage of Britain's National Health Service, disparities in grade level of occupation correlated with significant disparities in health outcomes and life expectancy (Marmot 2000).

2. See Mullahy, Robert, and Wolfe (2004). For problems with the position, see King (chapter 8, this volume). My own argument does not rest on the accuracy of the position. What is important for my claim is only that socioeconomic factors, such as level of income, race, ethnicity, disability, etc., *track* health disparities, not that they directly *cause* them.

3. See Shim et al. (chapter 9, this volume). Shim et al. speak of "cultural health capital" as "a repertoire of skills, competencies, resources, and styles" that both patients and health providers deploy and which include "at this historical moment . . . elements like medical knowledge and health literacy; an enterprising, proactive, instrumental attitude towards one's own health; and the ability to adapt one's interactional style" (240).

4. The medical/bioethical conception of autonomy is a thin conception, while the philosophical conception discussed below is far thicker. Nonetheless, the thinner conception relies on a set of presumptions that get buried in the assumption that a person is capable of making her own medical decisions. It presumes that one has a significant measure of control over one's life and that one is in command of the cultural resources required to speak with physicians as equals—understanding the language and concepts used, having the confidence to challenge the physician, pose questions, and trust that the physician is really concerned with one's well-being and not simply the bottom line, that the physician truly does respect them as individuals who have the right to determine their own life course and will speak openly and honestly to them, etc.

5. This is John Rawls's famous "Original Position" in which we are under a "Veil of Ignorance."

6. Rawls writes: "The principles of justice specify the form of background justice apart from all particular historical conditions. What counts is the workings of social institutions now, and a benchmark of the state of nature—the level of well-being (however specified) of individuals in that state—plays no role" (Rawls 1958, 54–55).

7. The reader may wonder whether the terms "independent" and "autonomous" are interchangeable and if so redundant. The term "independent" can refer variously to political independence, wherein a person has full rights of inclusion and self-determination in the political process; to economic independence, wherein a person is not beholden to another to provide for material sustenance; to independence in functioning, wherein a person can carry out basic tasks of living without another's assistance; or to independence in decision making. "Autonomy" can be used to refer to independence in any of these spheres, but is most particularly used to designate independence in decision making—in other words, self-determination. Autonomy generally presumes a level of rational capacity and reliance on practical reasoning. In the medical context "independence" is generally used as a way of speaking of functioning, but "autonomy" is generally used in contexts of decision making. But these different uses are not always consistent, and the terms are sometimes used interchangeably. When independence is freedom from the influence of others, or independence in judgment, particularly with the presumption that the judgment is based on rational considerations, then it pretty much coincides with autonomy. When independence refers to financial independence or general functioning, it is less so. But much of the thesis that I am defending is that while one might presume that autonomy in medically relevant decision making can be considered apart from political and material factors, such autonomy is in fact dependent on the various sorts of independence I outlined here.

8. But see King (chapter 8, this volume) for a dose of healthy skepticism that this conclusion is warranted. King argues that all that has been proven is an association, not a causal link, between social inequalities and health inequalities and that there is no evidence that intervening upstream—rather than, say, making more health care available—would be the best way to reduce these disparities.

9. Daniels would reply that this is not necessarily a health inequity if such distribution of health resources was open to a deliberative process, which he identifies as one that meets what he holds to be four conditions of an "ethic of accountability": publicity, relevance, appeals, and enforcement. These conditions specify that decisions about the distribution of resources must be open to public scrutiny; that the principles need to be relevant to those subject to them; that there must be a way to challenge and revise decisions in light of further evidence; and that there must be a way to enforce that the first three conditions are met. But who is to engage in this deliberative process? Not those who are subject to the illnesses that would be low on the list, as they are unlikely to be able to be self-advocates; and probably not their familial caregivers, if they have such, since they are likely to be overburdened by their care. Once again, for those who cannot function as autonomous subjects, the process is stacked against them, and they are unlikely to fare well. See Daniels and Sabin 1997.

10. See Meyers 1989. Also see Meyers 2002, 20–21. Notions of self-discovery, self-definition, and self-direction are not merely procedural, as they direct one to a certain set of possible lives and not others.

11. I believe, but have not been able to verify, that it was not until the passage of the Hazardous Labeling Act, passed in the 1960s, that all prescription medicines were labeled with the actual name of the medication.

12. Oken 1961, cited in Buchanan 1978.

13. Interestingly, all three at first refused the ambulance. It may well be that fear of the severity of a problem may make us irrationally engage in denial.

REFERENCES

Beauchamp, Tom L., and James F. Childress. 2001. *Principles of Biomedical Ethics*. New York: Oxford University Press.

Buchanan, Allen. 1978. "Medical Paternalism." *Philosophy and Public Affairs* 7 (4): 370–90.

Buss, Sarah. 2002. "Personal Autonomy." *Stanford Encyclopedia of Philosophy*. Winter. http://plato.stanford.edu/archives/win2002/entries/personal-autonomy/. Accessed 25 August 2015.

Corruccini, Robert S. 1984. "An Epidemiologic Transition in Dental Occlusion in World Populations." *American Journal of Orthodontics* 86 (5): 419–26.

Daniels, Norman, Bruce Kennedy, and Ichiro Kawachi. 1999. "Why Justice Is Good for Our Health: The Social Determinants of Health Inequalities." *Daedalus* 128 (4): 215–51.

Daniels, Norman, and James Sabin. 1997. "Limits to Health Care: Fair Procedures, Democratic Deliberation, and the Legitimacy Problem for Insurers." *Philosophy and Public Affairs* 26 (4): 303–50.

Friedman, Marilyn. 2003. *Autonomy, Gender, Politics*. Studies in Feminist Philosophy Series. New York: Cambridge University Press.

Mackenzie, Catriona, and Natalie Stoljar. 2000. *Relational Autonomy: Feminist Perspectives on Autonomy, Agency, and the Social Self*. New York: Oxford University Press.

Marmot, Michael. 2000. *The Whitehall Study*. http://www.workhealth.org/projects/pwhitew.html. Accessed 14 December 2012.

Mayberry, Robert M., David A. Nicewander, Huanying Qin, and David J. Ballard. 2006. "Improving Quality and Reducing Inequities: A Challenge in Achieving Best Care." *Proceedings of Baylor University Medical Center* 19 (2): 103–18.

Meyers, Diana T. 1989. *Self, Society, and Personal Choice*. New York: Columbia University Press.

———. 2002. *Gender in the Mirror: Cultural Imagery and Women's Agency*. New York: Oxford University Press.

NCD (National Council on Disability). 2009. *The Current State of Health Care for People with Disabilities*. http://www.ncd.gov/publications/2009/Sept302009#Self-Assessed%20Health. Accessed 27 September 2013.

Nedelsky, Jennifer. 2011. *Law's Relations: A Relational Theory of Self, Autonomy, and Law*. New York: Oxford University Press.

Oken, Donald. 1961. "What to Tell Cancer Patients: A Study of Medical Attitudes."
    Journal of the American Medical Association 175 (13): 1120–28.

O'Neill, Onora. 2002. *Autonomy and Trust in Bioethics*. Cambridge: Cambridge
    University Press.

Rawls, John. 1958. "Justice as Fairness." *Philosophical Review* 67 (2): 164–94.

Scott, Janny. 2005. "Life at the Top in America Isn't Just Better, It's Longer." *New York
    Times*, May 16. http://www.nytimes.com/2005/05/16/us/class/life-at-the-top-in-
    america-isnt-just-better-its-longer.html. Accessed 25 August 2015.

Wilkinson, Richard G. 1992. "Income Distribution and Life Expectancy." *British Medical
    Journal* 304 (6820): 165–68.

———. 1996. *Unhealthy Societies: The Afflictions of Inequality*. London: Routledge.

Wolfe, Barbara, John Mullahy, and Stephanie Robert. 2003. "Health, Income, and
    Inequality: Review and Redirection." Russell Sage Foundation Working Paper Series.
    Russell Sage Foundation. http://www.russellsage.org/research/reports/health-
    inequality. Accessed 25 August 2015.

PART II

Disrupting Assumptions and Expanding
Perspectives through Cases

5

Embodied Inequalities

An Interdisciplinary Conversation on Oral Health Disparities

Sarah Horton and Judith C. Barker

ABSTRACT

This chapter combines ethnographic and social epidemiological approaches to analyze the causes of Latino children's high rates of oral disease as well as their cumulative effects. Social epidemiological approaches suggest the complex interplay of biology and social structure at multiple levels in creating health inequalities. How can we use ethnography to operationalize this model, illustrating the varying role of familial, clinical, and sociopolitical contexts in creating farmworker youths' health inequalities? Moreover, how can social epidemiology heed the insights of ethnography, and what happens when we assign equal truth status to parents' "local" knowledge and to expert knowledge of epidemiological reports? We use this chapter both as a lens for understanding the roots of farmworker children's poor oral health and as a thought experiment for considering the provocative methodological and epistemological questions posed by an interdisciplinary dialogue on health inequalities. The study of oral disease is intriguing not only because oral disease is often caused by inequality itself, but also because its visibility to the naked eye makes it symbolic of Latino youth's depreciated social position. Severe early childhood caries can leave lasting effects on children's physical development, including malformed oral arches and crooked permanent dentition. Farmworker youth perceived such lasting effects as obstructing their plans and preventing their social mobility. Using a life course perspective, we examine the way that farmworker young adults' poor oral health feeds back into a system of social inequality. Using the lens of oral health, this chapter presents a vivid argument for why health inequalities are cause for policy intervention—that is, why they are a matter not only of fairness but also of equity and justice.

INTRODUCTION

Epidemiological reports consistently show that Latino children have worse oral health than African American and white children. Among Latino sub-groups, Mexican American children have the highest mean number of decayed teeth and unfilled cavities. While acknowledging barriers to receipt of dental treatment, the dental public health literature tends to zero in on Mexican immigrant parents as the primary cause of their children's poor health outcomes. It portrays immigrant caregivers as "bad parents," suggesting that they frequently put their children to bed with sweetened beverages (Shiboski et al. 2003) and fail to take their children for preventive dental checkups (Scott and Simile 2005).

In an ethnographic study of the issue in California's Central Valley, we found that Mexican immigrant parents echoed experts' concerns about the epidemic of early childhood caries (ECC) affecting their children. In their interviews, parents often puzzled over the causes of their children's "cracked" and "stained" teeth. "It's odd that children's teeth go bad so early here" was a common refrain. We found that immigrant parents often attributed their children's high rate of cavities—a stark contrast from their own oral health profiles as children—to the different diets and environments children encountered in the United States. Yet a vocal group of immigrant parents were most concerned about a different matter, complaining that their children's *dientes picados* (rotten teeth) seemed to permanently blight their smiles as young adults. These parents reported that children who had had their decayed primary teeth extracted often found that as they matured, their permanent teeth came in *torcidos*, or crooked.

This chapter explores the gulf between the epidemiological evidence and parents' own complaints and considers whether and how interdisciplinary research might forge an analytical bridge between them. It explores the challenges of combining epidemiological and ethnographic approaches to uncover the concrete pathways through which social inequality translates into decayed and "crooked" teeth. What epidemiological models exist to explain how inequality is embodied, and how do factors at the level of the individual, the family, the clinical encounter, and public policy contribute to Mexican American children's high rates of cavities? How might we use ethnography to operationalize the insights of multilevel epidemiological models and pinpoint the specific processes that produce oral health inequalities?

We use this chapter not only as a lens onto the practical matter of understanding the roots of immigrant children's poor oral health but also as a thought experiment considering the broader methodological and epistemological quandaries posed by an interdisciplinary dialogue on health inequalities. We raise the following questions: What priority should we assign to unraveling the causes behind epidemiological reports of Latino children's high rates of oral disease and—by contrast—to exploring the reasons for immigrant parents' own reports about their children's malformed permanent dentition? How should we identify and treat the value of each kind of evidence, and what happens when we assign equal validity to epidemiological reports and parents' own observations? What criteria should we use to weigh whether oral health disparities for farmworker children are not only unfair but unjust (see Braveman, chapter 1, and Kelleher, chapter 3, this volume)? In considering these questions, we attempt to "lift the blinders" imposed by discipline-specific analysis (Singer 2009, 28) in order to reveal the contributions of interdisciplinary analysis to unraveling the root causes of health disparities and illuminating the material effects of social inequality.

EPIDEMIOLOGICAL APPROACHES TO HEALTH INEQUALITIES

Two new ecosocial approaches—one coined by a social epidemiologist and one by a medical anthropologist—offer powerful new insights into the processes through which social inequality "become[s] biology" (Gravlee 2009). Departing from the premise that membership in marginalized social groups is intimately tied to health inequalities that must be redressed (see also Braveman, chapter 1, this volume), both direct attention to the cumulative interplay between biology and social structure that yields long-term effects. The social epidemiologist Nancy Krieger, for example, uses the concept of "embodiment" to examine how individuals "literally incorporate, biologically, the social and material world in which we live" (Krieger 2001, 672). For Krieger, the concept of "embodiment" levels the perceived opposition between the "social" and the "biological." In focusing solely on endogenous biological responses, she argues, biomedical and psychosocial approaches neglect the social determinants of health. Meanwhile, exclusively political economic approaches to health lack fine-grained attention to the physiological channels through which illness materializes. Krieger's concept of "embodiment" thus provides a powerful yet nuanced conceptual tool to examine the way the human body is nested within overlapping domains of biology, ecology, and social organization (Krieger 2001, 671).

While the approach of "embodiment" directs attention to the conjoint biological and social determinants of health, the lens of "syndemics"— proposed by the medical anthropologist Merrill Singer—offers critical insights into the additive burden of disease among marginalized populations. Positing the interaction between social inequality and disease as a physiological process, Singer points to the way that the synergistic interaction of diseases at the cellular level creates qualitatively distinct phenomena. For example, researchers have found that the herpes simplex virus and the most common variants of the human papilloma virus correlate with greater immunosuppression in HIV-positive women than other sexually transmitted diseases. The insight of a "syndemics" approach is to provocatively question biomedicine's partitioning of diseases into discrete, bounded categories, proposing that the clustering of distinct diseases together may constitute evidence of a "higher order phenomenon" (Singer and Clair 2003, 431) greater than and distinct from each disease alone.

Both ecosocial models suggest a "multilevel" framework, urging attention to the interplay between the biological and the sociopolitical at multiple levels. They attempt to pinpoint the specific and measurable physiological channels through which social disadvantage materializes as illness. Krieger shows, for example, how the excess risk of hypertension among African Americans is the physical embodiment of myriad social and material factors—including residential and occupational segregation, exposure to toxic substances, interpersonal discrimination, the targeted marketing of commodities, and inadequate health care (2001). Meanwhile, Singer places social inequality on equal footing as disease as cofactors in syndemics, suggesting that inequality exerts a measurable physiological effect through proxies such as malnutrition and stress. A "syndemics" approach thus resocializes biology, arguing for the importance of the social determinants of health in a language that epidemiologists can understand.

Both models unmask population patterns of health and disease as what Krieger calls "biological expressions of social relations" (Krieger 2001, 672), revealing illness as the mutable and embodied expression of inequality itself.

Yet even more provocatively, both models take a developmental perspective, directing attention to the cumulative interplay between biology and social structure over the life course. Singer, for example, draws on epidemiological studies showing that early childhood disadvantage may materialize as illness later in life, suggesting that the synergistic result of disease interaction may in fact be delayed (Singer 2009, 143–44; see also Krieger 2001, 673).

Oral disease provides a ripe opportunity to examine the cumulative interplay between biology and social structure. Indeed, children's oral disease has important lasting effects on both systemic health and their long-term physical development. Periodontal disease alone has been linked to heart disease, stroke (Beck et al. 1996), and, most recently, pancreatic cancer (Michaud et al. 2007). Severe ECC may adversely affect a child's self-esteem, speech development, and ability to eat (USDHHS 2000). Less well documented, however, are the cumulative effects of severe ECC, as the literature in physical anthropology suggests that the premature loss of primary teeth may also affect the permanent shape of the oral cavity itself (Corruccini 1984; Miyamoto, Chung, and Yee 1976; Oppenheim 1964). What, then, are the causes of Latino children's oral health disparities, and what are their long-term effects?

Placing Immigrant Children's Health Disparities in Context

Let us first place immigrant children's oral health disparities in a broader context. Latino children have poorer oral health than children from all other racial and ethnic groups other than Native Americans (Dye, Li, and Thornton-Evans 2012). Among all Latino subgroups, Mexican American children have the highest rates of oral disease, and evidence suggests that children of immigrant parents—and of farmworkers in particular—are especially at risk (Chaffin, Pai, and Bagramian 2003; Lukes and Simon 2005; Quandt et al. 2007). There is a great deal of analysis in the dental public health literature about the behaviors that may lead to this high prevalence of oral disease among Latino children. Most of this research fingers individual caregivers as the culprits, suggesting that Latino parents may be more likely to give children bottles or sweetened beverages at bedtime (Huntington, Kim, and Hughes 2002; Shiboski et al. 2003; Weinstein et al. 1992). It suggests that Latino parents do not engage in preventive oral health behaviors because they fail to appreciate the value of children's primary teeth or their importance to the health of children's permanent dentition (Hilton et al. 2007). Yet very little research explores the sociopolitical contexts that mediate immigrant caregiver practices, nor their own understandings of the oral health consequences of their dietary and feeding practices.

Ecosocial models suggest we examine the multiple domains that shape children's oral health, including their home environments, their treatment in dental offices, and dental public health policy. The original study we discuss here, funded by the National Institute of Dental and Craniofacial Research (a branch of the National Institutes of Health), specifically focused on caregiver beliefs and behaviors regarding their children's oral health. To provide a more holistic understanding of the factors that affect Mexican American children's oral health, we broadened our focus to address questions neglected in the dental public health literature. We asked: What are immigrant parents' feeding practices, and how are they shaped by the different biocultural environment within which they were raised? How do state dental insurance policies ameliorate or exacerbate the incidence of oral disease for farmworker children? And, finally, what might be the long-term effects of such poor oral health for farmworker children?

This chapter is the result of two related studies on the causes of oral health disparities for Latino farmworker children in Mendota, a rural farmworking community in California's Central Valley.[1] Dubbed the "Cantaloupe Capital of the World," Mendota is a predominantly Latino and largely immigrant community. The town's population is about eleven thousand people, although this number more than doubles during the summer harvest season. According to the 2010 census, the population is 97 percent Hispanic, and 51 percent are "foreign-born." The average household income is $25,807. Because of its poverty and large immigrant population, some social service providers pejoratively refer to the town as a "port of entry" for Mexican immigrants; others call it a "migrant labor camp."

In the first study, the first author conducted nine months of intensive fieldwork on the familial and social contexts that contribute to Mexican American children's high rates of ECC. To understand caregivers' beliefs and behaviors regarding oral disease, she conducted interviews with twenty-six Mexican immigrant parents. Criteria for participation included being a Mexican immigrant and a primary caregiver for a focal child under the age of six (see Barker and Horton 2008; Horton and Barker 2010a, 2010b). Interview questions included caregivers' understandings of the causes of oral disease, their oral hygiene and infant feeding practices, and their children's dental experiences. Because parents' own upbringings shaped their oral hygiene behaviors toward their children, questions also included parents' own experiences with oral disease and their dietary practices in their countries of origin.

Because caregiver behaviors did not single-handedly create their children's poor oral health, a comprehensive study of the issue also required tracking the effects of dental public policy on children's access to care. The first study included interviews with twelve dentists within a forty-five-mile radius of Mendota who accepted California's dental Medicaid insurance program, or Denti-Cal. Because these interviews revealed how Denti-Cal reimbursement policies exerted a profound influence on clinical practice and dentists' treatment strategies, we decided to design a second study to explore this issue in greater depth. To better understand the policy context behind Denti-Cal reimbursements, we conducted seven interviews with officials within the California State Office of Oral Health. We also conducted interviews with ten additional dentists, twelve office managers and billing clerks, and two clinic directors within Fresno County.

Finally, to gain insight into the long-term effects of farmworker's children's high rates of ECC, the first author conducted interviews with four farmworker young adults. These interviewees were chosen randomly with the goal of finding youths with backgrounds comparable to those of the children of immigrant caregivers. In short, we intended these interviews to provide us with a glimpse of the potential cumulative effects of children's poor oral health; we attempted to select farmworker young adults who might represent the future of the children discussed in our first set of interviews.[2]

THE BIOCULTURAL TRANSITION: IMMIGRANT CAREGIVERS' DIET AND INFANT-FEEDING PRACTICES

If a comprehensive understanding of children's oral health requires examining multiple overlapping domains, let us start with a discussion of children's home environments and their parents' feeding practices. We found that immigrant parents' child-feeding behaviors could not be understood without a grasp of the distinct environment in Mexico in which they were raised. The majority of parents came from the classic sending states in western and central Mexico—Michoacán, Jalisco, Zacatecas, and Guanajuato. Rural communities in central and western Mexico have long been linked to the Central Valley through migration networks, yet such routes were institutionalized during the Bracero Program of 1942–64. During this period the United States imported 4.6 million Mexican laborers—many of them small landholders and peasants—to work as temporary "guestworkers" in agriculture and the railroads (Ngai 2004). In short, migration networks from

rural parts of western and central Mexico generally provide the labor sup-
ply to feed the demands of California agribusiness. Thus, all but four of the
Mexican caregivers the first author interviewed were from small rural towns
they described as *ranchos* or *ranchitos*—towns of fifteen thousand people or
less. Because of their rural origins and recent arrival, they were less familiar
with American biomedical understandings of the causes of oral disease and
its proper treatment.

Caregivers' oral health experiences were shaped by the environments in
which they were raised in Mexico—environments that contrasted sharply
with those their children faced in the United States. Diet, especially one high
in carbohydrates or sugar, is a major factor in the etiology of dental caries. An
examination of the diets and infant-feeding practices caregivers described as
being common to rural Mexico illustrates the biocultural transition they un-
derwent on arriving in the United States. All but two of twenty-six caregivers
had grown up on family farms in which their diets depended on subsistence
agriculture. Yet the relatively uncariogenic diet of rural Mexico strongly contrasted with the diet they encountered in the United States—one in which
sodas, candies, and processed and refined foods were the norm (see Horton
and Barker 2010a).

On their arrival in the United States, immigrant caregivers' socioeconomic circumstances shaped a dramatic change in infant-feeding practices
from breast-feeding to bottle-feeding. Because it is low-paid work, few farmworking families can survive without mothers themselves entering the work-
force. Immigrant mothers found themselves newly navigating a contradiction
between the tasks of farmwork and mothering (see de la Torre 1993). The
rhythms of industrial farmwork in the United States do not accommodate
childcare; none of the women we interviewed simultaneously worked in the
field and breast-fed their children. In fact, women reported that the amount
of time they breast-fed their children was directly shaped by the seasonal
schedule of farmwork. Most women worked during the lucrative summer harvest season and rested during the winter. Thus a child born directly after the
harvest season might be breast-fed for six months, whereas one born in the
late spring or summer might not be breast-fed at all. In short, the structure of
farmwork demanded that working mothers bottle-feed their children; breast-
feeding was a luxury few farmworking mothers could afford.

Immigrant women themselves had predominantly been breast-fed when
they were children—partly due to custom and partly due to the high expense
of formula. Yet because immigrant mothers were first-generation bottle-feeders,

they were unprepared for the oral health consequences of prolonged bottle-feeding. Studies have linked the consumption of sugary liquids in bottles for prolonged periods of time leads to a specific form of ECC called "baby bottle tooth decay"—or the decay of the anterior teeth (Shiboski et al. 2003). Unaware of such consequences, some immigrant caregivers placed juice or Nesquik-flavored milk in bottles and allowed their children to feed at night. In short, the structure of farmwork and the availability of infant formula had encouraged immigrant caregivers to abandon breast-feeding in favor of bottle-feeding. Yet because they were unaccustomed to the more stringent oral hygiene requirements of the new cariogenic environment they found in the United States, their adoption of appropriate health behaviors lagged behind their adoption of new infant-feeding practices.

THE POLICY CONTEXT: CREATING EMBODIED INEQUALITIES

Although caregiver dietary and feeding practices helped create a high incidence of decay among children of farmworkers, they are not the only factors that contribute to such embodied inequalities. Although parents seek care for their children's dental problems, California's dental Medicaid—or Denti-Cal—policies constrain the kinds of treatment available to children and play just as large a role in shaping their physical development. Low Denti-Cal reimbursement rates led to disparate treatment patterns for rural low-income children, particularly for those whose severe ECC made them difficult to treat. Thus the biocultural transition immigrant caregivers undergo combines with underinsurance to create a specific form of embodied inequality.

Because farmwork is temporary and seasonal work, it typically does not offer health insurance benefits. Instead, farmworking families are dependent on government health insurance programs for low-income families such as Medi-Cal and Denti-Cal. While farmworker children with legal status may qualify for Medi-Cal or Denti-Cal, undocumented residents must resort to a county health insurance program or to emergency Medicaid, a federal program open to the undocumented family members of citizens. These programs pay only for emergency dental treatment such as extractions. Because their parents were uninsured farmworkers, the children in our sample were forced to rely on Denti-Cal or limited emergency services. Thus Mendota served as a kind of perverse "natural laboratory" in which to view the effects of underinsurance on children's health.

Let us first explain why a market-based dental insurance system may leave a particularly lasting imprint on a child's oral health. Oral health is less of a public priority than general physical health. Oral disease is the most common chronic childhood illness; dental care accounts for roughly 25 percent of total health-care spending for children in the United States. Yet it comprises only 2.3 percent of Medicaid funding nationwide (Milbank Memorial Fund 1999), and only 2 percent of California's Medicaid budget. Because of their limited funding, public dental health insurance programs are underfunded and understaffed. Thus a Medicaid system that underfunds dental treatment disproportionately affects low-income children.

Ninety-eight percent of patients with Denti-Cal receive treatment in private practice (CHCF 2007, 19). Yet barriers to access and obstacles to quality treatment for Denti-Cal patients are particularly pronounced in private clinics. Denti-Cal currently reimburses private dentists at 30–40 percent of the rates they receive from private insurers. Low reimbursement rates compound preexisting barriers to access for young children, whose behavioral issues frequently make dentists consider them especially difficult to treat. This narrows the field of available dentists. Within a fifty-mile radius of Mendota—a catchment area serving a population of roughly eight hundred thousand—only five dentists accepted children under five insured by Denti-Cal. The underfunding of California's Denti-Cal system in turn translates into reduced reimbursement rates for participating dentists, and obstacles to access for its beneficiaries.

Those private dentists who did accept young children on Denti-Cal viewed themselves as having a "mission" to help the underserved. One described his decision to treat this population as a "commitment to the Lord." Another— who performed oral surgery—explained that he had decided to "focus on the small ones" because of their need: "Ninety percent of my practice is kids on Denti-Cal. Because by the time they get here, they all have such bad problems that the other dentists can't treat them." Yet despite these dentists' ethic of care, low Denti-Cal reimbursement rates translated into strict limitations on the treatment for such patients. Revenues from privately insured patients and those with Healthy Families[3] kept these dentists "afloat," subsidizing the treatment they provided those on Denti-Cal. Thus private dentists who accept patients with Denti-Cal had to adopt specific strategies of treatment in order to remain financially viable.

Private dentists reported two distinct treatment strategies they employed in order to continue to treat patients with Denti-Cal. One was to hold constant the percentage of their patients on public insurance. One dentist only saw children Denti-Cal on Tuesdays; another limited Denti-Cal patients to no more than 40 percent of his patient base. This strategy resulted in restricted access to care for Denti-Cal patients, and longer wait times for a first appointment. A second strategy—a "Medicaid mill" approach—was to economize on the time spent on Denti-Cal patients. Under this approach, dentists screened and treated Denti-Cal patients en masse, attempting to perform as many services as possible within a single visit in order to maximize reimbursements. As one dentist explained: "I try to do all the treatment in one sitting. . . . I can do twelve crowns on a kid in one hour and he's playing and having a good time an hour later." Because such dentists specialized in an unprofitable niche market—one with greater demand than availability— they treated young children with Denti-Cal in an assembly-line manner.

Because private dentists felt they were "racing against the clock"—as one put it—many avoided performing time-extensive procedures that were covered by Denti-Cal but reimbursed poorly. Two of the ten private dentists we interviewed in the county did not perform pulpotomies, a children's version of a root canal. Although dental school guidelines recommend that all precautions be taken to save children's teeth to ensure the health of their permanent teeth, Denti-Cal's high standards for proof of service in order to receive reimbursements make children's restorations prohibitive. As one dentist who had left private practice to work in the county mobile van put it, the public insurance frequently denies reimbursements for pulpotomies on which insurance officials deem that the radiographs of the roots show they are "not filled adequately." "So when you keep sending in your X-rays and get your reimbursements denied, you get frustrated. As a result, there are very few dentists who do pulpotomies on Denti-Cal patients in the area," she said. In short, onerous reimbursement regulations and heavy caseloads—the very circumstances faced by private dentists participating in Denti-Cal—may encourage them to extract rather than restore low-income Latino children's teeth.

DISPARATE DENTAL TREATMENT FOR FARMWORKER CHILDREN

An ecosocial study might have ended with this conclusion, but parents' complaints of children's cracked baby teeth yielding crooked permanent teeth demand as charitable a hearing as experts' concerns over their high rates of oral disease. Indeed, taking parents' reports seriously adds another layer of complexity to the interplay between biology and social structure. As it turns out, parents' intuitions were supported by the scientific literature. Children's premature extractions may, over time, permanently affect their oral cavities; they may in fact produce the malocclusions, or "crooked teeth," that some parents lamented.

To understand how caregiver practices interact with the dental public policy to produce farmworker children's marked physiognomies, let us take the case of Isabel, an older child in our sample.[4] Isabel's mother, Maria, first told me about her older daughter's oral health history when I inquired about the oral health of her five-year-old, Elsa, who suffered from extensive decay in her anterior teeth. While Maria was concerned about Elsa's cavities, she was most concerned about what they portended for her future. "I'm worried she's going to look like her older sister," Maria confided. She dispatched Elsa to corral Isabel, who had been watching TV, to serve as a living cautionary tale. Squirming with embarrassment, the nine-year-old reluctantly opened her mouth to reveal her shame—two anterior teeth stubbornly splayed outward.

Maria launched into Isabel's oral health history. Isabel's story of dental misfortune began when she was barely two years old, Maria said. "They were kind of black, near the gum and below as well," Maria remembers. Maria had never seen a child's teeth rot; she says she thought they were stained from the iron drops her doctor gave Isabel for her anemia. When she discussed Isabel's decay with staff at the federal Women, Infants and Children nutritional program, they told Maria she should not allow Isabel to bottle-feed at night. Maria took away the child's bottle, but even that did not stop the advancing decay.

When Maria brought Isabel for a medical checkup, the doctor told Maria that the girl required an urgent dental visit. He referred Isabel to one of the few dentists in the area who accept children with dental Medicaid. Maria was prepared for her daughter to emerge from her appointment with what children at Isabel's nursery school called "the silver teeth"—the stainless steel crowns for which Denti-Cal reimburses. In Maria's school, children displayed "the silver teeth" like a charming accessory; they were a status symbol differentiating children who had Denti-Cal from undocumented children, who did not. However, when the dental assistant walked Isabel out, Isabel had nothing but a hole where her three upper front teeth had once been. To Maria, Isabel's treatment was symbolic of low-income migrant families' second-class citizenship. "They just pulled them out like she was a little animal," Maria says bitterly.

For years, Maria and Isabel had awaited the arrival of Isabel's permanent teeth. Maria imagined them as white and straight; they would grow to fill the hole the dentist had left. Yet when Isabel entered middle school, her front teeth emerged crooked. To Maria, it seemed that Isabel's smile was permanently blighted by her premature extractions. "People say it's because they didn't give her *plaquitas* [false teeth] that her teeth came out the way they did," Maria says. She points to Isabel's school photos on the dining room shelf, showcasing her pursed, wan smile. "She says the kids stare at her at school when she opens her mouth," Maria says.

Isabel was not alone in her misfortune. Four of our interviewees had also brought their small children to a single private dentist in town only to hear that several of the child's front teeth had to be extracted. In two cases, parents took their children to a different dentist for a second opinion, and their children received pulpotomies to save the structure of their teeth. Yet not all parents were so savvy. Like Isabel, those children who had had their front upper teeth extracted also found that the arrival of their permanent teeth did little to assuage their chagrin—they too came in crooked.

As it turns out, Maria may have been correct in intuiting the source of Isabel's "curse"; Isabel's crooked smile may indeed be chalked up to her early extractions. Research in physical anthropology suggests that dental crowding—or "crooked teeth"—is largely limited to populations in industrialized societies due to the effect of environmental factors on the development of the jaw. The premature loss of a child's front teeth and the consumption of soft, processed foods may understimulate the jaw, leading to its uneven development (Corruccini 1984; Lombardi 1982). Crooked teeth thus derive from insufficient jaw space to accommodate tooth size, as normal-sized teeth emerge within an insufficiently developed jaw (Begg 1954). In short, the premature extraction of children's front teeth—the very teeth often affected by "baby bottle tooth decay"—may lead to underbites, overbites, and "crooked teeth" (Oppenheim 1964).

Isabel's story reveals that an underfunded dental public health-care system leaves lasting imprints on children's bodies; children's structural disadvantage is incorporated into their physical development in enduring ways. Parents' complaints of "cracked" baby teeth yielding "crooked" permanent teeth are not whimsical "folk beliefs" but are supported by the expert literature. Children's early childhood caries set them up for the potential for a lifetime of oral disease, yet the premature extraction of their front teeth ensured that their permanent teeth came in crooked. The clustering together of ECC and dental malocclusions among poor Mexican American children may constitute a local syndemic—one that, as we have seen, is iatrogenically mediated.

METHODOLOGICAL REFLECTIONS: THE POWER
OF THE "ETHNOGRAPHIC IMAGINATION"

What can we learn from this interdisciplinary conversation? Perhaps most obviously, ethnography and social epidemiology differ in the value they accord different types of evidence. While the dental public health literature statistically documents the existence of an epidemic of ECC among Latino children, immigrant parents' experiences suggest that the early extraction of such decayed teeth may have long-term embodied effects. Immigrant parents in the Central Valley themselves brought to light the potential existence of a syndemic that had escaped the attention of dentists and epidemiologists alike. Thus one of the strengths of what we call the "ethnographic imagination" (see Mills 1959) lies in its ear placed squarely on the ground—its accord of as much importance to the data provided by individuals as to that abstracted from surveys.

Anthropology's committed epistemological stance demands that we take parents' knowledge seriously, serving as a corrective in a world that privileges "expert knowledge." Science studies scholars remind us that although "expert knowledge" is viewed as "authoritative" because of its presumed decontextualization from local experience and contexts, it is in fact just as "local" as "lay knowledge." Like parents' own knowledge, "expert knowledge" is constructed by specific agents operating in a particular and unique sociocultural environment (Latour and Woolgar 1979). In this particular case, the act of methodologically validating parents' knowledge and placing it on equal footing with that produced by epidemiologists helped unsettle the hierarchy of value that privileges "experts" over "laypeople." Equally importantly, it also generated productive new insights. The textual dialogue we created between the knowledge of two different kinds of "experts"—epidemiologists and immigrant parents—helped produce new understandings of the factors that shape farmworker youths' distinct oral health profiles.

Finally, it is important to note that experts and immigrant parents not only provided different kinds of knowledge, but also revealed quite different priorities regarding Mexican American children's health. While dental public health experts focused on the high rates of cavities among Mexican American children, parents expressed particular concern about the potential long-term effects of children's oral disease on their appearance and sense of self. Parents added important variables such as social stigma and identity to a conversation dominated by a focus on physical health; as we shall see, they expressed special concern about the meaning of children's marked physiognomies in local social systems. Heeding parents' perspectives helps add nuance and complexity to a dialogue on health disparities that revolves primarily around narrowly defined and statistically documentable health outcomes. Until vulnerable populations are fully engaged as stakeholders in the research process, ethnography can help stake a place at the table for them in a conversation dominated by public health and policy experts.

Embodied Inequalities

Finally, ethnography can help reveal additional dimensions that are missing from ecosocial frameworks. The case of oral disease adds an additional layer of complexity to models of how social inequality is embodied. Severe oral disease shapes not only children's physiologies but also their physiognomies; the effects of severe oral disease are visible to the naked eye. Farmworker youths perceived their countenances as irrevocably marked with the signs of their disadvantaged childhoods; their faces permanently bore the marks of their second-class citizenship. Yet social epidemiological models see disease, not illness; their etic approach neglects the subjective dimensions of the lack of well-being. Thus the study of oral disease shows that ill health has not only material but also symbolic significance.

The oral health histories the first author conducted with farmworker young adults who attempted to leave Mendota provide a glimpse of this. In their interviews, these young adults—who represented children's potential future selves—spoke of the time and money they invested in dentistry. It was not uncommon for such youths to become more concerned about the appearance of their teeth once they left the Central Valley and attempted to find jobs (see Horton and Barker 2010b for more examples). One such youth—an honor's student in high school—was concerned that the visible black stain on his front teeth would interfere with his dream of eventually becoming a newscaster. Another—who eventually paid $13,000 to erase his history of decay—used to wrap his front teeth in toilet paper to cover over his shame. To explore this phenomenon, we will begin with the story of Roberto. An aspiring politician, Roberto found that his teeth stood in the way of his dreams, constraining his upward social mobility. Roberto's story illustrates not only the lasting imprint left by Denti-Cal policies on young farmworking children's bodies, but also their cumulative effects.

ROBERTO: ATTEMPTING TO BLEND INTO THE MIDDLE CLASS

Roberto was born outside Mendota in 1977; he was one of seven children raised by a single farmworking mother. He remembers that his mother was not particularly concerned about his oral health when he was a child. "[Oral health] was beyond their concerns. Their concerns were how they were going to put food on the table tomorrow," he says. By the time he was two, his front five teeth had become brown and cracked. Because of his pain, Roberto refused to open his mouth during his dental visits. Roberto badly needed dental treatment, but he was deemed "uncooperative." He had to be referred to a dentist who performed oral sedation, an hour's drive away. It's unclear whether these five teeth could have been saved with pulpotomies, but the dentist extracted them all.

Roberto's negative dental experiences would lead to a lifetime of dental fear and poor oral hygiene. By the time he entered middle school his permanent teeth had come in crooked—probably because of his premature extractions. Yet while Denti-Cal's low reimbursement rates may encourage some dentists to perform extractions rather than restorations, the program does not pay for the orthodontry that would fix the long-term problems such extractions create. Denti-Cal only covers braces only in cases of "medical necessity"—that is, if children's crooked teeth hinder their bite or prevent their eating. Thus while Roberto's early dental experiences had led to a lack of preventive care, his extractions may have set him up for visibly crooked teeth as an adult.

While Roberto was embarrassed about his crooked front teeth during high school, it wasn't until he left Mendota and went to college that he became acutely self-conscious. "[In high school], you just looked like everyone else," he says. Yet Roberto had started college far from home at California State University, Sacramento; he was doing well and was considering a career in politics. He was overseeing a welfare-to-work program at the time and was concerned he might be mistaken for a participant. So he went to an orthodontist to be fitted for braces and learned that he would first have to attend to the issues he had neglected as a child. Roberto first had four root canals and five fillings, for which he paid a total of $5,000 out-of-pocket. The braces cost him an additional $4,000.

Thus for Roberto, dental care is clearly linked with social mobility; teeth have become a means through which to signal his distance from his farmworking roots. Indeed, Roberto has since become one of Mendota's more successful sons. He has interned for Sacramento's congressman in Washington,

DC, and now is a member of the local city council. Yet while Roberto has a gleaming smile, he plans to get more dental work. He wants to have his four front teeth shaved down and restored with new caps and to have his twelve amalgam fillings replaced with porcelain ones. For Roberto, "bad teeth" were the most visible signal of his humble origins, and dentistry was his ticket into a new class bracket. In short, self-funded dental treatment is the price adult children of farmworkers pay to overcome their histories of decay and blend into the professional world.

ERLINDA: MARKED BY UNDERINSURANCE

While Roberto has paid to successfully blend into the middle class, Erlinda, an adult of twenty-five, finds that her presentation of self has precluded her ability to similarly "disappear." Instead, Erlinda has borne the marks of her lack of insurance as a child all her life. Born in Mexico to migrant farmworking parents, Erlinda was the only child of eleven who was not a U.S. citizen, and thus the only child without health insurance. She felt this sense of stigma most acutely in regard to her teeth.

As a child, Erlinda could only rely on emergency Medi-Cal and the county's limited indigent program for dental care, both of which only pay for extractions. Thus while Erlinda began brushing her teeth when she entered preschool, she never visited a dentist as a child. Her farmworking parents, who supported the family of thirteen on a combined salary of roughly $14,000, couldn't afford the visit. This set up a pattern of care in which Erlinda visited the dentist only when in extreme pain, at which point she would have to have her teeth extracted.

When she was about ten, two molars began hurting her greatly. Several days each year, she left school early because of her pain. Finally, at twelve, Erlinda's pain had become too much to bear. The dentist offered her parents a choice: he could extract five of her permanent teeth or he could charge her parents $125 a filling. Her parents didn't want her to have her teeth extracted, so they decided to wait. "My mom said, 'We'll find a way to fix your teeth,'" she remembers. But year after year went by, and they still weren't able to pay for her restorations; she eventually had the teeth extracted three years later.

Yet more damaging to Erlinda's sense of self was the social stigma she felt due to her crooked and decayed teeth. When she entered junior high school, the division between children with dental insurance and those without it became more pronounced. Many of the girls in Erlinda's class—whose own mothers worked in the field with hers—were getting braces through Denti-Cal. "They would say, 'I want to get the blue ones next time.' 'I think I'm going to get the pink ones,'" she says with envy. For her friends braces were an accessory, but for Erlinda they were a privilege she didn't have. She once asked her mother whether she could leave school for a year to work for money for her braces, but her mother said no.

At fourteen, having only once received a preventive cleaning, Erlinda began having more problems. Besides the mounting pain in several teeth, she developed severe decay on a front tooth—a visible black stain. She tried to brush it frequently to make it less visible. She saw the movie *Beetlejuice*, in which a girl puts Wite-Out on her teeth to make them look whiter. That gave Erlinda the idea of putting white nail polish on her teeth to try to hide the decay.

Other than such sporadic treatment, Erlinda has relied on visits to Mexico, where dental care is cheaper. Her big break came when she was eighteen and had moved to L.A. to work. She was having a hard time getting a job in an office; a friend had told her that she should try to "straighten out" her teeth. Her sister told her there was a good dentist in Tijuana, so she decided to get all her restorative work done at once. She paid USD $2,800 over a series of weekends for an extraction, two root canals, twelve fillings, and a crown—work that would have cost her three times as much in the United States. Yet while Erlinda has finally been able to receive the dental treatment she could never have as a child, her childhood dental experiences have left long-lasting effects on her appearance and sense of self.

DISCUSSION

The stories of Roberto and Erlinda illustrate how the interaction between caregiver practices and insurance policies yield concerns regarding heightened visibility for farmworker young adults. As Brackette Williams argues (1989), national community is seen as synonymous with an unmarked ethno-racial group that has the unacknowledged privilege of effortlessly blending in with national culture. Roberto's and Erlinda's complaints of difference highlight their embodied inequality, or their perceived sociocultural and bodily distance from this unmarked norm. Both see their teeth as a marker of their social vulnerability—a visible sign of their farmworking past. Understandably, their complaints of visibility intensify with the distance they hope to travel from their roots in Mendota—whether to news studios in Fresno or the halls of Congress in Washington.

For farmworker youths, disfigurement assumes the status of an involuntary bodily marking, one that others can read as a sign of depreciated social status. For both Roberto and Erlinda, their poor oral health is perceived to mark them as irrevocably "different," serving as an obstacle to upward social mobility. This is apparent in Roberto's heightened self-consciousness about his teeth with the distance he traveled from his farmworking roots, adopting behaviors excessive even for members of the middle class. Yet the exorbitant price tag for the dental work that Roberto would require illustrates the prohibitive cost of reversing a childhood of poor oral health. While Roberto is able to project elite citizenship by continuously working on his teeth, Erlinda's story shows that resources are necessary simply to disappear into the category of the "unmarked."

METHODOLOGICAL REFLECTIONS: HEALTH AND SOCIAL INEQUALITY AS A DIALECTIC

Let us consider the implications of our study first for methodological approaches to unraveling the causes of health disparities, and ultimately for the question of when health inequalities become a matter of social justice. Recent ecosocial models draw attention to the multiple domains within which the physical body is nested, proposing that we examine the diverse contributions of children's home environments, treatment in dental offices, and public policy to their poor oral health. With its gaze trained narrowly on health indicators, social epidemiology is ill prepared to connect broad sociopolitical circumstances with specific health indicators. Ethnography can help operationalize the insights of both "embodiment" and "syndemics" approaches by producing fine-grained analyses of the processes in various domains that shape children's embodied difference.

Yet beyond grounding epidemiological insights, ethnographic analysis identifies a missing factor in both ecosocial frameworks of health disparities. In focusing on the corporeal imprint left by the social world, an "embodiment" framework explicitly views ill health as a static end product. Similarly, a "syndemics" approach suggests that we treat social conditions and disease as equal cofactors in contributing to health disparities, but fails to explicitly examine how such disparities themselves contribute to the dynamic. Illness is both material and symbolic; affliction has not only subjective but also social meaning.

Our analysis suggests we must examine health inequalities and social conditions as a dialectic: children's poor oral health is not only the end product of social inequalities but is also, as a factor itself, contributing to the perpetuation of a system of social disparity.

Finally, this case has implications for the important question of under what circumstances are health inequalities are a matter of social justice. Kelleher (chapter 3, this volume) raises the question of whether the goal of reducing health inequalities is an intrinsic good, and what rationale justifies prioritizing this goal over that of ameliorating the health of all. Examining this question through the lens of syndemics provides an intriguing answer. A syndemics approach argues that health inequalities have greater repercussions than meet the eye because they interact to create an additive burden of disease for the poor. It proposes that diseases assume a qualitatively distinct form in conditions of social inequality. In arguing that social inequality is a cofactor in causing and exacerbating disease, a syndemics approach makes what Kelleher calls a "causal relationist" argument for the need for social intervention. Because social inequality itself is the cause of children's oral health disparities, intervening to reduce oral health disparities among the poor becomes a social obligation—a matter not merely of fairness but of justice.

Yet social inequality is not merely a cause of such health inequities; farmworker youths' oral disease in turn reproduces their social disadvantage. Mexican American youths' blighted smiles are in fact symbolic of their depreciated social position. This case study thus makes what Kelleher calls a "relational egalitarian" argument for intervening to ameliorate these visible health inequities. Farmworker youths' marked physiognomies are a matter of social concern because they "frustrate [their] realization of relational ideals" (101) such as being treated as social equals and effortlessly blending into the middle class. Thus, this study not only demonstrates biology and society as cofactors in the disease process; it also provides a powerful argument for why farmworkers' marked physiognomies are not only a concern of public health but also a matter of social justice.

NOTES

1. The research on which this article was based was supported through a cooperative agreement between the National Institute of Dental and Craniofacial Research (Grant U54 DE 014251) and the Center to Address Children's Disparities in Oral Health (J. A. Weintraub, DDS, MPH, PI). The grant was titled "Hispanic Oral Health: A Rural

and Urban Ethnography," and Judith C. Barker was PI. The first author reanalyzed the original data produced from this grant and wrote the article; the second author read drafts and offered comments.

2. Although our aim in interviewing adult children of farmworkers was to gain an understanding of the long-term social effects of oral health disparities for farmworker children, we cannot assume that such adults precisely represent the adult selves of the children who were the focus of interviews in our first study. A full understanding of the long-term consequences of oral health disparities for farmworker children would require a longitudinal study, which we were unable to do. However, we do feel it is reasonable to infer that the focal children in our first study might face similar social consequences of their pronounced oral decay once they reached young adulthood.

3. Healthy Families is a program that provides health insurance to children whose families do not qualify for Medicaid but whose incomes fall below 250 percent of the federal poverty level.

4. The names of all interviewees have been changed to protect their privacy.

REFERENCES

Barker, Judith C., and Sarah B. Horton. 2008. "An Ethnographic Study of Latino Preschool Children's Oral Health in Rural California: Intersections among Family, Community, Provider and Regulatory Sectors." *BMC Oral Health* 8 (1): 8.

Beck, James, Raul Garcia, Gerardo Heiss, Pantel S. Vokonas, and Steven Offenbacher. 1996. "Periodontal Disease and Cardiovascular Disease." *Journal of Periodontology* 67 (10s): 1123–37.

Begg, P. Raymond. 1954. "Stone Age Man's Dentition: With Reference to Anatomically Correct Occlusion, the Etiology of Malocclusion, and a Technique for Its Treatment." *American Journal of Orthodontics* 40 (6): 298–312.

CHCF (California HealthCare Foundation). 2007. *Denti-Cal Facts and Figures: A Look at California's Medicaid Dental Program.* Oakland: California HealthCare Foundation.

Chaffin, Jeffrey G., Satish Chandra S. Pai, and Robert A. Bagramian. 2003. "Caries Prevalence in Northwest Michigan Migrant Children." *Journal of Dentistry for Children* 70 (2): 124–29.

Corruccini, Robert S. 1984. "An Epidemiologic Transition in Dental Occlusion in World Populations." *American Journal of Orthodontics* 86 (5): 419–26.

de la Torre, Adela. 1993. "Hard Choices and Changing Roles among Mexican Migrant Campesinas." In *Building with Our Hands: New Directions in Chicana Studies*, edited by Adela de la Torre and Beatriz Pesquera, 168–80. Berkeley: University of California Press.

Dye, Bruce A., Xianfen Li, and Gina Thornton-Evans. 2012. *Oral Health Disparities as Determined by Selected Healthy People 2020 Oral Health Objectives for the United States, 2009–2010.*" NCHS Data Brief No. 104. Hyattsville, MD: National Center for Health Statistics. http://www.cdc.gov/nchs/data/databriefs/db104.htm. Accessed 26 August 2015.

Gravlee, Clarence C. 2009. "How Race Becomes Biology: Embodiment of Social Inequality." *American Journal of Physical Anthropology* 139 (1): 47–57.

Hilton, Irene V., Samantha Stephen, Judith C. Barker, and Jane A. Weintraub. 2007. "Cultural Factors and Children's Oral Health Care: A Qualitative Study of Carers of Young Children." *Community Dentistry and Oral Epidemiology* 35 (6): 429–38.

Horton, Sarah B., and Judith C. Barker. 2010a. "A Latino Oral Health Paradox? Using Ethnography to Specify the Biocultural Factors behind Epidemiological Models." In "Anthropological Perspectives on Migration and Health," special issue, *National Association of Practicing Anthropologists Bulletin* 34 (1): 68–83.

———. 2010b. "Stigmatized Biologies: Examining the Cumulative Effects of Oral Health Disparities for Mexican American Children." *Medical Anthropology Quarterly* 24 (2): 199–219.

Huntington, Noelle L., Il Joon Kim, and Christopher V. Hughes. 2002. "Caries Risk Factors for Hispanic Children Affected by Early Childhood Caries." *Pediatric Dentistry* 24 (6): 536–42.

Krieger, Nancy. 2001. "Theories for Social Epidemiology in the 21st Century: An Ecosocial Perspective." *International Journal of Epidemiology* 30 (4): 668–77.

Latour, Bruno, and Steve Woolgar. 1979. *Laboratory Life: The Social Construction of Scientific Facts*. Beverly Hills: Sage.

Lombardi, A. Vincent. 1982. "The Adaptive Value of Dental Crowding: A Consideration of the Biologic Basis of Malocclusion." *American Journal of Orthodontics* 81 (1): 38–42.

Lukes, Sherri M., and Bret Simon. 2005. "Dental Decay in Southern Illinois Migrant and Seasonal Farmworkers: An Analysis of Clinical Data." *Journal of Rural Health* 21 (3): 254–58.

Michaud, Dominique S., Kaumudi Joshipura, Edward Giovannucci, and Charles S. Fuchs. 2007. "A Prospective Study of Periodontal Disease and Pancreatic Cancer in U.S. Male Health Professionals." *Journal of the National Cancer Institute* 99 (2): 171–75.

Milbank Memorial Fund. 1999. *Pediatric Dental Care in CHIP and Medicaid: Paying for What Kids Need, Getting Value for State Payments*. New York: Milbank Memorial Fund.

Mills, C. Wright. 1959. *The Sociological Imagination*. London: Oxford University Press.

Miyamoto, W., C. S. Chung, and P. K. Yee. 1976. "Effect of Premature Loss of Deciduous Canines and Molars on Malocclusion of the Permanent Dentition." *Journal of Dental Research* 55 (4): 584–90.

Ngai, Mae M. 2004. *Impossible Subjects: Illegal Aliens and the Making of Modern America: Illegal Aliens and the Making of Modern America*. Princeton, NJ: Princeton University Press.

Oppenheim, M. 1964. "The Importance of Preserving the Primary Dentition." *Pennsylvania Dental Journal* 31: 38–42.

Quandt, Sara A., Heather M. Clark, Pamela Rao, and Thomas A. Arcury. 2007. "Oral Health of Children and Adults in Latino Migrant and Seasonal Farmworker Families." *Journal of Immigrant and Minority Health* 9 (3): 229–35.

Scott, Gulnur, and Catherine Simile. 2005. "Access to Dental Care among Hispanic or Latino Subgroups: United States, 2000–03." *U.S. Centers for Disease Control and Prevention: Advance Data from Vital and Health Statistics* 354 (May): 1–16.

Shiboski, Caroline H., Stuart A. Gansky, Francisco Ramos-Gomez, Long Ngo, Robert Isman, and Howard F. Pollick. 2003. "The Association of Early Childhood Caries and Race/Ethnicity among California Preschool Children." *Journal of Public Health Dentistry* 63 (1): 38–46.

Singer, Merrill. 2009. *Introduction to Syndemics: A Critical Systems Approach to Public and Community Health*. San Francisco: Jossey-Bass.

Singer, Merrill, and Scott Clair. 2003. "Syndemics and Public Health: Reconceptualizing Disease in Bio-Social Context." *Medical Anthropology Quarterly* 17 (4): 423–41.

USDHHS (U.S. Department of Health and Human Services). 2000. *Oral Health in America: A Report of the Surgeon General*. 00-4713. Rockville: U.S. Department of Health and Human Services, National Institute of Dental and Craniofacial Research, National Institutes of Health.

Weinstein, Philip, Peter Domoto, Kyoko Wohlers, and Mark Koday. 1992. "Mexican-American Parents with Children at Risk for Baby Bottle Tooth Decay: Pilot Study at a Migrant Farmworkers Clinic." *ASDC Journal of Dentistry for Children* 59 (5): 376–83.

Williams, Brackette F. 1989. "A Class Act: Anthropology and the Race to Nation across Ethnic Terrain." *Annual Review of Anthropology* 18: 401–44.

6

Chasing Virtue, Enforcing Virtue

Social Justice and Conceptions of Risk in Pregnancy

Debra DeBruin, Anne Drapkin Lyerly,
Joan Liaschenko, and Mary Faith Marshall

ABSTRACT

Judgments about risk of harm raise issues of profound moral significance. In this chapter, we criticize prevailing assumptions about risk management in pregnancy. While bioethicists tend to focus on beneficence when analyzing issues of risk, we argue that beneficence does not exhaust the moral significance of risk and that judgments about risk also raise issues of social justice. Our analysis thus dovetails with Kittay's chapter (this volume), which demonstrates that matters of autonomy also raise social justice challenges. We begin our chapter by highlighting criteria for adequate understanding of social justice. Importantly, we view social justice as transcending the distribution of harms and benefits standardly thought to constitute justice. We then consider how culture shapes the normative significance of risk: how we think about risk, what measures we feel justified taking to manage risks, whose interests are promoted by various approaches to risk, whom we hold responsible and for what. Our analysis moves beyond criticism to propose reform of cultural attitudes toward pregnancy and its management. We assess recent claims that "fetal origins" research provides a basis for such reform, and we highlight opportunities for a more just approach to risk management in pregnancy. Drawing on Braveman's work (this volume), we argue that recognition of the significance of social determinants of health plays a critical role in transforming the management of risk in pregnancy. Overall, our analysis engages foundational philosophical questions about the nature of social justice in concert with attention to cultural context.

INTRODUCTION

Conceptions of risk raise issues of profound moral significance. Since the notion of risk always involves concern with possible harm (of whatever variety—not all harms are physical) or compromise of a person's or group's good, bioethicists tend to think about questions of risk as matters of beneficence. However, we will argue that beneficence does not exhaust the moral significance of risk—that conceptions of risk also raise issues of social justice. In itself, this is a noteworthy deviation from typical understandings of the application of the canonical principles of bioethics. Our analysis thus dovetails with that provided by Eva Feder Kittay (chapter 4, this volume), who argues that discussions of autonomy also raise significant social justice challenges. Further, the concerns regarding social justice in our analysis transcend considerations of *distribution* of risks and benefits standardly discussed; matters of justice often transcend concerns about distribution. In particular, we attend to how culture shapes the normative significance of risk: how we think about risk, what measures we feel justified in taking to manage risks, whose interests are promoted by various approaches to risk, whom we hold responsible and for what. We focus in particular on the moral significance of conceptions of risk in pregnancy, though the analysis of risk and social justice presented here could perhaps be applied to other situations as well, such as the ways that race influences judgments about risk, as in debates about use of deadly force by police or by citizens invoking "stand your ground" justifications. Unlike foundational philosophical work, this analysis will provide "a normative reflection that is historically and socially contextualized" (Young 1990, 5). As such, it requires an interdisciplinary approach.[1]

We begin by exploring the predominant approach to managing risk in pregnancy. We proceed to consider the cultural significance of risk and use the discussion of culture as a springboard for an analysis of social justice as it relates to the perception and management of risk in pregnancy. This analysis highlights some criteria for an adequate understanding of social justice. We then consider recent claims that "fetal origins" research—multidisciplinary research concerning the fetal environment's long-term impact on health and well-being of offspring—provides a basis for reform of our conception of risk in pregnancy. We focus on the popular culture conversation about fetal origins research rather than the scientific literature, because the social uptake of the science has tremendous power to affect the cultural conception of risk. We argue that this popular conversation—preoccupied as it is with women's responsibilities for making lifestyle choices designed to protect their offspring from risks of harm not only during gestation but throughout their lifespan into adulthood—is mired in the predominant conception of risk that it wishes to discard. It thus largely misses what may be the truly transformative power of fetal origins research: its growing data-based support for the critical importance of the social determinants of health and the resulting acknowledgment of the deep significance of social (in)justice. Finally, we highlight opportunities for a more just approach to risk management in pregnancy.

MANAGING RISK IN PREGNANCY AND CHILDBIRTH

In a series of articles, a multidisciplinary research group addressing distortions of risk related to reproduction (the Obstetrics and Gynecology Risk Research Group, OGRRG) analyzes judgments about risk during pregnancy, examining standard advice about risk management in the context of pregnant women's daily behaviors (e.g., diet, activities) as well as the choices of clinicians and pregnant women regarding interventions during pregnancy and birth (Lyerly et al. 2009; Kukla et al. 2009; Lyerly et al. 2007). These authors note certain general patterns in risk management during pregnancy and childbirth. While there may be exceptions to these patterns, they nevertheless comprise cultural tendencies that affect pregnant women and their fetuses. For instance, they describe the tendency in American medicine to avoid interventions for pregnant women's nonobstetrical health needs such as depression or asthma and instead focus on purported dangers these interventions pose to fetuses. This occurs even in the absence of evidence and is characterized in particular by a tendency to ignore or fail to investigate the potential harms to pregnant women and their fetuses of forgoing clinical interventions. Unfortunately, those harms are all too often realized: for example, when a physician hesitates to provide lifesaving intervention for a pregnant woman for fear of teratogenic harm to a fetus, when a woman who is pregnant eschews her asthma medication and ends up in the emergency room with a severe asthma attack, or when a woman with severe depression heeds advice to forgo antidepressant medication and attempts suicide (Lyerly et al. 2009, 34–37; cf. Little 2011).

Notably, this tendency is not limited to the clinic and choices about medical intervention, but extends into women's everyday lives. In many instances, aspects of daily life are subsumed under the veil of medical surveillance, even when the medical implications of such are unknown. But advice likewise flows from strangers, friends, family, and nonmedical practitioners and is manifest in public counsel, rules, and popular discourse. The OGRRG authors observe that pregnant women are subjected to a "torrent of advice advanced in the name of safety" (Lyerly et al. 2009, 38). They describe the overall approach to managing risk during pregnancy as "an exercise of caution, restraint and fear" (Lyerly et al. 2009, 38).

This tendency also emerges at the level of public policy. For instance, decades of "protecting" women and fetuses from the possible harms of participating in research by routinely excluding women of childbearing age from clinical studies resulted in significant inequities in data-based understanding of women's health vis-à-vis men's health and denied women the potential benefits of research participation (Mastroianni, Faden, and Federman 1994; see also DeBruin 1994). Recognition of the social injustices inherent in these practices led to the adoption of policy requiring the inclusion of women in clinical research in 1993 (NIH ORWH 2013). Nevertheless, pregnant women continue to be routinely excluded from research, resulting in a dearth of information about how to safely and effectively treat illness during pregnancy (cf. Lyerly, Little, and Faden 2008; Chambers, Polifka, and Friedman 2008). Shielding pregnant women and their fetuses from the risks of research does not effectively spare them from risk. Rather, it shifts those risks to the domains of both clinical practice and public advice, which as a consequence entails the management of illness during pregnancy without a robust evidence base. In short, the ways we perceive and manage risk in the context of pregnancy have often and paradoxically put women and the children they bear in harm's way.

In contrast, there is a tendency, particularly among practitioners of obstetrics, to embrace intervention during childbirth. The tendency seems to reflect a technological imperative (I can, therefore I must), with responsibility linked to action, even when data indicate that intervening is associated with excess harm (Lyerly et al. 2009, 38). One example is the use of episiotomy, which became routine in the United States in the twentieth century, when women began giving birth in hospitals rather than at home, due to the presumption that it reduces risks of perineal trauma and helps the fetus by facilitating delivery (ACOG 2006). Yet data now indicate that episiotomy may in fact increase the risks of perineal injury to women and provide no fetal benefit. Episiotomy rates have slowly declined in the past two decades, but the procedure is still performed in several hundred thousand births per year. Similar patterns are seen with other interventions before or during birth, such as bed rest, routine fetal heart monitoring, and labor induction (Klein et al. 2007). Indeed, so ingrained is the inclination to intervene that new professional guidelines urging expectant management over intervention in longer labors made national headlines (AP 2014; referring to ACOG and SMFM 2014). The inclination toward intervention in labor, manifest in professional guidelines and clinical practice, reflects (and perhaps reifies) conceptions of risk during pregnancy and childbirth evident in the popular culture.

At first blush, these tendencies may appear to be unproblematically grounded in a cultural commitment to protect babies and children. Given limited research and thus uncertainty about how best to manage fetal risk, a "better safe than sorry" cultural practice of extreme caution may seem quite reasonable. However, an exploration of the cultural significance of risk and the social justice implications of our risk management practices in pregnancy suggests otherwise.

THE CULTURAL SIGNIFICANCE OF RISK

Bioethicists would typically respond to dominant practices of risk management in pregnancy by analyzing how the demands of beneficence apply to them. Risks of harm to affected individuals would be weighed against possible benefits to them, and scholars would insist that our understanding of both risks and benefits be grounded in data to the extent possible. Such an analysis provides a valuable contribution. The OGRRG authors push the analysis further. Building on the work of the anthropologist Mary Douglas (1966) and others, they suggest that the aversion to perceived risks of interventions for pregnant women's health concerns during pregnancy discussed above is grounded in cultural themes of purity and control. Arguably, the overall cultural expectation of self-sacrifice during pregnancy reflects the former: the purity of the pregnant woman's body must be maintained to protect the fetus from harm. While we may not speak explicitly in terms of "purity" in contemporary U.S. society, we do tend to think of supposed risk behaviors as vices or moral failings and characterize the self-sacrificing abstinence of pregnant women as virtuous behavior (Jos, Marshall, and Perlmutter 1995). Current rituals and beliefs about harms in pregnancy are expressed and made manifest in the discourse and practices of risk management (Lupton 1999). As such, aversion to risks of intervening in clinical or research settings as well as practices of everyday self-sacrifice during pregnancy often lack empirical grounding and "reflect a form of magical thinking rather than evidence-based reasoning about actual harms and dangers" (Lyerly et al. 2009, 39).

In contrast, the OGRRG contends, the enthusiasm for intervention during birth reflects a theme of control (Lyerly et al. 2009, 39). While the theme of control is often pronounced in liminal states such as birth and death, one way it manifests itself has been in the medicalization of childbirth in which expert knowledge is given priority over the knowledge of childbearing women, whose preferences and experiences are often marginalized or absent from consideration (Barker 1998). Medicalization in this case involves the enactment of expert knowledge in the form of various medical interventions seen as necessary to protect the fetus. Thus care is characterized by constant surveillance of the fetus and the woman who "is like a ship upon a stormy sea full of white-caps, and the good pilot who is in charge must guide her with prudence if he is to avoid a shipwreck" (Mauriceau quoted in Barker 1998, 1067).

The theme of control also emerges in counternarratives to the "medical model" of childbirth—in which advocates argue that childbirth is normal, natural, and intrinsically safe and minimize the potential for maternal or infant morbidity that childbirth (not just its medical management) can entail. Narratives of birthing women both associate control with a panoply of notions of the "good" and often acknowledge it—either due to institutional structures or physiologic realities—as unattainable (Namey and Lyerly 2010). However, women who express a desire for control tend to seek control that supports their dignity and empowerment. They seek self-determination, self-respect, the respect of care providers for them, personal security, trusting relationships with their care providers, and knowledge. Yet the enthusiasm for intervention on the part of maternity care providers all too often reflects a pursuit of control of the woman and her birthing experience, contrary to the respectful, empowering control sought by women themselves. If the pregnant woman is "like a ship upon a stormy sea" (Mauriceau quoted in Barker 1998, 1067), she is the object of intervention, not the subject of her birthing experience.

The apparently stark contrast between reticence to intervene to address women's health concerns during pregnancy and enthusiasm for intervention during childbirth may seem puzzling. How should we understand the divergent themes of purity during pregnancy and control during childbirth?

An anthropological analysis of risk sheds further light on these approaches and their moral significance. We supplement the analysis provided by the OGRRG by delving more deeply into the work of Mary Douglas, who argues that the cultural meaning of "risk" has changed over time. Originally, risk "meant the probability of an event occurring, combined with the magnitude of the losses or gains that would be entailed" (Douglas 1990, 2). Contemporary scientists and academic ethicists likely assume that the term continues to carry this meaning (absent, perhaps, the inclusion of gains in addition to losses, given current tendencies to talk about "risks and benefits"). However, Douglas contends that "a culture needs a common forensic vocabulary with which to hold persons accountable, and that 'risk' is a word that admirably serves the forensic needs of a new global culture" (Douglas 1990, 1). Cultures need a way to signify judgments of responsibility for (avoidance of) undesirable outcomes. Religious cultures use terms such as "sin" and "taboo," but our more secular culture needs a different term. "Danger" could serve, but "risk" predominates because it carries the pretense of scientific authority, a fitting secular parallel for the role of divine authority in religious cultures.

As a forensic term, "risk" is infused with moral significance. It is associated with cultural norms about acceptable versus condemnable behavior and attributions of responsibility. We may puzzle over the tendency to focus on the dangers various actions may hold for fetuses during pregnancy despite the absence of data, or in the face of data indicating the safety of those actions. We may decry the common use of interventions during childbirth that data show to be unduly risky or of unproven benefit. Appeals to data (or the lack thereof) cannot suffice to counter a cultural conception of risk that is fundamentally forensic rather than merely probabilistic. As Douglas explains, "It is futile to study risk perception without systematically taking the cultural bias into account" (Douglas 1990, 11).

RISK AND SOCIAL JUSTICE

The social justice significance of this cultural conception of risk emerges when the norms associated with this forensic notion are identified. Of particular salience are norms linked with pervasive notions of what makes a "good" mother: "The dominant idea of a 'good mother' in North America requires that women abjure personal gain, comfort, leisure, time, income, and even fulfillment; paradoxically, during pregnancy, when the woman is not yet a mother, this expectation of self-sacrifice can be even more stringently applied. The idea of imposing any risk on the fetus, however small or theoretical, for the benefit of a pregnant woman's interest has become anathema" (Lyerly et al. 2009, 40). Claire Dederer poignantly describes the pervasive and moralizing character of this notion of a "good mother" in her memoir about the struggles she and other women engaged with their gender roles: "We were a generation of hollow-eyed women, chasing virtue.... [We] were consumed with trying to do everything right" (Dederer 2010, 19).

The dominant conception of risk in pregnancy raises profound issues of social justice: it reflects oppressive professional and cultural norms that are *central* to our cultural conception of motherhood. As Young has forcefully argued, social justice relates fundamentally to the eradication of domination and oppression, which are not necessarily linked to unfairness in distribution of social benefits and burdens (Young 1990). Young maintains that "the scope of justice . . . is not limited to distribution, but includes all social processes that support or undermine oppression, including culture" (Young 1990, 152). To say our practices are oppressive does not imply that they purposefully or intentionally aim to discriminate against or subordinate women. It is now quite commonly accepted that unreflective cultural practices or institutional structures can be oppressive in the sense that these systems effect the subordination, diminishment, constraint, deprivation, or harm of members of particular social groups (Frye 1983). Ehrenreich and English posit that "the medical system is . . . strategic to women's oppression. . . . Justifications for sexual discrimination—in education, in jobs, in public life—must ultimately rest on the one thing that differentiates women from men: their bodies" (Ehrenreich and English 2011, 31–32).

To help specify the injustices inherent in cultural norms concerning risk and pregnancy, we turn to Powers and Faden's theory of social justice. It is beyond the scope of this chapter to argue in support of this theory against alternatives. We find the view developed by Powers and Faden particularly powerful for our analysis because when women are asked to offer their perspectives about what constitutes a good birth experience, the considerations they describe roughly parallel the essential elements of well-being delineated by these scholars (Namey and Lyerly 2010, 771). Very simply, Powers and Faden maintain that "well-being is best understood as involving plural, irreducible dimensions, each of which represents something of independent moral significance. We maintain further that justice is concerned with six essential dimensions of well-being. . . . We contend that each of these dimensions is an essential feature of well-being, such that a life substantially lacking in any one is a life seriously deficient in what is reasonable for anyone to want, whatever else they want. Each is thus a separate indicator of a decent life which it is the job of justice to facilitate" (Powers and Faden 2006, 6). Powers and Faden identify the six essential dimensions of well-being that are the concerns of justice as health, personal security, reasoning, respect, attachment, and self-determination (Powers and Faden 2006, 16–29).

We have already discussed the health impacts of our dominant cultural conception of risk management in pregnancy. The tendency to avoid interventions for women's health needs during pregnancy occasions excessive and often troubling risk for pregnant women and their fetuses. The practice of excluding pregnant women from clinical research in an effort to shield fetuses from risk shifts risk to the larger domain of clinical practice. The enthusiasm for intervention during childbirth expresses a commitment to "do everything" to protect fetuses (and sometimes women) even when evidence suggests that intervention may do more harm than good. In general, the ways we perceive and manage risk in pregnancy have often and paradoxically put women and the children they will bear in harm's way. In addition to health as narrowly and traditionally construed, views about risk also have consequences for other items on Powers and Faden's list of essential dimensions of well-being.

Consider, for instance, how childbearing women characterize their need to feel safe in birth: the need comprises both physical safety and the emotional and psychological attributes of personal security (Namey and Lyerly 2010, 773). Arguably, if the ways we perceive and manage risk in pregnancy carry undue risk of harm for women and their fetuses, then pregnant women's personal security is undermined. Moreover, the intense pressure placed on pregnant women themselves to safeguard their fetuses despite vexing uncertainty about how to do so surely undermines women's emotional and psychological security. As the journalist Annie Murphy Paul compellingly conveys, the focus on women carries an oppressive valence: "Always, it seems, the influence wielded by a pregnant woman is of a negative kind; always she is one slipup away from harming her fetus. Today's pregnant woman could be forgiven for feeling that there's a vast conspiracy afoot, bent on controlling her every action, stripping her of every pleasure, and inducing guilt at every turn" (Paul 2010a, 3).

However, the most troubling violation of pregnant women's personal security stems from our culture's enduring—and shocking—willingness to enforce the norms inherent in our forensic notion of risk by using coercive measures, even when case law and standards of professional ethics should preclude it. In a 2013 report, Paltrow and Flavin document more than four hundred cases of state-supported coercive interventions in pregnancy in forty-four states, the District of Columbia, and federal jurisdictions from 1973 (the year of the *Roe v. Wade* ruling) to 2005 (the latest date for which there were records of cases that had reached their legal conclusion at the time the article was published) (Paltrow and Flavin 2013, 300–301). They argue that, although their report provides the most comprehensive documentation of such cases, there is compelling reason to believe that it underestimates the prevalence of such coercive interventions (Paltrow and Flavin 2013, 300, 304–5).

Paltrow and Flavin's review of cases leads them to "challenge . . . the idea that arrests, detentions, and forced interventions of pregnant women are extremely rare and occur only in isolated, exceptional circumstances against a narrowly definable group of women. Quite to the contrary, cases documented in this study make clear that arrests, detentions and forced interventions have not been limited to pregnant women who use a certain drug or engage in a particular behavior. Our research shows that these state interventions are happening in every region of the country and affect women of all races . . . [although] clear racial disparities [are] identified" (Paltrow and Flavin 2013, 333). Notably, approximately 59 percent of cases involved women of color, mostly African American women. The review of cases also evidences socioeconomic disparities, with 71 percent of women qualifying for indigent defense (Paltrow and Flavin 2013, 311).

Paltrow and Flavin describe cases to illustrate the cultural phenomenon they document. In one case, a woman was convicted of homicide by child abuse when her pregnancy ended in stillbirth. Authorities alleged that her drug use caused the stillbirth, although they did not present credible data to support that allegation, and it was later shown that an infection caused the stillbirth. After she served eight years of her sentence, an appeals court overturned her conviction on grounds that her counsel failed to present relevant evidence for her defense. However, fearing that she would be retried and sent back to prison, she pled guilty to manslaughter and was released from prison given time served. In another case, a woman was forced to undergo cesarean delivery when physicians insisted that her decision to attempt a vaginal birth after a previous cesarean delivery posed a risk to her fetus. In this case, "a sheriff went to Pemberton's home, took her into custody, strapped her legs together, and forced her to go to a hospital," where she was subjected to a cesarean section against her will (Paltrow and Flavin 2013, 306–7). The woman in question successfully delivered subsequent pregnancies vaginally, casting serious doubt on the state's risk assessment in this case. In yet another case, when a woman voluntarily sought help for her addiction to Oxycontin, she was involuntarily committed to a psychiatric facility where she received no prenatal care. She lost her job as a result of her detention (Paltrow and Flavin 2013, 306–8).

Consistent with our analysis of the "magical thinking" associated with the dominant perception and management of risk in pregnancy, Paltrow and Flavin note that coercive interventions lack grounding in evidence.

> Although deprivations of women's liberty are often justified as mechanisms for protecting children from harm, we found that in a majority of cases the arrest or other action taken was not dependent on evidence of actual harm to the fetus or newborn. . . . In two out of three cases no adverse pregnancy outcome was reported. . . . In cases where a harm was alleged (e.g., a stillbirth), we found numerous instances in which cases proceeded without any evidence, much less scientific evidence, establishing a causal link between the harm and the pregnant woman's alleged action or inaction. In other cases, we found the courts failed to act as judicial gatekeeper to ensure, as they are required to do, that medical and scientific claims are in fact supported by expert testimony based on valid and reliable scientific evidence. (Paltrow and Flavin 2013, 317–18)

Oppressive cultural norms concerning pregnant women's responsibilities and the intolerability of posing risk to fetuses, as well as racism and classism—not scientific evidence—underlie these coercive interventions. The standard cultural expectation that requires compelling evidence to justify violations of personal security appears not to apply to pregnant women, especially if they are African American or poor.

As many have noted, these coercive interventions are premised on assumptions of maternal-fetal conflict, marked by divergence rather than alignment of maternal and fetal interests (Jos, Marshall, and Perlmutter 1995, 120; Nelson and Marshall 1998). As such, they also contravene another of Powers and Faden's dimensions of well-being—attachment (see, e.g., ACOG 2005). Indeed, they presume that the most intimate of attachments, namely gestation, is paradigmatically adversarial. Even when coercive legal intervention is not involved, negative experiences during childbearing, such as diminishment of women's epistemic authority and blaming and shaming women for perceived violations of risk-managing expectations, can strain connectedness to the fetus or neonate as well as others. In a series of in-depth interviews with Swedish women, Forssén found that such experiences were forcefully alienating for many of the women she interviewed, who experienced over decades "feelings of failure as mothers, of guilt, and of shame, which influenced their self-esteem and their future childbearing. This might also have influenced their attitude to seeking health care" (Forssén 2012, 1543). Beck's metaethnography of qualitative studies of traumatic birth notes that women may experience as traumatic births that clinicians view as routine and normal. She describes similar experiences to those highlighted by Forssén: "Women felt abandoned, stripped of their dignity, and not cared for as an individual who deserved to be treated with respect. Obstetric staff neglected to communicate with mothers. Women often felt invisible" (Beck 2011, 304). Beck notes that such traumatic birth experiences can negatively affect the women's relationships with their children as well as maternal-fetal bonding in subsequent pregnancies (Beck 2011, 306–8). Long-term psychological consequences of childbearing experiences may affect a host of alliances—ranging from intimate bonds with partners and children to relationships with care providers.

Another of Powers and Faden's core dimensions of well-being is reasoning. They focus on the development of intellectual and practical reasoning abilities that promote well-being. We can point to no special threat to the development of women's reasoning capacities as a result of pregnancy. However, Powers and Faden acknowledge that the social justice concern about reasoning extends to cultural norms about epistemic authority. They note that "such authorities may or may not be deserving of their trusted status, and their beliefs can be false, distorting, or self-serving, such as when they reinforce beliefs about ethnic or gender differences, undervalue the epistemic credibility of some groups, or exaggerate the epistemic credibility of those in dominant institutions and positions of cultural authority" (Powers and Faden 2006, 22).

State institutions that enforce coercive interventions against pregnant women without compelling evidence of harm to fetuses constitute illegitimate, untrustworthy epistemic authorities. Others have argued that the medicalization of pregnancy and childbirth elevates the epistemic authority of health professionals over that of pregnant women, although failure to respect women's informed decisions to embrace rather than eschew technology in birth suggests that an array of approaches to maternity care can entail challenges to women's epistemic authority. Regan and Liaschenko found that the degree to which nurses acknowledged the epistemic authority of pregnant women affected those nurses' views about risk in the birthing context and "influenced the use of technologies to augment, manage or expedite birth" (Regan and Liaschenko 2007, 617). It is also worth noting that the widespread exclusion of pregnant women from clinical research in an effort to protect fetuses undercuts the development of knowledge about pregnancy and so undermines women's ability to exercise their reasoning skills in this domain.

Our dominant perception and management of risk in pregnancy also undermines respect for pregnant women, another of Powers and Faden's core dimensions of well-being. Our tendencies to avoid intervention during pregnancy to shield fetuses from risk and to embrace intervention during childbirth to do everything possible for fetuses are not simply bad medicine or temporary burdens for women while pregnant. Rather, our norms regarding risk management reflect cultural assumptions about whose interests matter: women's interests (and sometimes their basic rights) are subordinated to concerns about avoidance of fetal risk, especially in situations involving coercive interventions. Forssén and others have demonstrated that even in less dramatic circumstances, the diminishment of women's epistemic authority involved in blaming and shaming women for perceived violations of risk-managing expectations undermines respect for women and their autonomy. Such violations of respect raise serious moral concerns regardless of their (in this case, very real) consequences. Forssén reports that "treatments in prenatal and maternity care were experienced [by women] as violations of their dignity and abuse, and posed lifelong threats to their health and well-being" (Forssén 2012, 1543; cf. Beck 2011). Moreover, the OGRRG authors point out that double standards inhere in our cultural judgments about risk/benefit trade-offs in pregnancy. For example, despite "inadequate data and plausible physiologic reasons for concern," women are assured that they need not abstain from intercourse during pregnancy—the "better safe than sorry" gospel is not preached to their male partners (Lyerly et al. 2009, 40). The point is not that the question of whether intercourse is safe should become a research priority. Rather, the issue is that, in the absence of adequate data to inform recommendations, gendered norms shape our culture's expectations concerning personal sacrifice as a means to manage risk in pregnancy.

Powers and Faden's final dimension of well-being is self-determination. To the extent that our norms concerning risk in pregnancy undergird coercive interventions, these norms clearly violate women's self-determination. However, even the mundane enactment of these norms infringes upon women's self-determination. The norm of purity inherent in the meticulous avoidance of anything that might risk harm to fetuses during pregnancy, along with the norm of control inherent in the vigorous embrace of intervention during birth, culturally compel women to sacrifice their own interests in an effort to protect their fetuses. The cultural pressure to comply with these norms is often so intense, the guilt over the prospect of being a "bad mother" so distressing, the scrutiny of women's behavior so intrusive, that is quite fitting to speak here of cultural compulsion. It is ironic, indeed, that pregnant women are simultaneously the object of penetrating surveillance and nearly invisible as concern with the fetus obstructs women's interests from view.

Thus, our perception and management of risk during pregnancy pose a threat to each of the core dimensions of well-being identified by Powers and Faden. These cultural norms are harmful both because they often result in worse outcomes for women and children and because they reflect and reify sexist assumptions. We often look to medical experts to identify and advise about risks, but the judgments of experts too often either lack grounding in data or ignore the paucity of available data, at the same time that they minimize the epistemic authority of pregnant women. Women are subjected to intense pressure to safeguard their fetuses, although the lack of research findings undermines their ability to make reasonable judgments about how to manage risks. Our society strives to avoid risks to fetuses and newborns, largely ignoring costs to pregnant women, and instead holds them primarily responsible for the safety of their fetuses and newborns. And all too frequently it employs arrests, detentions, and forced coercive interventions to enforce these cultural norms, despite the lack of justifying evidence. In short, these norms raise profound concerns about social justice. These injustices include inequities in the distribution of risks and benefits in this context—a very standard account of (in)justice. But the recognition of these inequities fails to fully capture the injustices involved in this context. An adequate account of justice must include but move beyond concerns regarding distribution, attend to culture (and so bring in the multidisciplinary expertise needed to do so), highlight domination and oppression as injustices, and confront overlapping, intertwined systemic forces creating structural inequalities—or, as Paul Farmer and his colleagues name them, structural violence (Farmer et al. 2006).

Our culture's conception of risk in pregnancy is sorely in need of transformation. Some have contended that new data emerging about fetal origins of adult disease ("fetal origins research") provides grounding for such a revisionist agenda. We will examine this claim below.

FETAL ORIGINS RESEARCH: TRANSFORMING
CONCEPTIONS OF RISK IN PREGNANCY?

In 2010, the journalist Annie Murphy Paul's book *Origins: How the Nine Months Before Birth Shape the Rest of Our Lives* caught the attention of the public and media. The book attends to what has come to be known as "fetal origins research"—a body of work aimed at understanding the impact of life before birth on long-term health and well-being, such as implications for incidence of heart disease, obesity, and mental illness in adulthood. The book aims to provide an introductory survey of fetal origins research that is accessible to a general, nonspecialist audience. Paul infuses her presentation of fetal origins research with personal musings on her experience of her own pregnancy.

Paul traces the beginnings of fetal origins research to the work of the British physician David Barker, who investigated why the highest rates of heart disease in England and Wales were found among those countries' poorest regions. His research demonstrated a correlation between low birth weight and heart disease in middle age. The finding—which Paul emphasizes has been amply replicated—established the influence of the prenatal "environment" on long-term health prospects, stunning many who attributed health risks to a combination of genetics and lifestyle factors (Paul 2010a, 24–28).

Paul discusses a number of other findings in fetal origins research, including incidence of PTSD in children whose mothers experienced trauma during pregnancy; links between stress experienced by pregnant women and premature delivery, low birth weight, and risks of mental illness in offspring; the effects of pregnant women's environmental exposures on their developing fetuses; links between depression and anxiety in pregnant women and emotional and behavioral health concerns in their children; and correlations between pregnant women's illness with pandemic influenza in 1918 and their children's educational attainment, income, socioeconomic status, disabilities, and height (Paul 2010a). Paul describes fetal origins research in general as demonstrating "that the lifestyle that influences the development of disease is often not only the one we follow as adults, but the one our mothers practiced when they were pregnant with us as well" (Paul 2010a, 8). She recognizes that this research risks being "cast as one long ringing alarm bell" (Paul 2010a, 9), warning pregnant women about the multitude of harms they pose to their fetuses, and acknowledges that fetal origins research appears to heighten the strength of our culture's expectations of pregnant women's intensive vigilance and self-sacrifice to safeguard their fetuses.

Yet Paul argues that despite these appearances, fetal origins research holds the power to transform our conception of risk in pregnancy. The research is not "full of dire warnings," but rather full of "hope," focused on the positive contributions that pregnant women can make to the health and well-being of their children (Paul 2010b, 52; cf. Paul 2010a, 9). She illustrates the point with common exhortations about pregnant women's diets, attending to issues concerning pregnant women's diets a great deal in the book. (She discusses them in seven of nine chapters.) She describes the positive approach that can be taken regarding the importance of healthy diet during pregnancy as "joyous affirmation, not anxious rejection or grim self-denial" (Paul 2010a, 37). Indeed, she contends, "'I'm doing it for my baby' is often uttered with a sigh of resignation, but it could just as easily be a slogan of liberation . . . I'm doing it for my baby!" (Paul 2010a, 38).

Paul talks repeatedly about revelations concerning the positive impact that pregnant women's choices can have on the children they birth. This, she contends, is the transformative power of fetal origins research. Pregnant women no longer need to worry about the harmful impact they may have on their fetuses. Instead, they can celebrate the positive contributions that their lifestyle choices can make to the health and well-being of their children.

This positive spin may be a psychological balm for some pregnant women, but it is hardly a revolution in our cultural conception of risk in pregnancy. Paul's central message about the vital importance of pregnant women's "lifestyle choices" does nothing to undermine the cultural norms inherent in the dominant model of risk in pregnancy. Pregnant women continue to be exhorted to "chase virtue" (Dederer 2010, 19), but to do so as "joyous affirmation, not anxious rejection or grim self-denial" (Paul 2010a, 37). Indeed, the expectation that pregnant women be joyous about their pursuit of virtue may simply add to the oppressive nature of the conception of risk.

The cultural uptake of Paul's work reveals that it does more to perpetuate the dominant model of risk in pregnancy than to spark a revolution against it. Reviews of the book note its importance as follows: "Focusing on how to minimize harm and maximize benefit during the nine months before birth, Paul's thought-provoking text reveals that this pivotal period may be even more significant and far-reaching than ever imagined" (*Publisher's Weekly* 2010). In the *New York Times Book Review*, Groopman relates the significance of the book to his own life: he confesses that after the birth of each of his children, he and his wife "breathed a deep sigh of relief." He affirms that they had been "meticulous in following our obstetrician's advice," but worried until each child was born healthy, at which point they felt they "had successfully skirted the perils of pregnancy." But, he notes, Paul's account of fetal origins research reveals that such a sense of relief may be premature, as "we do not put fetal life so readily behind us" (Groopman 2010, 1). Blog posts about the book echo these themes (see, e.g., Kirshenbaum 2010; cf. Slothers 2010). Fetal origins research is thus viewed as demonstrating that pregnant women's lifestyle choices are more important than ever before appreciated. It is not surprising, then, that Paul's account of the research has been described as "a useful, if not essential, addition to any pregnancy library" (Springen 2010), a "must read for anyone pregnant or planning on getting pregnant" (Jones 2010).

THE POSSIBILITY OF GENUINE TRANSFORMATION

Far from providing reform of the dominant conception of risk in pregnancy, central themes in the public conversation on fetal origins research serve, rather, to perpetuate it and its sexist norms. Fetal origins research does nevertheless contain the seeds of a more appropriate conception of risk in pregnancy. A transformed conception of risk will find its basis neither in more positive spins on women's lifestyle choices during pregnancy, nor in the mere infusion of data into the conversation about risk, since, as we have seen, data interpreted through the lens of the dominant conception of risk cannot ground transformation.

Indeed, at the heart of the issue concerning the public uptake of fetal origins research is the myopic focus on lifestyle as a determinant of health. As seen throughout the discussion above, Paul and others identify women's lifestyle choices as both critical to human health and the central substrate for translating data from fetal origins research into improving the health of future generations. Yet recall that Paul traces the beginnings of fetal origins research to the work of the British physician David Barker, who investigated why the highest rates of heart disease in England and Wales were found among those countries' poorest regions. His research demonstrated a correlation between impoverished women's nutritional status, low-birth-weight babies, and heart disease in middle age. Indeed, much of the research about nutrition discussed in *Origins* involves impoverished populations and/or famine events. The research documents long-term health effects of such nutritional disadvantage for those who were so affected in utero, including increased rates of obesity, diabetes, heart disease, and mental health concerns. While the research relates directly to often dire social circumstances, Paul focuses instead on maternal food choices, even seeking out the help of a nutritionist at Harvard Medical School to "help me with my grocery list" (Paul 2010a, 39).

Of course not everyone has access to a nutritionist—much less one from a top medical school. Even if they did, we know that access to nutritional food is far from a given, particularly among groups where perinatal and other health outcomes are the worst. The media has brought attention to these problems of late, highlighting a number of poor communities whose only source of food is a local convenience store where fresh produce is a rarity and high-calorie, high-sodium, sugar-laden packaged and processed foods are the only real options (Gonzalez 2008). This is among the messages advanced by another growing body of literature addressing broad factors affecting human health—the "social determinants of health"—and highlights the idea that health is not simply a matter of lifestyle choice, but a product of social structures beyond any individual's control. As Irwin et al. put it, "Modifiable risk factors for chronic illness—such as poor diets, alcohol abuse, and smoking—are often seen as individual 'lifestyle choices.' But such choices are conditioned by patterns of material deprivation and social exclusion. Health-compromising behaviors are disproportionately concentrated in socially disadvantaged groups, both in developed and in developing countries. Effective policy to tackle health challenges must address the underlying social conditions that make people who are disadvantaged more vulnerable" (Irwin et al. 2006). As Braveman explains (chapter 1, this volume), approaches to defining and measuring health differences among social groups that genuinely capture the connections to social disadvantage and social justice can lead to such effective policy approaches and social change.

Yet somehow the tenets of social determinants of health research have not substantively penetrated public discussions of fetal origins research, even now that women's bodies are perceived as "one of the most influential environments on Earth" (Blum, Review of *Origins*, in Paul 2010a, ii). Indeed, despite her focus—and, as we've seen, the focus of the public conversation about her work—on women's lifestyle choices, much of the research that Paul discusses relates *directly* to social determinants of health. In addition to the work regarding nutritional disadvantage noted above, Paul also presents research concerning the correlation between pregnant women's exposure to air pollution (vehicle exhaust, factory emissions) and premature birth, low birth weight, heart defects, increased cancer risk, and cognitive delays in their offspring. She describes the connection between pregnant women's experience of violent social conditions and increased risk of schizophrenia in their sons and daughters.

In the context of her discussion of that quintessential "lifestyle choice" concerning use of alcohol in pregnancy, she notes, without commentary, that "even among women who drink heavily during pregnancy . . . not all will deliver a baby with fetal alcohol syndrome. In fact, one study reports, while 71 percent of the babies of poor alcoholic women had FAS, that was true of only 4.5 percent of the infants of more affluent alcoholics, probably because of their more nutritious diets" (Paul 2010a, 93). Our individualistic American culture tends to focus on lifestyle choices and matters of personal responsibility and ignore the critical importance of social factors (i.e., issues of collective responsibility).

It is interesting how forcefully and exclusively the focus on lifestyle is manifest in discussions of fetal origins research in particular, though perhaps not surprising when we consider that it is *mothers* (or mothers-to-be) whose lifestyle is being discussed. After all, if they are to be thought of as "good," pregnant women are expected to subordinate their interests to efforts to reduce or eliminate fetal risk. In fact, much of the language around fetal origins research—referencing women and their bodies as "influential environments" (Blum, review of *Origins*, in Paul 2010a, ii)—suggests that it is not just women's interests that are subsumed by efforts to reduce fetal risk, but women themselves. Again, Mary Douglas sheds light on these cultural phenomena. She contends that one of the functions of "risk" as a forensic notion is to support an individualistic culture:

> Danger in the context of taboo is used in a rhetoric of accusation and
> retribution that ties the individual tightly into community bonds
> and scores on his mind the invisible fences and paths by which the
> community coordinates its life in common. By grace of their concern
> for these lines and boundaries, they can share their territory and
> muster resources to protect it. The modern risk concept, parsed now
> as danger, is invoked to protect individuals against the encroachments
> of others. It is part of the system of thought that upholds . . . individ-
> ualist culture. . . . The dialogue about risk plays the role equivalent to
> taboo or sin, but the slope is tilted in the reverse direction, away from
> protecting the community and in favor of protecting the individual.
> (Douglas 1990, 7)

Moreover, Douglas maintains that individualistic cultures commonly render the oppressed invisible: "Each culture discriminates, but the hierarchical one does it overtly, handing out group badges of difference; the individualist one does it covertly, by ignoring the powerless" (Douglas 1990, 14).

Braveman's chapter in this volume provides profound insights on these issues. She explains that while there is a "massive" amount of evidence supporting the significance of such health disparities, debates remain about how to best define and measure differences in health outcomes. Some approaches embrace the cultural commitment to individualism and study health differences in isolation from their connections to social disadvantage. She powerfully argues that only approaches that explicitly examine the connection between differences in health outcomes and social disadvantage can reveal the social justice issues that must be addressed and so motivate fitting social and policy approaches to ameliorate these issues.

TOWARD A MORE JUST CONCEPTION OF RISK IN PREGNANCY

Taking seriously evidence of the long-term significance of the social determinants of health has the potential to radically shift our cultural perspective of conceptions of risk in pregnancy. It will also promote justice. Powers and Faden argue that "inequalities in the health of children are among the most morally urgent for public health to address" and thus should be recognized to be a priority for social justice (Powers and Faden 2006, 94). They discuss what they call the "life course" approach to understanding health: "Some events that occur during critical developmental periods produce adverse effects on health over the course of a life time. Poor nutrition and environmental exposures before and soon after birth can produce permanent and sometimes irreversible damage to organs, tissues, and body systems that can predispose people to such conditions as cardiovascular disease, developmental disabilities, noninsulin-dependent diabetes, and hypertension" (Powers and Faden 2006, 77). Powers and Faden argue that this life course approach to health—which critically includes fetal origins research as we have been discussing it—has significant implications for social justice for children (Powers and Faden 2006, 77–78).

A social justice concern about women dovetails with that regarding children in this context. A shift in cultural perspective from an obsession with women's lifestyle choices to a focus on social determinants of health and their attendant health disparities would provide a promising foundation for reform of our sexist, puritanical, and controlling conceptions of risk and motherhood. Such a shift grounds a move away from unattainable expectations that pregnant women completely subordinate their well-being in an attempt to avoid any risk (however small or hypothetical) to their fetuses, to a dialogue about what social changes need to occur to appropriately support pregnant women and provide for the well-being of the children they will bear. We do not intend to create a false dichotomy here; we recognize that both social determinants and lifestyle choices matter for a responsible approach to risk management in pregnancy. But our current cultural conception of risk and its management during pregnancy focuses almost exclusively on lifestyle choices—that is to say, most if not all risks are treated as though they are attributable to women's lifestyle choices, and so women are held responsible for the avoidance of risks, when in reality many important risks relate to social determinants of health and are thus beyond women's control.

Recognition of the significance of social determinants of health thus plays a critical role in this transformation of our cultural conception of risk in pregnancy. Other changes will also be needed. For example, as we have seen, research concerning pregnancy is critical, so that judgments about how to manage risk can be informed by science rather than grounded in sexist norms. Of course, research must be approached responsibly. It is beyond the scope of this analysis to propose an approach to such research; others have addressed the issue more centrally (Lyerly, Little, and Faden 2008). However, as we have also seen, research will not suffice to prompt cultural change, since it will be interpreted through the cultural norms concerning pregnancy. Those norms must be addressed head-on. Women should be accorded respect, not rendered invisible while subordinated to concerns about their fetuses and subjected to unjust treatment to enforce those concerns. As the OGRRG explains in reference to the clinical context, "It is the physician's obligation not to eliminate risk, but to help patients weigh risk, benefit, and potential harm, informed by best scientific evidence and guided by a patient-centered ethic" (Lyerly et al. 2007, 982). In addition, the moral centrality of relationships should be recognized, to ground acknowledgment of the pregnant woman's primacy as the advocate for her and her fetus's well-being and undermine all-too-typical adversarial constructions of maternal-fetal relations. In general, the oppression of women must be recognized and resisted.

A good deal of work has yet to be done to describe a just conception of risk in pregnancy. Young insists that "only changing the cultural habits themselves will change the oppressions they produce and reinforce. . . . This is cultural revolution" (Young 1990, 152). Eva Feder Kittay also recognizes the critical importance of such revolution in her chapter in this volume, concluding that fundamental cultural changes are needed for the health-care system to respect autonomy and promote good care. Yet as Douglas recognizes, we tend to be blind to our own cultural assumptions and habits: "A special effort of sophistication is necessary to see our own culture" (Douglas 1990, 4). We hope that the analysis we offer here helps to bring into focus matters of culture that will help to support cultural revolution and thereby promote social justice. Of course, academic work alone will not promote social justice—such is the nature of justice.

NOTE

1. In his fascinating chapter in this volume, Paul Brodwin offers commentary on our chapters' similarities and differences in methodological approach, particularly as they attend to questions of textual interpretation, or hermeneutics. Specifically, Brodwin appeals to Paul Ricoeur's analytical framework contrasting what he calls the hermeneutics of faith and the hermeneutics of suspicion. Brodwin maintains that his analysis proceeds on the former, while ours primarily relies on the latter. He intends to imply not a criticism, but a distinction in approach (personal communication, June 11, 2015). We agree that our analysis aims at uncovering deeper truths, consistent with his characterization of a hermeneutic of suspicion. However, we would offer that the contrast Brodwin makes is not so stark. Indeed, research that figures centrally in support of our analysis uses the interpretive strategy of a hermeneutic of faith to explore the views and experiences of women about pregnancy, taking seriously the role of women interviewed as experts in their own right (see, e.g., Forssén 2012; Beck 2011; Namey and Lyerly 2010).

REFERENCES

ACOG (American College of Obstetricians and Gynecologists). 2005. "Maternal Decision Making, Ethics, and the Law. ACOG Committee Opinion No. 321." *Obstetrics and Gynecology* 106: 1127–37.

———. 2006. "ACOG Practice Bulletin No. 71: Episiotomy." *Obstetrics and Gynecology* 107: 956–62.

ACOG (American College of Obstetricians and Gynecologists) and SMFM (Society for Maternal Fetal Medicine). 2014. "Obstetric Care Consensus No. 1: Safe Prevention of the Primary Cesarean Delivery." *Obstetrics and Gynecology* 123 (3): 693–711. doi:10.1097/01.AOG.0000444441.04111.1d.

AP (Associated Press). 2014. "Guidelines to Reduce C-Section Rates Urge Waiting." http://www.npr.org/templates/story/story.php?storyId=279747276. Accessed 19 February 2014.

Barker, Kristin K. 1998. "A Ship upon a Stormy Sea: The Medicalization of Pregnancy." *Social Science and Medicine* 47 (8): 1067–76.

Beck, Cheryl Tatano. 2011. "A Metaethnography of Traumatic Childbirth and Its Aftermath: Amplifying Causal Looping." *Qualitative Health Research* 21 (3): 301–11.

Chambers, Christina D., Janine E. Polifka, and Jan M. Friedman. 2008. "Drug Safety in Pregnant Women and Their Babies: Ignorance Not Bliss." *Clinical Pharmacology and Therapeutics* 83 (1): 181–83.

DeBruin, Debra. 1994. "Justice and the Inclusion of Women in Clinical Studies: A Conceptual Framework." In *Women and Health Research: Ethical and Legal Issues of Including Women in Clinical Studies,* edited by Anna C. Mastroianni, Ruth Faden, and Daniel Federman, 2:127–50. Washington, DC: National Academy Press.

Dederer, Claire. 2010. *My Life in Twenty-Three Yoga Poses.* New York: Farrar, Straus and Giroux.

Douglas, Mary. 1966. *Purity and Danger.* New York: Routledge.

———. 1990. "Risk as a Forensic Resource." *Daedalus* 119 (4): 1–16.

Ehrenreich, Barbara, and Deirdre English. 2011. *Complaints and Disorders: The Sexual Politics of Sickness.* 2nd ed. New York: Feminist Press at CUNY.

Farmer, Paul E., Bruce Nizeye, Sara Stulac, and Salmaan Keshavjee. 2006. "Structural Violence and Clinical Medicine." *PLoS Medicine* 3 (10): e449.

Forssén, Annika S. K. 2012. "Lifelong Significance of Disempowering Experiences in Prenatal and Maternity Care Interviews with Elderly Swedish Women." *Qualitative Health Research* 22 (11): 1535–46.

Frye, Marilyn. 1983. *The Politics of Reality: Essays in Feminist Theory.* Trumansburg, NY: Crossing Press.

Gonzalez, David. 2008. "The Lost Supermarket: A Breed in Need of Replenishment." *New York Times,* May 5, New York Region section. http://www.nytimes .com/2008/05/05/nyregion/05citywide.html. Accessed 26 August 2015.

Groopman, Jerome. 2010. "Book Review: *Origins.*" *New York Times,* September 30, Books section. http://www.nytimes.com/2010/10/03/books/review/Groopman-t.html. Accessed 26 August 2015.

Irwin, Alec, Nicole Valentine, Chris Brown, Rene Loewenson, Orielle Solar, Hilary Brown, Theadora Koller, and Jeanette Vega. 2006. "The Commission on Social Determinants of Health: Tackling the Social Roots of Health Inequities." *PLoS Medicine* 3 (6): e106. doi:10.1371/journal.pmed.0030106.

Jones, K. 2010. "Must Read for Anyone Pregnant or Planning on Getting Pregnant." Reader review of Paul 2010a. October 3. http://www.amazon.com/Origins-Months-Before-Birth-Shape/dp/B004Z4M1A4/ref=sr_1_1?ie=UTF8&qid=1376671211&sr=8-1&keywords=origins+how+the+nine+months+before+birth+shape+the+rest+of+our +lives. Accessed 16 August 2013.

Jos, Philip H., Mary Faith Marshall, and Martin Perlmutter. 1995. "The Charleston Policy on Cocaine Use during Pregnancy: A Cautionary Tale." *Journal of Law, Medicine and Ethics* 23 (2): 120–28.

Kirshenbaum, Sheril. 2010. "Discussion: *Origins: How the Nine Months before Birth Shape the Rest of Our Lives.*" *The Intersection.* October 5. http://blogs.discovermagazine.com/ intersection/2010/10/05/origins-how-the-nine-months-before-birth-shape-the-rest-of-our-lives/. Accessed 16 August 2013.

Klein, Michael C., Murray W. Enkin, Andrew Kotaska, and Sara G. Shields. 2007. "The Patient-Centered (R) Evolution." *Birth* 34 (3): 264–66.

Kukla, Rebecca, Miriam Kuppermann, Margaret Little, Anne Drapkin Lyerly, Lisa M. Mitchell, Elizabeth M. Armstrong, and Lisa Harris. 2009. "Finding Autonomy in Birth." *Bioethics* 23 (1): 1–8.

Little, Margaret Olivia. 2011. "Treating Important Medical Conditions during Pregnancy." In *Enrolling Pregnant Women: Issues in Clinical Research*, 23–26. Bethesda: National Institutes of Health.

Lupton, Deborah. 1999. *Risk*. New York: Routledge.

Lyerly, Anne Drapkin, Margaret Olivia Little, and Ruth Faden. 2008. "The Second Wave: toward Responsible Inclusion of Pregnant Women in Research." *International Journal of Feminist Approaches to Bioethics* 1 (2): 5–22.

Lyerly, Anne Drapkin, Lisa M. Mitchell, Elizabeth M. Armstrong, Lisa H. Harris, Rebecca Kukla, Miriam Kuppermann, and Margaret Olivia Little. 2007. "Risks, Values, and Decision Making Surrounding Pregnancy." *Obstetrics and Gynecology* 109 (4): 979–84.

———. 2009. "Risk and the Pregnant Body." *Hastings Center Report* 39 (6): 34–42.

Mastroianni, Anna C., Ruth Faden, and Daniel Federman, eds. 1994. *Women and Health Research: Ethical and Legal Issues of Including Women in Clinical Studies*. Vol. 1. Washington, DC: National Academy Press.

Namey, Emily E., and Anne Drapkin Lyerly. 2010. "The Meaning of 'Control' for Childbearing Women in the U.S." *Social Science and Medicine* 71 (4): 769–76.

Nelson, Lawrence J., and Mary Faith Marshall. 1998. *An Ethical and Legal Policy Analysis of State Compelled Loss of Liberty as an Intervention to Manage the Harm of Prenatal Substance Abuse and Drug Addiction*. Research Program Report. Robert Wood Johnson Foundation Substance Abuse Policy.

NIH ORWH (National Institutes of Health Office of Research on Women's Health). 2013. *Background: Inclusion of Women and Minorities in Clinical Research*. May 13. http://orwh.od.nih.gov/research/inclusion/background.asp. Accessed 12 August 2013.

"Nonfiction Reviews: Review of *Origins*." 2010. *Publisher's Weekly*, August 2.

Paltrow, Lynn M., and Jeanne Flavin. 2013. "Arrests of and Forced Interventions on Pregnant Women in the United States, 1973–2005: Implications for Women's Legal Status and Public Health." *Journal of Health Politics, Policy and Law* 38 (2): 299–343.

Paul, Annie Murphy. 2010a. *Origins: How the Nine Months before Birth Shape the Rest of Our Lives*. New York: Free Press.

———. 2010b. "How the First Nine Months Shape the Rest of Your Life." *Time Magazine*, September 22. http://www.aimsusa.org/library/Time%20-%20How%20the%20First%209%20Months%20Shape%20the%20Rest%20of%20Your%20Life.pdf. Accessed 26 September 2013.

Powers, Madison, and Ruth Faden. 2006. *Social Justice: The Moral Foundations of Public Health and Health Policy*. Issues in Biomedical Ethics. New York: Oxford University Press.

Regan, Mary, and Joan Liaschenko. 2007. "In the Mind of the Beholder Hypothesized
     Effect of Intrapartum Nurses' Cognitive Frames of Childbirth Cesarean Section Rates."
     Qualitative Health Research 17 (5): 612–24.
Slothers, M. 2010. Comment on "A Womb with a View." December 28. *Motherlode:
     Adventures in Parenting* (blog). *New York Times*, September 27, 2010. http://parenting
     .blogs.nytimes.com/2010/09/27/a-womb-with-a-view/. Accessed August 16, 2013.
Springen, Karen. 2010. "Review of *Origins*." *Booklist*.
     September 1. http://www.booklistonline.com/ProductInfo.
     aspx?pid=4269402&AspxAutoDetectCookieSupport=1. Accessed 16 August 2013.
Young, Iris Marion. 1990. *Justice and the Politics of Difference*. Princeton, NJ: Princeton
     University Press.

7

Justice, Respect, and Recognition in Mental Health Services

Theoretical and Testimonial Accounts

Paul Brodwin

ABSTRACT

This chapter raises a key question for the interdisciplinary study of health and justice: is dialogue possible between theoretical models and first-person testimony about the harms caused by injustice? To consider this question, I examine the claim that disrespect is a form of injustice. The philosopher Stephen Darwall and social theorist Axel Honneth conceptually elucidate the links between justice, respect, and recognition. Their normative arguments offer a high-order conceptual framework for recognizing people's equal worth as human beings. This chapter compares their abstract frameworks with a landmark autobiography by a founder of the psychiatric survivor movement. The search for commensurability between these texts exposes the precise difference between experience-far and experience-near genres of ethical expression. This chapter adopts a similar approach as DeBruin et al. (this volume) in examining popular cultural discourses in light of formal theory. Both chapters take seriously the lay narratives and forms of ethical argumentation that circulate outside the academy. Both envision a plural ethics of justice and health that acknowledges how ordinary people interpret and respond to institutionalized oppression.

INTRODUCTION

Posing questions about justice and inequality in the realm of mental health services opens up two very different lines of analysis. A long tradition of social epidemiology demonstrates the disproportionate burden of mental illness associated with poverty, migration, and membership in stigmatized ethnic and racial groups (Ngui et al. 2013; Kessler et al. 2012; Martins et al. 2012).[1] This approach begins with objective epidemiological data and then launches a normative argument about the psychiatric sequelae of social injustice. The inequalities documented in this literature arise from large-scale social arrangements, including class hierarchy, global imbalances of resources and opportunities, and symbolic violence against historically marginalized populations. The increased prevalence of psychiatric disorders and the limited access to treatment are unjust because they afflict people already inhabiting the lower rungs of inegalitarian societies. This line of analysis makes an implicit promise to health planners and policy makers. Explaining how social hierarchies and cultural discrimination overproduce psychiatric symptoms is clinically useful. This effort and the knowledge it supplies can inform new types of outreach and more finely targeted interventions with the ultimate goal of lessening the unequal burden of illness (Eaton 2012).

A second line of analysis frames injustice not as the unfair burden of risk, but as the denial of full legal and civil rights. This second approach focuses on the denigration and abuse suffered by people simply because they are recipients of mental health services (Callard et al. 2012). It begins with a normative perspective about rights and fundamental freedoms that people often lose when they are diagnosed, hospitalized, or placed under formal and informal clinical surveillance. Unlike the first line of analysis, this approach does not focus on large-scale social inequities or the interaction of psychiatric illness with other factors (such as migration or poverty). Instead of a broad population-based coverage, it investigates more narrowly the very apparatus of psychiatric treatment. It interrogates the legitimacy of coercion, the rationale for treating people against their will, and whether some types of interventions are incompatible with patient rights (Dennis and Monahan 1996; Kallert, Mezzich, and Monahan 2011). It frames injustice as the imbalance of power between clinicians and patients that is arguably built into the ideology and clinical routines of contemporary psychiatry (Peele and Chodoff 1999).

This chapter concerns the second line of analysis. It takes up debates about imposed treatment in the contemporary mental health system. It engages with the voice of ex-patients who claim that the system disrespects them and does not recognize their civil, legal, and human rights. The chapter thereby tries to broaden the discussion about social justice and health by introducing ideas from the philosophy of recognition and respect. Moreover, it draws a comparison between high-order conceptual approaches and the voice of people with lived experience of forced psychiatric treatment. The presentation tacks back and forth between theoretical models of respect from Stephen Darwall (1977) and Axel Honneth (1995), on the one hand, and the landmark autobiographical testimonial by Judi Chamberlin (1978), on the other. The theoretical models, of course, are pitched at a general level and never mention the particular conflicts and ethical problems associated with mental health services. The autobiography, by contrast, is drenched in the details of the author's experience as a patient and activist. The chapter enacts a dialogue between these divergent positions about respect, recognition, and justice.

THE CHALLENGE OF PERSONAL TESTIMONIES ABOUT INJUSTICE

Judi Chamberlin's *On Our Own: Patient-Controlled Alternatives to the Mental Health System* (1978) is a foundational text of the U.S. psychiatric survivors' movement. The book harshly criticizes the contemporary U.S. mental health system, and it centrally concerns justice, respect, and society's obligation toward people struggling with extreme personal crises. The author, however, does not write from the position of a professional academic. The warrant and rhetorical strategy of her truth claims are autobiographical, and they reflect her personal experience with forced hospitalization and mandated medication. Her strongest demand is couched as an activist political project. And her ethical vision comes through testimony: a textual witness to the subjective experience of disrespect and the scars it leaves on psyche and body.

Listening to the anguished voices in this text raises a key question for interdisciplinary conversations about justice and health care. Is a coherent conversation even possible between moral philosophers, on the one hand, and people who base their authority upon the personal experience of suffering, on the other? What are the conditions of possibility for dialogue, or at least mutual intelligibility, between such divergent frameworks about social justice? In this chapter, the question turns on the precise difference between two subject positions—the psychiatric survivor and the academic theorist—and their respective arguments about respect and recognition.

One way to parse this difference would contrast the immediacy of testimony to the distance and formality of philosophical frameworks. Some medical anthropologists would label the first "moral talk" and the latter "ethics" (Brodwin 2008; Kleinman 1999; Hoffmaster 1992). "Moral talk" refers to the untheorized normative claims made by ordinary people on the basis of their immediate, personal, and embodied experience. Moral talk emerges in the informal rush of everyday life and gets expressed idiomatically. Even when written down and published as narrative or polemic, it bears the marks of its origins. Ethics, by contrast, gets expressed in formal systematic language and is bound by disciplinary rules of evidence and proof. Moral talk enables mutual understanding in one's own circle of intimates, friends, and fellow sufferers. Ethics is the preferred medium of communication among academics, policy makers, and other acknowledged experts. Precisely because moral talk is so raw and spontaneous, anthropologists tend to regard it as a surer guide to the local experience of injustice and inequality (Brodwin 2013). Stories of harm that one has personally suffered are anchored in particular events and places. Such subjective reports are unfiltered by disciplinary canons, and for that reason, personal narratives about directly experienced harms are often held up as uncontestable reflections of the real (Scott 1994).

The authors of first-person testimonies of injustice in the mental health system extend this argument about the unique legitimacy of their voice. For them, personal testimony is not just epistemologically more accurate; it is politically more privileged. For example, Judi Chamberlin champions the liberating effect of developing an account of one's suffering independent of expert categories (Chamberlin 1978, 63). She believes that articulating one's direct experience of injustice and sharing these accounts publicly is counterhegemonic. Telling a personal story in one's own words, she asserts, resists a frequent assumption among mental health clinicians that patients are untrustworthy chroniclers of their lives and that their perspectives are merely symptomatic of the illness.

The braiding of personal veracity and political efficacy has persisted over the decades, despite numerous changes in the makeup and agenda of the psychiatric survivor movement (McLean 2000, 2009). David Oaks, director of the advocacy group Mind Freedom International, lived through five psychiatric hospitalizations before becoming an organizer and activist. Many years later, he collaborated with national and international ex-patient organizations to write the Declaration of Dresden against Coerced Psychiatric Treatment. This formal and carefully crafted political document is obviously not an instance of moral talk. But it draws its warrant for authority, once again, from the authors' personal experience: "Our organizations are in a unique position to speak on this issue because we have experienced forced psychiatry and know the damage it has done to our lives. . . . We believe that people who have been coerced by psychiatry have a moral clam to make the definitive statement concerning such coercion" (Oaks 2011, 197).

Taking a similar position, British activists who identify as "self-harmers" (who engage in nonfatal self-mutilation and self-poisoning) regard personal testimony as a crucial political maneuver. Self-harm, according to this movement, is not a symptom or suicidal gesture, but an expression of inner hurt. To proclaim that personal and experiential truth in print or at public gatherings is a rhetorical *force majeure* that demands validation from the listener and corrects the imbalance of power between self-harmers and clinicians who would pathologize them (Cresswell 2005). For all these survivor-activists, testimony as such not only has greater validity than professional categories and concepts. It also advances their political struggle. By demanding to be taken seriously, the speakers stake a claim to full equality with mental health providers and push back against professional privilege and its potential for abuse.

At the extreme, survivor-activists claim exclusive authority for their testimonial voice. They argue that without the personal experience of hospitalization or forced treatment, other people (philosophers or bioethicists, for example) cannot truly understand the harms caused by such common features of psychiatric patienthood. This argument makes the strongest possible claim about the authenticity of experience, but it has a troubling implication. If people who have never been committed or forcibly medicated cannot truly understand the depth of survivors' suffering, then the possibility of dialogue between the two groups shrinks almost to zero. Nothing could bridge the irreconcilable positions of academic theorists and the psychiatric survivor community, even if both are deeply concerned with reforming today's mental health system (Estroff 2004). The general type of discussion inaugurated by this book would be hopelessly irrelevant, from the perspective of those who directly feel the sting of injustice.

THE SEARCH FOR COMMENSURABILITY

The present chapter steps back from that conclusion and tries to reopen a space for productive conversation. It sets the two subject positions—philosophical and testimonial—side by side and searches for hidden resonances and possible translations, even those unintended by the authors themselves. The search, however, requires a certain humility. Given the passion and rhetorical power of the survivors' testimonies, dialogue is not at all guaranteed. In the end, perhaps the two positions are truly incommensurable and cannot be productively compared without severely distorting the meaning of one or the other (Povinelli 2001). In cases of true incommensurability, comparison is an empty exercise with meager results. Holding two texts or worldviews side by side may point out chiefly their fundamental difference and mutual irrelevance. The conceptual mismatch would make further discussion futile.

To acknowledge that two approaches to social justice—one authorized by academic canons and the other by the evidence of experience—might be incommensurable yet nevertheless proceed to compare them demands a spirit of charity. To make an analogy to normal human conversation: it proceeds through an interpretive generosity, that is, the willingness of both parties to seek out and even create areas of shared relevance. Finding such areas can proceed in various ways. Most simply, each speaker accepts the other's voice as self-enclosed, and they search for point-to-point correlations between what each of them has said. The shared relevance, if it occurs at all, is a happy accident. More complexly but more productively, both speakers proceed by enlarging their horizons of understanding until they meet and overlap. This second framework, indebted to twentieth-century philosophical hermeneutics (Ricoeur 1981), insists that any human conversation is potentially a creative act. New spaces of shared understanding can emerge through the willingness to interpret what the other person says as a partial revelation of truth.

Trying to commensurate two kinds of texts is similarly a creative act. The act of interpretation leans forward into a new formulation of the various authors' main preoccupations. Taking suggestions already made by each author, the interpretation develops them in new directions in order to construct a workable shared discursive space. The task demands careful negotiation. The texts examined in this chapter use the same words in different ways. The authors rely on different warrants for their authority and their truth claims. They advance their arguments through different rhetorics and strategies of persuasion (Chandler, Davidson, and Harootunian 1994). The task of commensuration in such cases relies on the hope (but without guarantees) that we can align radically different texts, based on the intuition that they address similar human concerns.

That hope animates both this chapter and that of DeBruin and colleagues (same volume). Both chapters examine the distance between formal philosophical arguments about health and justice and the types of ethical reasoning that circulate outside the academy. Both chapters examine popular cultural discourses through a conceptual theoretical lens. At a finer level, however, the two chapters rest on different hermeneutic orientations. Paul Ricoeur (1970) clarifies the difference through his well-known contrast between the hermeneutics of faith and of suspicion. The interpretive strategy of faith aims at restoring the meaning of a text, narrative, or cultural symbol. It implies a willingness to listen as well as the assumption that producers of texts are legitimate experts in their own experience (Josselson 2004). The hermeneutics of suspicion aims at demystifying the text. It assumes that surface meanings hide deeper truths and that the producers of a text are likely caught up in self-deception and insufficient awareness of their own motives.

The present chapter follows the hermeneutics of faith. It accepts that the foundational text of the psychiatric survivor movement apprehends something true about the contemporary experience of people with severe mental illness. This chapter regards Chamberlin's analysis of the predicament of patienthood as plausible. Admittedly, her ethical claims are unsystematic and polemical, but they grow from her legitimate experience of harm. By contrast, the chapter by DeBruin et al. largely relies on the hermeneutics of suspicion. The authors delve into the broad cultural conversation about the morality of medical intervention during pregnancy and the ways it shapes women's subjective experience. But their argument then takes a more skeptical turn. They interpret lay conceptions of the risks of pregnancy as a mystified ideology that sustains an oppressive social order. Paradoxically, and despite women's goals, the lay discourse on risk often puts women and children in harm's way. The authors thus launch a normative critique of popular notions. In the end, they give interpretive priority to systematic philosophies of social justice over lay understandings. Taken together, these two chapters lay out divergent ways that ethical theory can engage with non- or pretheoretical forms of moral talk. Starting from the hermeneutics of faith, this chapter sheds new light on the landscape of interdisciplinary bioethics. In particular, it offers a promising strategy to negotiate between lay and expert frameworks about social justice and health.

The hermeneutics of faith, however, encounters a thorny problem when applied to testimonies of psychiatric survivors. Interpreting such texts requires careful handling of an explosive topic: the legitimacy of involuntary treatment. Debates surrounding the topic are already polarized, and they draw in people with starkly opposed political and personal interests. Testimonials such as

Chamberlin's book or the first-person accounts on websites such as MindFree-dom.org (an advocacy group for people with lived experience of forced hos-pitalization) are filled with stories of the denial of rights by abusive clinicians, imposed medications that incapacitate one's willpower, the bodily violations of electroconvulsive therapy (ECT), and other forms of coercion and humili-ation masquerading as care. Arguing forcefully from the opposite side, leading psychiatrists claim that about 50 percent of people with schizophrenia do not know they have an illness, and their poor insight is a major barrier to accepting and staying in treatment (Arango and Amador 2011). From this mainstream standpoint, schizophrenia (and, to a lesser extent, other illnesses with possi-ble psychotic features such as schizoaffective disorder, bipolar disorder, and major depressive disorder) distort people's subjective view of their own con-dition. Lack of insight makes people with schizophrenia uniquely ill-suited to speak the truth about their experience.

The debate also gets carried out in competing books written by psychi-atrists and aimed at a popular readership. Allying himself with self-help ad-vocates and psychiatric survivors, Peter Breggin writes that people treated against their will mainly learn "how to adjust to being bullied . . . and to be 'good patients' in order to avoid punishment and stay out of trouble" (Breggin 1991, 378). By contrast, the prominent psychiatrist E. Fuller Torrey endorses assisted treatment, including commitment and the threat of legal proceedings or incarceration to compel treatment, as legitimate options for people who re-fuse medication (Torrey 2001, 306). Torrey also considers the survivor move-ment as an impediment to better mental health services and Breggin's book as one of the fifteen worst ever written about schizophrenia (Torrey 2001, 427).

The shrill polarization is unfortunate. It threatens to drown out the more nuanced view that involuntary treatment is occasionally necessary while at the same time corrosive to people's dignity and their sense of personal effectiveness. According to the psychiatrist Ron Diamond, for example, court-ordered treat-ment indicates a failed relationship between patients and clinical staff. Potentially helpful in the short run to avoid danger and to start a medication regime, coer-cive relationships nevertheless undercut patients' ability to take more control of their lives (Diamond 1996, 61). Acknowledging the inherent ethical problems of commitment and its potential long-term antitherapeutic effects, Diamond urges clinicians to minimize this form of coercive treatment, in part by building long-term and respectful relationships (Diamond 1996, 68). The psychiatrist Tomer Levin (2001) makes a similar argument but in a very different genre. In his raw eyewitness account of physical coercion on an in-patient unit, he describes a woman crying uncontrollably after being placed in four-point restraints because of her hostile assaultive behavior. Looking at her on the ward, Levin had to remind himself that physical restraints have a therapeutic intent (to calm psychotic patients and facilitate a forced rest). But he also acknowledged the unintentional humiliation and degradation that they cause. In his sensitive narrative, he interprets physical restraints as both clinically effective and harmful to the woman's dignity. Significantly, neither interpretation rules out the other. Levin maintains a dual vision of the woman as both a patient (requiring treatment, even against her will) and a person (requiring respect).

Reading Chamberlin's book through the hermeneutics of faith requires a similar double perspective. She issues a strong call for respect, and readers can acknowledge it as a partial revelation of her true experience without needing to agree with all her critiques of biopsychiatry. To commensurate her experience-near account of the harm caused by the denial of respect with the experience-far accounts by moral philosophers necessarily moves beyond the polarized debates about involuntary treatment. This chapter mainly shows how personal narrative and theoretical arguments can, in fact, complement each other, but it also suggests a new approach to the problematic of coercion in mental health services. Illuminating the subjective and social dynamics of respect contributes a nuanced view of the ambivalent effect of psychiatric power in the lives of people under treatment (compare Brodwin and Velpry 2014).

THEORETICAL MODELS OF RESPECT AND RECOGNITION

Respect and recognition are fundamental components of a just social order in the writings of Stephen Darwall and Axel Honneth. Darwall begins with a commonplace of modern moral philosophy: the obligation to regard all persons as entitled to respect (Darwall 1977). He then establishes recognition and appraisal as two distinct kinds of respect. He defines the former as an absolute moral obligation. In any encounter or relationship, one must take seriously the irreducible personhood of the other individual. Other people share the same human essence as oneself, and for that reason one must regard their claims for dignity and worth as fundamentally legitimate. The attitude of respect that unfolds from this mutual recognition exerts a normative demand: that is, it rules out certain behaviors toward others as morally unacceptable. Appraisal respect is a different matter altogether. People are entitled to this second kind of respect by developing their character or achieving certain kinds of value (symbolic, material, intellectual, divine, etc.) that are celebrated by local norms. Respect based on appraisal (unlike recognition respect) depends on biographical details, personal traits, or social roles and identities. Different people, therefore, appropriately deserve greater or lesser amounts of appraisal respect from others.

Darwall's notion of recognition respect has several implications for theories of social justice. Respect of this sort—due to people simply because they belong to the all-encompassing human community—is obviously diminished when they are devalued because of their particular identities. Sexism and racism starkly illustrate the denial of recognition respect. In such forms of social stratification, members of the dominant group deny that people from subordinate groups have moral claims on par with other persons. In certain settings, moreover, the stratification becomes so hegemonic that it seeps into people's habitual self-regard. It can corrode people's ability to extend recognition respect even to themselves. Darwall states that such a deficit in "recognition self-respect" manifests itself as behaving in patently self-destructive ways and submitting without protest to degrading treatment from others.

Self-respect and its effects on personal behavior are matters of individual subjectivity. Nevertheless, they dovetail with theories of social justice in the following way. Recognition respect is a relational gesture: an attitude one holds toward another person. The attitude carries a normative force and provides a basis for evaluating face-to-face actions as morally permissible or impermissible. By extension, larger-scale social relations are bound by the same moral calculus. For a social order to be considered just, it must facilitate the development of recognition self-respect, and it must not force people to acquiesce in the denial of their own dignity. The lack of self-respect in a single individual can therefore signal the operation of injustice on the societal level. Recognition self-respect acts like a barometer, sensitive to the effects of large-scale injustice as they manifest themselves in the field of people's intimate self-regard. People's ordinary moral talk and their autobiographical narratives bear witness to this relation between larger structures of social injustice and personal feelings of abjection.

Respect and recognition are also key words in Axel Honneth's account of social justice (Honneth 1995). Honneth is a theorist in the critical tradition of the Frankfurt school, and his account seems a good fit for the conflicts laid out by psychiatric survivors' narratives because both the theoretical and the testimonial accounts turn on questions of liberation and counterhegemony. Honneth's entire project rests on a nonatomistic vision of society. Human beings are not intrinsically self-sufficient monads. To the contrary, self-realization and autonomy grow only through experiencing the recognition of others. His theory of justice, therefore, does not begin with a view of isolated individuals who defend or advance their self-interest, nor does it end by proposing principles for the fair distribution of goods to individual citizens. It begins instead with the community or *polis* within which individuals recognize each other through various kinds of intersubjective gestures. Human flourishing depends fundamentally on sustained social relations, and Honneth places himself in the context of a broad group of thinkers who explore various sorts of ideal-type relationships and their effect on self-realization. His project thus resonates with, for example, Hirschmann's analysis of children's early concept of self that flows from experiencing their mothers' care (Hirschmann 1989), and Taylor's essay about new forms of collective identity created by state-level acknowledgment of the authenticity of particular groups (Taylor 1992).

Honneth's model has an important sociological implication. Processes of recognition unfold within structures as small as families and as large as nation-states, but at whatever scale, they enable a rough harmony and accommodation between people who otherwise remain divided by personal interest, ideological commitments, or group loyalty. When a subject knows she is recognized, she can more easily accommodate the demands of life in community. Social cohesion thus results through the continually renewed process of relational affirmation, not the top-down imposition of order. Social conflict, by contrast, erupts when this process is interrupted—that is, when people's demands for recognition are denied. Indeed, people feel the absence of recognition acutely as a denial and even a violation, not just the lack of a desired good. Withholding recognition can cause real harm. Undercutting a claim to equal personhood denigrates and insults the people actually making the claim (Honneth 1995, 93).

At one level, the struggle for recognition is a social phenomenon, and at another level, its deepest motives lie in the operation of human subjectivity. People intrinsically desire to express themselves, and by necessity the expression involves others as witnesses and interlocutors. Expression is possible only when others take the speaker as a legitimate partner for dialogue and, reciprocally, as a worthy addressee for *their* subjective expressions. With this formulation, Honneth offers a baseline definition of recognition rooted in the social psychology of George Herbert Mead (1934). According to Mead, individuals become conscious of themselves only through observing how other people react to them. Self-consciousness is not a primordial experience. Indeed, Mead regards inner experience as originally amorphous and unorganized. Self-consciousness begins to take shape exclusively through the process of being perceived, listened to, and addressed by another person. A stable self-concept emerges because an individual becomes the relational object to his interactive partner. The very possibility of self-consciousness depends on experiencing oneself from the second-person perspective.

In this model, the search for recognition is not optional. To the contrary, people feel compelled to seek it out, because the stakes are so high. Honneth gives the example of the baseline needs of the developing child. In the ideal case, a child's claim on his parents for recognition of his emotional and physical needs immediately encourages the parents to confirm their child's legitimate dependency. In healthy affective relationships like the bond between parent and child or between lovers, the imperative for recognition strengthens and sustains social reciprocity at several levels at once (meeting concrete needs, confirming each other's personal worth, guiding the other into a larger social network, etc.).

An immense pressure drives the search for recognition, but the process does not always flow smoothly. The reason again derives from the nature of human subjectivity. Subjective experience is dynamic, forever unfolding as people engage with the world in new ways. They continually seek to express themselves and the novel quality of their experience and therefore require new forms of mutual recognition on both the interpersonal and collective level. On the face-to-face level, people seek recognition by finding new partners for interpersonal dialogue. When individuals form or join collective groups on the basis of similar life experiences, they pitch their demand for recognition on the collective level. They seek endorsement of their own group's legitimacy and distinctive experience, and this sort of endorsement can come only from other nearby groups. Intersubjective recognition (at any level), however, is never guaranteed. The routine interactions that already exist in the immediate social milieu may simply not fit the claimants' need for dialogue or an affirming witness. Even worse, long-standing hierarchies may lead people to refuse to listen to new articulations of experience and reject a group's claims to enter the public discourse on equal terms. In such cases, a fault line opens between the subject and the others who withhold recognition. Blocking a claim for recognition has several consequences for the subject's self-awareness and political identity. When a bid for recognition is blocked, it typically does not fold back upon itself or wither away. To the contrary, the claimant becomes acutely aware of the refusal. Honneth states that the refusal actually provokes greater, if more painful, self-awareness. The claimant is often spurred to articulate her

Figure 7.1. Respect, Recognition, and Justice

	Love	Rights	Solidarity
Mode of recognition	emotional support	cognitive respect	social esteem
Dimension of personality	needs and emotions	moral responsibility	traits, abilities
Forms of recognition	primary relationships	legal relations	communities with shared values
Practical relation to self	basic self-confidence	self-respect	self-esteem
Forms of disrespect	abuse and rape	denial of rights, exclusion	denigration, insult
Threatened component of personality	physical integrity	social integrity	honor, dignity

Source: Adapted from Honneth 1995, 129.

experience more clearly and to reach for more creative interpretations of the situation she faces. The refusal thus lays bare the pressure behind every search for mutual recognition.

When the search for recognition fails, the pressure driving it can manifest itself as anger and outrage. The anger is absolutely fitting, since the refusal threatens the claimants' dignity and the very terms of their self-consciousness (born, by definition, in an intersubjective field). To deny the legitimacy of someone's experience can also be an act of social extrusion. It can forcibly remove that person from the world of shared meanings and discourses. In response, Honneth says, people try to resolve the dilemma of blocked recognition by moving into the political arena. His model shows how the imperative for recognition can ultimately fuel the demand for social justice (compare Goering 2009). The argument comes from one dimension of a ramifying model that extends far beyond the concerns of this chapter. The full model (see figure 7.1) integrates three different fruits of intersubjective recognition: self-confidence, self-respect, and self-esteem. Each of these desirable forms of self-consciousness flows from a different type of social reciprocity. Self-confidence is the outcome of emotional concern, typically enacted in

relationships of love and friendship. Self-respect is the product of legal recognition via the operation of formal laws and explicit discourse of universal
rights. Self-esteem comes from the approval of others who share the same substantive values and commitments. Each of these three relationships unfolds in
a separate sphere: the family, the state, and civil society, respectively.

In the schematic version presented in figure 7.1, the second column lays
out the dynamic links between respect and social justice. Honneth assumes
that for people living in a democratic society, self-respect is inseparable from
one's status as a rights-bearing person. That status depends fundamentally on
being recognized as a legitimate member of a given political community: a
bounded polity with a formal commitment to the full political enfranchise-
ment of all members. Conversely, being extruded from or denied membership
in this polity injures a person's "intersubjectively acquired relation-to-self"
(Honneth 1995, 94). Being treated as something less than a rights-bearing person undercuts self-respect, and Honneth mentions crippling feelings of social
shame produced by the effective denial of full citizenship to African Americans in the Jim Crow era. These feelings, in fact, drove the imperative for recognition that animated the U.S. civil rights movement.

In a similar vein, Larchanché (2012) describes the aura of illegitimacy
surrounding undocumented immigrants in France and its effects on their
self-consciousness. Larchanché portrays African immigrants who are stigmatized by dominant racist and nationalist ideologies; they live in fear and suspicion because of the threat of deportation and the disdain shown to them
by state workers. As a result, many regard themselves as undeserving of medical care, and their low self-esteem actually harms their health. The impact
of recognition on self-respect comes through in a comment to Larchanché
from an undocumented immigrant from Guinea-Conakry now living in Paris:
"See, this piece of paper (he waves the AME [State Medical Aid] form he just
received in front of me), this makes me feel real. I know it doesn't solve my
problems. But it makes me feel like I'm legitimate, that I'm honest. I'm here to
do things right. I'm not here to cheat. I work hard. I don't ask for anything but
respect" (Larchanché 2012, 862).

The need for self-respect thus compels people to confront those who
wield formal social power, whether bureaucrats or clinicians. It underlies the
compulsion to expand the space of mutual recognition and to assert legal
rights on behalf of oneself and others who are similarly disrespected. The
granting of rights not only changes one's juridical status. It also enables the
ability to regard oneself as a morally responsible person (a process that recalls

Darwall's argument about recognition self-respect). This linkage between political resistance and fundamental forms of self-regard is the engine of justice claims in Honneth's model. Possessing the same legal rights as all other citizens produces a desirable state of self-consciousness. One is able to respect oneself because one manifestly deserves (and receives) the respect of everyone else. Honneth's ambitious model connects the levels of subjective experience, interpersonal and intergroup relations, and political advocacy. In the end, he argues, people's claims for justice in a democratic society integrate all three levels. His model shows that behind the formal rights claims made in a courtroom, manifesto, or published testimonial lies a vast realm of subjective experience and a remembered history of the denial of recognition.

THE TESTIMONY OF DISRESPECT AND DENIED RIGHTS

The remainder of this chapter tries to commensurate the theoretical arguments of Darwall and Honneth with the testimonies, arguments, and political project of the early psychiatric survivors movement, as represented by Chamberlin's foundational book. To commensurate these three texts does not mean building point-by-point comparisons between them. The goal instead is to show how they complement and illuminate each other and how, as an ensemble, they clarify some of the most difficult debates about justice in the mental health system. Chamberlin's book dates to the earliest stage of the survivor movement in the 1970s. Around this time, individuals who had experienced forced hospitalization formed the first loose survivor organizations, such as the Psychiatric Inmates Liberation Movement in the United States and the Mental Patients' Union in the United Kingdom. Such groups rejected not only involuntary commitment and other forms of mandated treatment but also the medical model itself. They regarded mental psychiatric crises not as a disease but as an attempt to respond to difficult and oppressive life circumstances (Crossley 2006). The agenda of these early activists aimed minimally at basic civil rights for patients, notably the right to refuse treatment and the end of isolation rooms. Most went further and called for the abolition of the mental hospital and its replacement by a network of drop-in and live-in centers entirely under the control of the people utilizing them.

Compared to later developments in the survivor's movement, this first phase was the most radical in its rejection of biopsychiatric dogma (McLean 2000). The movement comprised activist political organizations that mobilized their members, offered them a new collective identity (as survivors or psychiatric inmates, instead of mere patients), issued manifestos, and built new social arrangements for mental respite and healing. Chamberlin's *On Our Own: Patient-Controlled Alternatives to the Mental Health System* is a product of this historical moment. The structure of the book parallels the course of the author's adult life. Her presentation begins with the story of her own string of psychiatric hospitalizations in 1966. It is a harrowing narrative of overmedication, locked wards, seclusion rooms, and other forms of overwhelming psychiatric power. Although Chamberlin mentions the internal distress (suicidal gestures and the misery of a failed marriage) that preceded her entry into the mental health system, she does not connect her suffering to an underlying biological disease. Her suffering, she writes, was caused by the specific conditions of institutionalization. Doctors and medical staff ignored her pleas to be discharged (she was a patient at several New York hospitals of the era, including Mt. Sinai, Gracie Square, Hillside, Bellevue, Montefiore, and Rockland State). Her movements were controlled by bureaucratic rules and rigid behaviorist schemes of granting greater privileges, such as short-term leaves from the hospital grounds, in return for docile compliance. Cold and impersonal clinicians, dehumanizing admission procedures, and the daily humiliations of de facto incarceration created the personal experience of massive disrespect: "The experience totally demoralized me. I had never thought of myself as a particularly strong person, but after hospitalization, I was convinced of my own worthlessness. I was told that I could not exist outside an institution. I was terrified that people would find out that I was an ex-patient and look down on me as much as I looked down on myself. . . . [The] system had locked me up, denied me warm and meaningful contact with other human beings, drugged me, and so thoroughly confused me that I thought of this system as helpful" (Chamberlin 1978, 6–7).

Several years after her final hospitalization, Chamberlin faced another painful personal crisis while living in Vancouver, but this time she entered the Vancouver Emotional Emergency Center, a short-term residence that explicitly refused the label of a treatment facility. The center was Chamberlin's first exposure to nonprofessional, client-controlled services where "no-one, no matter how poorly functioning, is looked down on as hopeless or as less than human" (Chamberlin 1978, 8). A group of ex-patients had founded the Vancouver center, and they operated it as a nonhierarchical collective with minimal distinction between residents and staff. After telling the story of her own crisis and recovery in the first half of the book, Chamberlin elaborates this organizational template in great detail. She develops a model for alternative drop-in and residential facilities that are completely voluntary and established outside of professional control. She compares several contemporary experiments and offers guidance about solving typical organizational and communication pitfalls as well as negotiating the larger political and fiscal obstacles to long-term sustainability.

Throughout the book, Chamberlin writes in the first-person voice as a participant in these efforts at massive reform. She described how the experience of entering the movement changed her:

> For several years before getting involved in mental patients' liberation, I had become increasingly angry about my hospitalization. There was no-one to share these perceptions with. . . . I didn't confide in most people that I was an ex-patient. My anger existed side by side with my acceptance of my own "mental illness." I thought that my story was an isolated example of poor treatment.
>
> My feelings began to change when I discovered the existence of the Mental Patients' Liberation Project in New York. . . . We talked about our experiences and discovered how similar they were. Whether we had been in grim state hospitals or expensive private ones, whether we were there voluntarily or involuntarily . . . [we] had experienced depersonalization, the stultifying effects of drugs, the contempt of those who supposed "cared" for us. . . . We also began to talk about the kinds of help troubled people need. . . . It quickly became clear that there was no way to fix up the current mental hospital system. (Chamberlin 1978, 66–67)

SEARCHING FOR COMMENSURABILITY BETWEEN ETHICAL THEORY AND PERSONAL TESTIMONY

The ethical arguments from Darwall and Honneth help illuminate the turning points in Chamberlin's autobiographical narrative. The imperative of recognition was blocked in several different ways during her young adulthood. Chamberlin traces her first psychiatric crisis to her difficulty recovering from a miscarriage. She says she needed to withdraw, "to lie in bed and pull the covers over my head [and] . . . to return to myself" (Chamberlin 1978, 23). But her husband didn't understand, and her psychiatrist told her to get back to work, spend more time with people, and take medication. The diagnosis of depression and a string of forced hospitalizations quickly followed. Key people in her immediate social world thus disconfirmed Chamberlin's subjective framing of her own suffering and replaced it by an interventionist and authoritative medical interpretation.

The medicalization itself then created a new and distinctive brand of suffering. For a time, Chamberlin accepted the "spoiled identity" of a psychiatric patient (Goffman 1963). She observed how people reacted to her—to borrow G. H. Mead's language, she experienced herself from the second-person perspective—and began to internalize their judgments of her as weak, dependent, and sick. People surrounding her prevented her from articulating the lived experience of forced and dehumanizing hospitalization. She thereby became subjectively engulfed in the unsympathetic gaze of others and in the patient role thrust upon her (compare Lally 1989). To adopt Darwall's terms, she stopped regarding herself as possessing the dignity and worth inherent in all persons. Her deficit of recognition self-respect manifested as a passive acceptance of her degraded status. In Chamberlin's autobiographical testimony, one type of disrespect paved the way for another. In the first instance, her husband and psychiatrist effectively invalidated her own way of framing her experience. Immersion in the social identity as a mental patient then inaugurated a second and more public type of devaluation. Her self-reported experience suggests how various types of disrespect can jointly produce an imprisoning self-consciousness that will arguably last as long as one's isolation from, and lack of communication with, other people similarly disrespected.

Chamberlin's book thus illustrates the on-the-ground dynamics of Honneth's and Darwall's general theories; it furnishes a case study of the absence of mutual recognition and recognition self-respect. The testimonial book, however, engages in detail with the specific ideology underlying the apparatus of disrespect, unlike the philosophical theories that are pitched at a more general level. Chamberlin traces the neglect and dehumanization that she experienced to a key ingredient of contemporary biopsychiatry: the notion that severe mental illness temporarily effaces core aspects of personhood and normal cognition and that it renders people unable to discern their best interests. She knows that this viewpoint justifies the use of involuntary commitment, seclusion rooms, and mandated medications. She presses her claim to full personhood and unimpaired subjective capacity as an oppositional move against such core tenets of biological psychiatry (Amador 2000).

When applying generic theories of ethics to particular lives and social circumstances, we must reckon with the content, not just the formal operation, of disrespect. Chamberlin's book pushes us precisely in this direction. Her story shows that the meaning of and rationale for disrespect affects the degree of harm that results. Withholding recognition of a person's subjective experience always damages self-regard, but some damage hits especially deep. To commensurate Honneth's and Chamberlin's books—that is, to read each one in light of the other—draws our attention to both the specific cultural meaning and the broader sociological function of disrespect, how they influence each other, and how the eventual outcome depends on the distinctive meanings of impaired or diminished personhood that dominate in a given society.

Chamberlin's decision to join the overtly political psychiatric survivor's movement stands as the redemptive moment in her life story. Her decision is the book's pivot point where it leaves off personal testimony and becomes a manual for organizers and activists. The interpretive recognition that Chamberlin received from her peers enabled her to develop a healthier self-concept and greater personal autonomy and creative potential (key desirable traits noted by Honneth 1995, 81–84). Significantly, this change in self-consciousness did not come about by reaching inward for hidden psychological resources. It happened, instead, when she mobilized with other to confront powerful institutions and push for full civil rights. Indeed, the book briefly takes on a manifesto quality when Chamberlin approvingly describes a fourteen-point mental patient bill of rights written by the New York–based Mental Patients' Liberation front. This document restates the rights guaranteed to all U.S. citizens and explicitly applies them to the conditions of psychiatric treatment.

The turn to the political in Chamberlin's book illustrates Honneth's notion that recognition means full acceptance as a member of the relevant wider community. In democratic states, the sine qua non of acceptance is the granting of rights (Honneth 1995, 79). Rights are usually enunciated at a formal level and invoke generic categories (for example, the citizen or the human). Nevertheless, the process of recognizing someone's rights claim has a profound effect on self-consciousness. It ushers in a new relationship to oneself, precisely because one is accepted as bearing the same worth as all others. The unfolding of Chamberlin's own life story illustrates Honneth's point that blocking the imperative for intersubjective recognition unleashes a normative demand for equal treatment under the law. The political agenda of the psychiatric survivors' movement also confirms Honneth's observation about the time frame for such demands. People make rights claims both to criticize the

present social order and to conjure up relationships of mutual recognition before they actually exist.

Chamberlin's embrace of a rights-based discourse (in her trajectory from
ex-patient to activist) illuminates another feature of the models of respect
from Darwall and Honneth. Both models draw an important distinction between the respect granted on the basis of a person's particular character or
achievements and that granted because of their fundamental status as human
beings. Recall that Darwall labels the first as appraisal respect and the second
as recognition respect. He regards the second as more fundamental. Refusals
to acknowledge the moral claims of members of a particular group may seize
on people's gender, race, sexual identity, or, for that matter, psychiatric diagnosis and functional capacities, and for Darwall, all such refusals are unjust. Darwall builds his view about appraisal and recognition respect on a deeper distinction between two subject positions. Appraisal respect flows to individuals
because of their own accomplishments, while recognition respect is accorded
simply on the basis of personhood as such. The idiosyncratic individual and
the universal human are the sole conceivable subjects of respect.[2]

Chamberlin, however, advocates for the rights of psychiatric survivors on
behalf of a third subject position: membership in a distinctive social group
that has a singular history of abjection. Her claims for respect are thus bound
up in the politics of recognition (Taylor 1992), in the following sense. The experience of coerced psychiatric hospitalization typically isolates and margin-
alizes people. Reframing treatment as oppression and organizing ex-patients
to establish self-help groups, drop-in centers, and the like creates a social
movement with its own ethos, mission, and markers of identity. Chamberlin's
book makes a bid for recognition on behalf of this collective movement. But
the very existence of such a group, and its distinctive voice and ethical claims,
is unpredicted by Darwall's notion of recognition respect. Undoubtedly, the
rhetoric of the patient bill of rights fits the outlook of recognition respect. The
bill explicitly addresses psychiatric survivors as American citizens who, on
that basis, have fundamental rights of autonomy, bodily integrity, and sovereign decision making. The bill nevertheless owes its social force and political
relevance to its origin in a particular group's shared experience, or, more precisely, to the small-scale processes of mutual recognition that made it possible
for people to articulate their individual experience in a collective voice.

The same question of commensurability between philosophical and
survivor-activist positions comes up with Honneth's model. His model dis-
tinguishes between the notions of respect and esteem, and the third column

of figure 7.1 schematically lays out the process of gaining social esteem. A key type of mutual recognition, Honneth writes, comes from communities of like-minded people who allow us to "relate positively to [our] concrete traits and abilities" (Honneth, 1995, 121). This sort of recognition does not burn away superficial differences in search of a universal moral core possessed by all human beings. Rather, it unites people who share distinctive orientations and values. It arises by definition in bounded social groups and precise historical periods. He gives several examples of the reciprocal dynamics of esteem, including the orientation toward honor held by European feudal nobility, the money-based prestige of the bourgeoisie, and the solidarity valued among oppressed classes in capitalist societies. In each case, individuals win recognition by embodying values held by a specific collective group, not humanity writ large.

Honneth says nothing about the order in which the three forms of recognition must be achieved. The model in figure 7.1 does not establish any precedence among love, rights, and solidarity. It does not tell a person or group where to start in the practical struggle for recognition. In Chamberlin's case, by contrast, social esteem necessarily came first and provided the groundwork to press for legal relations of respect. The key turning point in Chamberlin's autobiographical narrative occurred when she discovered a community of shared values and concerns. Only in the context of this community could she articulate her experience of denigration. That is, only the nascent psychiatric survivors' movement could grant her the dignity of having survived. The starting point in Chamberlin's transformation from dependent and demoralized ex-patient to survivor-activist could not have been the recognition of legal rights. As already noted, people typically make the claim for legal recognition in anticipation of rights not yet achieved and with no guarantee that they will ever be won. The necessary starting point for Chamberlin's passage toward self-respect was the social esteem from others who share the same values and social location. Only once that esteem sediments into self-consciousness and sparks collective solidarity can the imperative for recognition enter the political arena and fuel the demand for social justice.

CONCLUSION

This chapter explores the commensurability of radically different texts about respect, recognition, and justice. It compares experience-near and experience-far accounts and explores their resonance. The chapter suggests two general ways that testimonial and philosophical approaches complement each other. Testimonials report on specific instances of personal denigration, shame, abuse, and loss, but they typically do not offer a detailed positive portrait of respect. A generic ethics derived solely from testimonials would consist of a string of negative injunctions, that is, entreaties to avoid harming some closely held but never fully articulated quality of personhood. By reading testimonies through the lens of thinkers like Darwell and Honneth, we can tease out a richer and more explicit account of the very object of respect. In personal testimonials, the relationships between discrete dimensions of respect and recognition get blurred because of the sheer pressure to vindicate one's experience. Carefully mapping these dimensions builds up a robust theory of respect that is transposable to different cases.

The theoretical framings, for their part, can paint a falsely static picture. Respect is a relational concept. It has an inherently dialogical quality and depends on processes of give-and-take evident in the very vocabulary of making claims, accepting or denying them, providing or withholding recognition, and so on. These are social gestures that unfold over time, and people on the ground who actually pursue respect continually devise strategies, carry them out, evaluate the results, and try again. The task of theoretical analysis, however, must stabilize the notion of respect in order to parse it into dimensions like appraisal and recognition respect or love/rights/solidarity. Perhaps inevitably, experience-far theoretical models of respect have a static quality that removes the concept from the flow of social transactions. Reading these models through the lens of personal testimony can restore the dynamic and open-ended quality of respect. It is a temporal and relational concept that slowly reveals its various dimensions across the trajectory of a single individual's life or the history of a collective movement. The synoptic portrait of respect in figure 7.1 thus clarifies the concept but also imparts a false stability to the experience. In the end, high-order models may remain oblique to, and partially incommensurable with, personal testimony. But even this problematic shows the centrality of respect as a crucial ingredient in social life and a just social order.

NOTES

1. Kessler's research agenda is exemplary in demonstrating the correlation between poverty and mental illness. Bhugra and Gupta explore the influence of social inequality and discrimination on migrants' mental health. Membership in racial and ethnic groups that are culturally stigmatized and disadvantaged by forms of structural inequality is

correlated with higher prevalence of mental disorders, although Martins demonstrates that the types of vulnerability, precise pathways, and confounding variables are very complex.

2. This application of Darwall's framework raises the following question. He claims that recognition respect is owed to all persons, but does the category of "person" in his essay include people with lesser autonomy or rationality due to severe mental illness? Several passages suggest that he does intend an inclusive definition of personhood. To be entitled to respect, he writes, means to be "entitled to have other persons take seriously and weigh appropriately the fact that they are persons in deliberating about what to do" (Darwall 1977, 38). Rationality, emotional stability, and the capacity for self-governance are features that merit positive appraisal, and they arguably constitute "excellences of persons" (Darwall 1977, 45). But Darwall never states or implies that the absence or impairment of such features diminishes personhood as such. Indeed, to extend recognition respect for people means precisely that we do not appraise their specific features. "Rather," Darwall writes, "we are judging that the fact that he or she is a person places moral constraints on our behavior" (Darwall 1977, 46). An irreducible conception of personhood fits with both the tenor of Darwall's essay and the normative argument that an individual's diminished competence should not lessen others' acknowledgment of his or her agency (Kittay, chapter 4, this volume). It is also consistent with the nonpolarized view about the ethics of involuntary treatment advanced earlier. People with psychotic disorders, even when they are physically constrained or subject to court-ordered treatment, remain persons who on that basis alone deserve respect as ends in themselves.

REFERENCES

Amador, Xavier Francisco. 2000. *I Am Not Sick, I Don't Need Help!* New York: Vida.

Arango, Celso, and Xavier Amador. 2011. "Lessons Learned about Poor Insight." *Schizophrenia Bulletin* 37 (1): 27–28.

Breggin, Peter Roger. 1991. *Toxic Psychiatry: Why Therapy, Empathy and Love Must Replace the Drugs, Electroshock, and Biochemical Theories of the "New Psychiatry."* New York: Saint Martin's.

Brodwin, Paul. 2008. "The Coproduction of Moral Discourse in U.S. Community Psychiatry." *Medical Anthropology Quarterly* 22 (2): 127–47.

———. 2013. *Everyday Ethics: Voices from the Front Line of Community Psychiatry.* Berkeley: University of California Press.

Brodwin, Paul, and Livia Velpry. 2014. "The Practice of Constraint in Psychiatry: Emergent Forms of Care and Control." *Culture, Medicine, and Psychiatry* 38 (4): 524–26. doi:10.1007/s11013-014-9402-y.

Callard, Felicity, Norman Sartorius, Julio Arboleda-Flórez, Peter Bartlett, Hanfried Helmchen, Heather Stuart, José Taborda, and Graham Thornicroft. 2012. *Mental Illness, Discrimination and the Law: Fighting for Social Justice.* Hoboken: Wiley-Blackwell.

Chamberlin, Judi. 1978. *On Our Own: Patient-Controlled Alternatives to the Mental Health System*. New York: McGraw-Hill.

Chandler, James K., Arnold Ira Davidson, and Harry D. Harootunian, eds. 1994. *Questions of Evidence: Proof, Practice, and Persuasion across the Disciplines*. Chicago: University of Chicago Press.

Cresswell, Mark. 2005. "Psychiatric 'Survivors' and Testimonies of Self-Harm." *Social Science and Medicine* 61 (8): 1668–77.

Crossley, Nick. 2006. *Contesting Psychiatry: Social Movements in Mental Health*. New York: Routledge.

Darwall, Stephen L. 1977. "Two Kinds of Respect." *Ethics* 88 (1): 36–49.

Dennis, Deborah L., and John Ed Monahan, eds. 1996. *Coercion and Aggressive Community Treatment: A New Frontier in Mental Health Law*. New York: Plenum.

Diamond, Ronald J. 1996. "Coercion and Tenacious Treatment in the Community: Applications to the Real World." In *Coercion and Aggressive Community Treatment*, edited by Deborah L. Dennis and John Ed Monahan, 51–72. New York: Plenum.

Eaton, William W. 2012. *Public Mental Health*. New York: Oxford University Press.

Estroff, Sue E. 2004. "Subject/Subjectivities in Dispute: The Poetics, Politics, and Performance of First-Person Narratives of People with Schizophrenia." In *Schizophrenia, Culture and Subjectivity: The Edge of Experience*, edited by Janis Hunter Jenkins and Robert J. Barrett, 282–302. Cambridge: Cambridge University Press.

Goering, Sara. 2009. "'Mental Illness' and Justice as Recognition." *Philosophy and Public Policy Quarterly* 29 (1/2): 14–18.

Goffman, Erving. 1963. *Stigma: Notes on the Management of Spoiled Identity*. Englewood Cliffs, NJ: Prentice-Hall.

Hirschmann, Nancy J. 1989. "Freedom, Recognition, and Obligation: A Feminist Approach to Political Theory." *American Political Science Review* 83 (4): 1227–44.

Hoffmaster, Barry. 1992. "Can Ethnography Save the Life of Medical Ethics?" *Social Science and Medicine* 35 (12): 1421–31.

Honneth, Axel. 1995. *The Struggle for Recognition: The Moral Grammar of Social Conflicts*. Translated by Joel Anderson. Cambridge: Polity.

Josselson, Ruthellen. 2004. "The Hermeneutics of Faith and the Hermeneutics of Suspicion." *Narrative Inquiry* 14 (1): 1–28.

Kallert, Thomas W., Juan E. Mezzich, and John Monahan, eds. 2011. *Coercive Treatment in Psychiatry: Clinical, Legal and Ethical Aspects*. Hoboken, NJ: Wiley-Blackwell.

Kessler, Ronald C., Shelli Avenevoli, E. Jane Costello, Katholiki Georgiades, Jennifer Greif Green, Michael J. Gruber, Jian-ping He, et al. 2012. "Prevalence, Persistence, and Sociodemographic Correlates of DSM-IV Disorders in the National Comorbidity Survey Replication Adolescent Supplement." *Archives of General Psychiatry* 69 (4): 372–80.

Kleinman, Arthur. 1999. "Moral Experience and Ethical Reflection: Can Ethnography Reconcile Them? A Quandary for 'the New Bioethics.'" *Daedalus* 128 (4): 69–97.

Lally, Stephen James. 1989. "'Does Being in Here Mean There Is Something Wrong with Me?'" *Schizophrenia Bulletin* 15 (2): 253–65.

Larchanché, Stéphanie. 2012. "Intangible Obstacles: Health Implications of Stigmatization, Structural Violence, and Fear among Undocumented Immigrants in France." *Social Science and Medicine* 74 (6): 858–63.

Levin, Tomer. 2001. "A Psychiatric Resident's Journey through the Closed Ward." *Schizophrenia Bulletin* 27 (3): 539–47.

Martins, Silvia S., Jean Ko, Sachiko Kuwabara, Diana Clarke, Pierre Alexandre, Peter Zandi, Tamar Mendelson, Preben Bo Mortensen, and William W. Eaton. 2012. "The Relationship of Adult Mental Disorders to Socioeconomic Status, Race/Ethnicity, Marital Status, and Urbanicity of Residence." In *Public Mental Health*, edited by William W. Eaton, 151–97. New York: Oxford University Press.

McLean, Athena Helen. 2000. "From Ex-Patient Alternatives to Consumer Options: Consequences of Consumerism for Psychiatric Consumers and the Ex-Patient Movement." *International Journal of Health Services* 30 (4): 821–47.

———. 2009. "The Mental Health Consumers/Survivors Movement in the United States." In *A Handbook for the Study of Mental Health: Social Contexts, Theories and Systems*, edited by Teresa L. Scheid and Tony N. Brown, 461–77. New York: Cambridge University Press.

Mead, George Herbert. 1934. *Mind, Self, and Society: From the Standpoint of a Social Behaviorist*. Chicago: University of Chicago Press.

Ngui, Emmanuel M., Lincoln Khasakhala, David Ndetei, and Laura Weiss Roberts. 2013. "Mental Disorders, Health Inequalities and Ethics: A Global Perspective." In *Public Health and Social Justice*, edited by Martin T. Donohoe, 235–44. San Francisco: Jossey-Bass.

Oaks, David W. 2011. "The Moral Imperative for Dialogue with Organizations of Survivors of Coerced Psychiatric Human Rights Violations." In *Coercive Treatment in Psychiatry: Clinical, Legal and Ethical Aspects*, edited by Thomas W. Kallert, Juan E. Mezzich, and John Monahan, 187–211. Hoboken, NJ: Wiley-Blackwell.

Peele, Roger, and Paul Chodoff. 1999. "The Ethics of Involuntary Treatment and Deinstitutionalization." In *Psychiatric Ethics*, edited by Sidney Bloch, Paul Chodoff, and Stephen A. Green, 423–40. New York: Oxford University Press.

Povinelli, Elizabeth A. 2001. "Radical Worlds: The Anthropology of Incommensurability and Inconceivability." *Annual Review of Anthropology* 30: 319–34.

Ricoeur, Paul. 1970. *Freud and Philosophy: An Essay on Interpretation*. Translated by Denis Savage. New Haven, CT: Yale University Press.

———. 1981. *Hermeneutics and the Human Sciences: Essays on Language, Action and Interpretation*. Translated by John B. Thompson. Cambridge: Cambridge University Press.

Scott, Joan. 1994. "The Evidence of Experience." In *Questions of Evidence: Proof, Practice, and Persuasion across the Disciplines*, edited by James K. Chandler, Arnold Ira Davidson, and Harry D. Harootunian. Chicago: University of Chicago Press.

Taylor, Charles. 1992. *Multiculturalism and "the Politics of Recognition."* Princeton, NJ: Princeton University Press.

Torrey, E. Fuller. 2001. *Surviving Schizophrenia: A Manual for Families, Consumers, and Providers*. New York: HarperCollins.

PART III

Rethinking Evidence and
the Making of Policy

8

Justice, Evidence, and Interdisciplinary Health Inequalities Research

Nicholas B. King

ABSTRACT

This chapter examines the interplay between normative judgments and empirical research. Using a case study of recent work on the social determinants of health, I argue that three domains that are normally thought of as conceptually and disciplinarily independent—epistemology, scientific methodology, and normative judgment—are in fact closely intertwined. When considering issues related to health inequalities and social justice, keeping these domains separate leads to poor science, poor theorizing, and, ultimately, poor policy choices. I identify three problems with the claim—proposed to some extent in the chapters by Kittay, Braveman, and Shim et al. in this volume—that in order to reduce health inequalities and improve population health, we are morally compelled to address the social determinants of health, through interventions that redistribute social or economic resources in a more fair or just manner. The problems are (1) assuming that data are the neutral products of objective scientific investigations; (2) misunderstanding causality and counterfactual reasoning; and (3) blind belief in the consonance of the good.

INTRODUCTION: EPISTEMOLOGY, METHODOLOGY, AND JUSTICE

At the conclusion of their book *Social Justice: The Moral Foundations of Public Health and Health Policy*, the bioethicists Madison Powers and Ruth Faden reflect on the interdisciplinary nature of work on justice and health inequalities: "Theories of justice without data regarding the way inequalities interact cannot result in just health or other social policies. Any plausible theory of justice needs . . . data provided by social and biomedical researchers who seek to understand how complex social and economic relationships affect health and other essential dimensions of well-being" (Powers and Faden 2006, 193). With respect to their own theory, they argue: "Our theory invites a more fine-grained analysis of the specific causal mechanisms that connect differential income and wealth with health disparities. Our theory does not start with a fixed hypothesis regarding which of the various means or vectors is causally most responsible for health outcomes. As a consequence, what matters most will become, in part, an empirical question. What will matter most for our theory will depend on what the data show, and in particular, on what the data show with regard to how inequalities in health and other dimensions of well-being causally interact" (Powers and Faden 2006, 194).

In this chapter, I expand on these reflections, echoing Powers and Faden's sensitivity toward the interplay between theory and empirical research, but also arguing that this interplay is considerably more complex than their account intimates. Using a case study of recent work on the social determinants of health, I argue that three domains normally thought of as conceptually and disciplinarily independent—epistemology, scientific methodology, and normative judgment—are in fact closely intertwined. When considering the relationships between health inequalities and social justice, keeping these domains separate leads to poor science, poor theorizing, and, ultimately, poor policy choices.

BACKGROUND: THE SOCIAL DETERMINANTS OF HEALTH AND "THE ARGUMENT"

The World Health Organization's Commission on Social Determinants of Health introduced its landmark 2008 report, *Closing the Gap in a Generation: Health Equity through Action on the Social Determinants of Health*, by claiming that "social injustice is killing people on a grand scale." It continued: "Traditionally, society has looked to the health sector to deal with its concerns about health and disease. . . . But the high burden of illness responsible for appalling premature loss of life arises in large part because of the conditions in which people are born, grow, live, work, and age. In their turn, poor and unequal living conditions are the consequence of poor social policies and programmes, unfair economic arrangements, and bad politics. Action on the social determinants of health must involve the whole of government, civil society and local communities, business, global fora, and international agencies" (WHOCSDH 2008).

This report summarized a large body of research indicating that so-called social determinants of health (hereafter SDH) exert a strong influence on population health and health inequalities. SDH comprise a wide range of factors, including (but not limited to) socioeconomic status (House 2002; Lantz et al. 1998); racial and ethnic discrimination (House and Williams 2003; Williams and Jackson 2005; Williams and Collins 2001); occupation, workplace stress, and autonomy (Marmot 2004); residential segregation and neighborhood of residence (Diez Roux 2001; Diez Roux et al. 2001; Schulz et al. 2002); urban planning and the built environment (Northridge, Sclar, and Biswas 2003); access to nutritious food (Wrigley 2002); political empowerment (LaVeist 1993); social capital (Kawachi et al. 1997); and political ideology (Coburn 2000, 2004). Unequal distribution of these factors contributes to attendant health inequalities: poorer and less well educated individuals, racial/ethnic minorities, and residents of poorer countries generally live shorter and have worse health than richer and better-educated individuals, racial/ethnic majorities, and residents of wealthier nations. Moreover, some argue that economic inequality in itself may be an independent determinant of overall population health—that is, countries with greater income inequality may have poorer overall health outcomes in addition to greater health inequalities (Wilkinson 1996; Wilkinson and Pickett 2009; Daniels, Kennedy, and Kawachi 2000).

The SDH approach is frequently contrasted with more traditional healthcare interventions that are viewed as narrowly biomedical. Since the pioneering work of Thomas McKeown (McKeown 1979), many have argued that vaccines, therapeutics, and other medical technologies have been responsible for only a small proportion of the mortality decline and increase in life expectancy characteristic of the epidemiologic transition (McKinlay, McKinlay, and Beaglehole 1989; McKinlay and McKinlay 1977). Others have criticized overreliance on "downstream" health interventions that rely on pharmaceutical "magic bullets" and target individual health behaviors, urging us instead to focus on "upstream" social and policy interventions (McKinlay 1986). Thus, Mervyn Susser and Nancy Krieger have argued for an "ecosocial" theory of disease causation which incorporates a wide variety of potential causal factors at multiple levels (Krieger 1994, 1999, 2001; Susser and Susser 1996a, 1996b). Bruce Link and Jo Phelan have proposed perhaps the most far-reaching SDH theory, arguing that unequal distribution of material and social resources results in persistent health inequalities across history, regardless of the underlying disease mechanism

(Link et al. 1998; Link and Phelan 1995, 2002; Phelan and Link 2005). Even in countries with universal access to health care, significant health inequalities persist (James et al. 2007), with SDH such as income (Alter et al. 2006, 2004), aboriginal status (Adelson 2005), and neighborhood of residence (Frolich, Ross, and Richmond 2006; Ross, Tremblay, and Graham 2004), influencing health, health inequalities, and access to medical care.

While most SDH research emerged from scholars in public health, medicine, and health policy, scholars in other disciplines, including philosophers, bioethicists, and social scientists have begun to address this topic. There is a rich literature on the ethics of inequality in general, and health inequalities in particular. Much of this literature has focused on the allocation of health-care resources (Daniels 1985, 1982; Callahan 1995). In addition, considerable work has been done on distinguishing inequalities in health status from inequalities in health-care delivery or access (Marchand, Wikler, and Landesman 1998; Powers and Faden 2000), on whether health can be considered a special moral good in the realm of social justice (Sen 2002; Walzer 1983), and on distinguishing health inequalities from health inequities (Braveman and Gruskin 2003; Whitehead 1992; Smedley, Stith, and Nelson 2003; Peter and Evans 2001; Hausman 2007; Carter-Pokras and Baquet 2002).

More recently, philosophers and bioethicists have begun to consider the impact of nonmedical determinants of health and health inequalities (Daniels 2006; Brock 2000; Daniels, Kennedy, and Kawachi 2000; Goldberg 2009; Farmer 2003; Benatar 1998; House 2002; House and Williams 2003). In his early essay "Broadening the Bioethics Agenda" (2000), Dan Brock urged ethicists to "forge links with public health comparable to those that we have forged with clinical medicine, to draw on the best work in social and political philosophy not just personal morality, and to use our expertise and training in ethical analysis to help develop an ethical framework adequate for addressing health inequalities and their social determinants" (Brock 2000, 35). Norman Daniels has similarly proposed a "broader bioethics agenda" that grapples with the role of SDH (Daniels 2006) and has followed up this call with a more substantial treatment of SDH in *Just Health* (Daniels 2008), as well as a collaboration with epidemiologists Ichiro Kawachi and Bruce Kennedy, *Is Inequality Bad for Our Health?* (Daniels, Kennedy, and Kawachi 2000).

Philosophers and bioethicists have been fairly unified in their interpretation of the evidence on SDH and its implications for health and social policy. They generally support the following claims, which I will henceforth refer to as "The Argument":

In order to reduce health inequalities and improve population health, we are morally compelled to address the social determinants of health, through interventions that redistribute social or economic resources in a more fair or just manner.

In the remainder of this chapter, I will present several critiques of The Argument as it is mobilized in interdisciplinary research.

NORMATIVE AND EMPIRICAL CLAIMS

Powers and Faden are correct in arguing that translating their theoretical account into practical policy recommendations requires solid empirical work identifying the causal mechanisms underlying the social determinants of health and health inequalities. However, this contention is based on a false separation between theorizing about health and social justice, and empirically investigating the connections between social justice and health. In this they are not alone, as virtually all proponents of The Argument bracket off theoretical considerations from empirical questions regarding the exact mechanisms linking social justice with health outcomes.[1]

The Argument is a normative claim (we are morally compelled to redistribute social or economic resources in a more fair or just manner) supported by two empirical causal claims (unequal distributions cause poorer health and health inequalities; redistribution will cause the improvement of health and reduction of health inequalities). Note that the normative claim requires the following empirical claims to be true:

1. Social inequalities, health, and health inequalities have been *measured* in an accurate and value-neutral manner, in the sense that they do not depend on theoretically determined normative prejudgments.

2. Social inequality or injustice is *associated* with population health and health inequalities. That is, situations in which distributions are more unequal or unjust will be accompanied by poorer population health and/or greater health inequalities.

3. This association is unidirectionally *causal* in nature. That is, social inequality or injustice is an independent driver of health outcomes and is not confounded by a third factor; and health inequalities are not the cause of social inequalities or injustice.

4. Reducing social inequalities or injustice will produce improvements in
   health and/or reduction of health inequalities.

For example, a claim that individuals with lower household income suffer
higher rates of mood disorders (Sareen et al. 2011) requires (1) accurate assessment of household income and diagnoses of mood disorders, and (2) a
demonstration that there is an association between lower household income
and higher likelihood of mood disorders. However, the further claim that
reducing inequalities in household income will reduce inequalities in mood
disorders further requires (3) proof that the association between household
income and mood disorders is not the result of individuals with mood disorders selecting into lower-earning households (either because they earn less
or because they live with people who earn less), nor the result of some third
factor such as education or substance abuse. Finally, any argument for reducing income inequality in order to promote equity in mood disorders should
(4) offer some plausible explanation for why lower income would result in
higher risk for mood disorders, such as increased stress or reduced access to
health care, and why redistribution would actually reduce the incidence of
mood disorders among those with lower household income.

DATA ARE NOT NEUTRAL

Let us first address empirical claim number 1. *Inequality* is often thought to
be an objective numerical comparison and is commonly contrasted with
the more complex concept of *inequity*, which involves normative judgments
regarding justice and fairness. For example, Kawachi and colleagues contend
that "inequality and equality are dimensional concepts, simply referring to
measurable quantities. Inequity and equity, on the other hand, are political
concepts, expressing a moral commitment to social justice" (Kawachi, Subramanian, and Almeida-Filho 2002, 647). More generally, Iris Marion Young
observes that "judgments of equality or inequality . . . are simply factual
comparisons of amounts or degrees of some variables between or among
entities. Such comparisons by themselves do not yield judgments with the
moral force that claims about social, economic, or political equality usually
carry" (Young 2001, 6). In this view, measuring inequality is assumed to be
a value-neutral process whose goal is producing accurate and unbiased data.
This data is then subject to ethical analysis in order to determine whether a
particular inequality is unjust, unfair, or socially unacceptable.

In fact, normative judgments about inequity are often embedded in measures of inequality (Harper et al. 2010; Daniels 1982; Asada 2007; Temkin 1993; King, Harper, and Young 2012; King et al. 2010). Measurement—especially measurement of attributes with the goal of informing public policy—is an inherently value-laden enterprise (Porter 1995; Manski 2013). In particular, judgments about justness, fairness, and social acceptability are inextricably bound to the selection of measures and analytic strategies, and thus frequently precede determinations of the magnitude, direction, rate of change, and cause of inequalities (Harper et al. 2010).

As I illustrate below, the value-ladenness of inequality measures has important ramifications for The Argument, insofar as it relies on empirical claims about the existence, causes, and means of ameliorating health inequalities, as the objective foundation for moral claims about which policies and interventions we are morally compelled to undertake. To illustrate this problem, I will review a well-known example in observational epidemiology: the use of absolute and relative inequality measures.

Health inequalities can be expressed either absolutely, in the accepted units of a health outcome, or relatively, as a dimensionless ratio. For example, if Group A has a mortality rate of 10 per 1,000, and Group B has a mortality rate of 20 per 1,000, the inequality between the two may be expressed absolutely, as B having 10 excess deaths per 1,000 (e.g., 20 – 10), or relatively, as B having twice the mortality rate of A (e.g., 20 ÷ 10).

While both are valid measures, they can sometimes lead to strikingly different interpretations of the magnitude and significance of inequality. This is especially true when considering cases in which medical or public health interventions have led to overall declines in mortality. Consider, for example, the case of HIV/AIDS. The approval of highly active antiretroviral therapy (HAART) in the United States in 1995 has often been considered an unmitigated success: age-adjusted mortality per 100,000 population declined from a high of 16.2 in 1995 to 11.5 in 1996 and 6.0 in 1997; by 2006 it had dropped to 4.0 (NCHS 2010, 229). While only 44 percent of those diagnosed with AIDS between 1981 and 1992 survived at least two years, 85 percent of those diagnosed between 1996 and 2000 survived at least two years (Schneider et al. 2006). Moreover, the benefits of HAART have been widespread: between 1995 and 2006, mortality was cut in half for men and women under sixty-four in all racial categories (NCHS 2010, 229).

However, some observers have suggested that the fruits of this medical innovation have not been distributed justly. One *American Journal of Public*

Health study observed that, in the United States, "national Black-White dis-parities widened significantly after the introduction of HAART, especially among women and the elderly" (Levine et al. 2007, 1884). Similarly, a study of HIV/AIDS mortality in Barcelona concluded that "AIDS mortality in-equalities by SES group remained quite stable, in the sense that lower SES groups had higher mortality than the more privileged ones, and inequalities did not narrow after the introduction of HAART" (Borrell et al. 2006, 605). Finally, one recent essay concluded: "Once HAART, a life-prolonging medical development, became available, we saw significant exacerbations of inequali-ties in HIV/AIDS mortality by both SES and race. . . . If similar patterns are replicated for other lifesaving discoveries, the cumulative effect of the maldis-tribution of such benefits will leave our society with enduring, perhaps even growing, health inequalities" (Rubin, Colen, and Link 2010, 1057).

Given these empirical studies, it might appear that the introduction of HAART has been a failure in terms of social justice, as social inequalities in HIV/AIDS mortality have stayed the same or even increased. However, in each of these cases, this claim is based on measuring health inequalities solely in relative terms. When one uses absolute measures, a different picture emerges (figure 8.1).

Figure 8.1 plots absolute and relative measures of racial inequalities in HIV/AIDS mortality between 1987 and 2006. Following the introduction of HAART, both overall and absolute racial inequality in mortality declined, while relative racial inequality increased. Looking at the rate difference, we might conclude that the introduction of HAART was beneficial in terms of social justice: it benefited both whites and blacks, and it reduced the racial in-equality to roughly the rate it was in 1995. Alternatively, if we consider only the rate ratio, we would likely conclude that the introduction of HAART was pro-foundly unjust, as it dramatically increased racial inequality in a short period.

It is important to note here that both inequality measures are *technically* correct and uncontroversial. While there are some methodological reasons for preferring one or another, ultimately that choice requires normative judgments regarding whether equality has "independent normative significance"—that is, whether it is a valuable goal in itself, independent of other considerations (Harper et al. 2010a). In this example, one must consider whether or not a re-duction in HIV/AIDS mortality inequality per se is a moral good, independ-ent of other considerations, such as overall population health and the absolute rates of disease for each group. If one endorses a strict egalitarian position that what matters is inequality alone, independent of considerations of overall

Figure 8.1. HIV/AIDS Mortality Rate, United States, 1987–2005

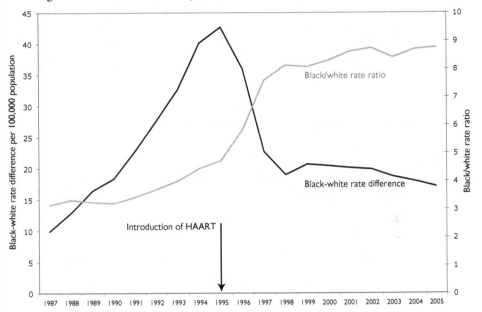

health, then relative measures (which measure inequality alone, insensitive to absolute disease rates and overall population health) are most appropriate. If, on the other hand, one endorses a more utilitarian position that places greater weight on overall population impact, then absolute measures are more appropriate.

The above example provides a simple illustration of a more pervasive problem in the measurement of health and social inequalities, and indeed in the production of ostensibly objective scientific knowledge. As Braveman's chapter in this volume notes, "Values inevitably play an important role in science, shaping the questions we ask and sometimes the methods we use" (35). To borrow the title of a recent edited volume, "raw data" is an oxymoron (Gitelman 2013). All data that may be relevant to The Argument, from information collected through censuses and routine surveillance, to the results of complex mathematical models, is informed by normative, political, and epistemological decisions. We thus cannot uncritically accept empirical claim 1. Health inequalities data are seldom if ever value-neutral; and if they are not value-neutral, then the proposition that a theory of justice can simply rely on them to guide normative decisions about acceptable health and social policies must be called into question.

CAUSALITY AND THE COUNTERFACTUAL TRAP

Let us now turn to empirical claims 2–4, which are frequently confused or conflated by proponents of The Argument. For example, in the introduction to his outstanding book, *Health, Luck, and Justice*, the philosopher Shlomi Segall argues:

> Even societies that feature universal and free access to health care may display considerable disparities in health. . . . It follows that if we care about equality and about health, providing free health care to all cannot possibly be enough. . . . Epidemiologists have been telling us over the past twenty years *that it is possible to mitigate disparities in health by redistributing some other goods, such as income, housing, employment, and workplace autonomy*. . . . This lesson, that inequalities in health itself ought to be of moral concern independently of inequalities in access to health care, and that they ought to be curbed by redistributing the social determinants of health, has now also been recognized by policy makers. (Segall 2010; emphasis added)

Here Segall conflates empirical claims 2–4, misreading evidence for *associations* between the distribution of social goods and health outcomes as evidence that *interventions* that redistribute social goods will improve health and/or reduce health inequalities. In fact, what epidemiologists have been demonstrating for (more than) twenty years is that disparities in health are *associated* with the distribution of other goods, such as income, housing, employment, and workplace autonomy (empirical claim 2). Few have demonstrated specific causal mechanisms explaining these associations (empirical claim 3), and fewer still have provided evidence for the impact of redistributive policies on health (empirical claim 4).

Segall is by no means alone in his conflation of evidence of association with proof of the efficacy of particular interventions. Consider, for example, Norman Daniels, whose Rawlsian approach comes under frequent criticism from Segall. In their 2000 essay, "Justice Is Good for Our Health," Daniels, Kennedy, and Kawachi present a strong case for investment in the social determinants of health. They conclude:

> Academic bioethics and popular discussions of health care reform have generally tended to focus on medicine at the point of delivery and have inadequately attended to determinants of health "upstream"

from the medical system itself. Empirical findings about the social determinants of health suggest that this is a serious mistake: upstream is precisely where we need to look. Put these findings together with a philosophical theory of justice that might apply in any society and we get this striking result: *In a just society, health inequalities will be minimized and population health status will be improved—in short, social justice is good for our health.* (Daniels, Kennedy, and Kawachi 2000, 33; emphasis added)

Daniels has repeated and extended this argument in several publications (Daniels 2006, 2008), and this essay has been extremely influential on, and widely cited among, ethicists and philosophers working on health inequalities. Yet, like Segall, Daniels, Kennedy, and Kawachi base their conclusion not on robust demonstrations of the specific *causal mechanisms* linking inequality and health, nor on evidence that *interventions* to promote justice will reduce health inequalities and improve population health, but rather on evidence of *associations* between greater income inequality, greater health inequality, and lower life expectancy. A more accurate conclusion to the above paragraph would be "More just societies appear to have fewer health inequalities and better overall health, though it is unclear whether this association is causal in nature and what specific interventions to improve social justice would reduce health inequalities and improve overall health."[2]

The conflation of empirical claims 2–4 reflects a conceptual and disciplinary division of labor between empirical health researchers and normative or theoretical bioethicists and philosophers. The Argument rests on empirical observations that are the end result of a long process of technical and normative choices. When specialists in empirical methods and epistemology read this literature, they can assess that process and decide for themselves whether to accept or reject the choices made. Nonspecialists seldom do so. To put it bluntly, specialists read the whole article and often care more about the methodology and results sections, while nonspecialists may only read the introduction and conclusion.

This is also due to the nature of social epidemiology, the discipline that produces most of the empirical data that The Argument rests on. As Sam Harper and Erin Strumpf have argued in a recent commentary on evidence regarding social determinants of health,

The discrepant readings of this evidence may be a consequence of
social epidemiologists generally answering descriptive questions
(whether socially disadvantaged individuals have poorer health), but
interpreting their findings causally (whether socially disadvantaged
individuals would have better health if they were to become advantaged, or vice versa). Such interpretation implies both an intervention
and a causal effect of that intervention. Social epidemiologists often
present their results in counterfactual terms that imply causation: if
clerical workers had the same mortality as administrators, if blacks had
the same mortality as whites, if everyone had the same mortality rates
as those with a university education, the reduction in disease burden
would be substantial. Furthermore, such counterfactuals often do
not correspond to any known or feasible interventions. (Harper and
Strumpf 2012, 796)

Nonspecialist readers of social epidemiology such as Segall frequently fall
into what we might call the "counterfactual trap," misreading observational
evidence of associations between social injustice and health outcomes (empirical claim 2) as causal claims about the specific mechanisms linking these
associations (empirical claim 3), and the efficacy of an intervention that
eliminates social injustice (empirical claim 4). Moreover, study conclusions
frequently make practice and policy recommendations that are unsupported
by, or do not logically follow from, the (observational) evidence contained in
the studies themselves (Prasad et al. 2013). Daniels and his coauthors are far
from alone in jumping from observational evidence of associations to policy
recommendations that simply do not follow.

Falling into the counterfactual trap is dangerous because it facilitates
unwise or potentially counterproductive policy recommendations regarding
justice and health. Consider, for example, a recent essay by the philosopher
Jonathan Wolff titled "How Should Governments Respond to the Social
Determinants of Health?" (Wolff 2011). Wolff draws on the well-known work
of epidemiologist Michael Marmot's Whitehall study, which identifies socioeconomic gradients in health among British civil servants. Marmot hypoth-
esizes that these inequalities are caused by psychosocial stressors including
lack of workplace autonomy and control (Marmot 2004). Arguing that "we
need to identify the ways in which our government is making us ill (or at least
not promoting our health)—especially the more disadvantaged among us—
and persuade the government to do things a different way" (Wolff 2011, 254),

Wolff suggests several social policies that will "make some use of the relation between stress and health" (ibid.), including government provision of domestic support, phased-in retirement for those who do physically demanding work, and allowing social welfare recipients to also earn income. Wolff claims that any costs for these policies should be borne by a "social determinants support budget" (ibid.), because their ultimate goal is to improve health.

Wolff's suggestions are clever, and I would support them as fair policies that improve general welfare. However, there is no reason to believe that they would have any particular impact on *health*, because Wolff has fallen into the counterfactual trap. Despite routinely stating his findings in the counterfactual terms that Harper and Strumpf discuss, Marmot's Whitehall work demonstrates only associations (empirical claim 2) between socioeconomic inequalities and health. It does not demonstrate that lower socioeconomic position *causes* worse health through psychosocial stress mechanisms (empirical claim 3), or that reducing psychosocial stress among the relatively worse-off will improve their health (empirical claim 3).

Researchers have in fact proposed an alternative reading of the Whitehall studies. Using the same data but different methods, they find that health may impact future occupational or employment status, rather than vice versa—that is, those who are relatively more healthy have better prospects for employment and promotion (Case and Paxson 2011). If this interpretation is correct, then Wolff's suggested policies may have little or no impact on health, because they target the *outcome* (socioeconomic inequalities) rather than the *cause* (health inequalities). They may even be counterproductive, as they will fail to help those most in need: the relatively less healthy who might benefit from an intervention that directly improves their health and thus their future employment status.

THE CONSONANCE OF THE GOOD

The conflation of empirical claims 2–4 may also result from belief in what I call "the consonance of the good"—that is, belief in the proposition that what we think of as good (or fair, or just) in one domain will lead to something good (or fair, or just) in other domains. Note here that what one considers "good" is an open question: regardless of whether one is a prioritarian, a Rawlsian, or a relational egalitarian,[3] what matters is the conviction that good begets good. So, for example, an egalitarian might hope that reducing income inequalities will also reduce health inequalities (or vice versa), while a libertarian might hope that increasing economic liberty will also promote other human rights (or vice versa). Wolff's suggestions, for example, seem to be driven by a conviction that policies that are in his estimation fair and just will also be good for health. There may be many ways to reduce psychosocial stress, including "technical fixes" such as distribution of antidepressants, or support of workplace meditation or psychological counseling, but Wolff chooses policies that also independently promote social justice.

While the consonance of the good might appeal to our intuitions by virtue of its apparent consistency, this appeal obscures the fact that whether good begets good is ultimately an *empirical* question about particular populations in particular times and places. Belief in the consonance of the good short-circuits Powers and Faden's invitation for "a more fine-grained analysis of the specific causal mechanisms that connect differential income and wealth with health disparities," because it simply assumes at the outset that good policies will inevitably result in good outcomes.[4] This belief also encourages a form of confirmation bias by making evidence that supports the consonance of the good appear prima facie more plausible than evidence that does not. Most of the major findings that proponents of The Argument cite—including the Whitehall study and the income inequality thesis referenced in this chapter—are sites of robust empirical debate, yet this debate is rarely if ever acknowledged or cited.

A "more fine-grained analysis" requires the ability to adjudicate different kinds of evidence and to tolerate empirical uncertainty when making difficult decisions about appropriate policies and interventions. Blind belief in the consonance of the good works against these intentions. It also diminishes our ability to confront the trade-offs that we must inevitably encounter in the real world. If what is good in one domain is inevitably good in another, then public policy is a trivial matter. Yet in the real world it is hardly so. In fact, those who make public policies must routinely consider trade-offs between different beliefs and values and, most importantly, trade-offs between things we hold good in one domain and things we hold good in another. What is needed is the ability to honestly and effectively confront these trade-offs, not blind faith in the hope that they simply do not exist.

Belief in the consonance of the good holds an additional danger. If one holds the belief that, given an association between the two, reduction of social inequalities will *inevitably* produce reductions in health inequalities, then it becomes all too easy to justify reduction of social inequalities solely on the basis of the resulting effects on health—thus replacing an argument that values social equity on the basis of its *intrinsic goodness* with one that values social equity merely for its *instrumental effects*. In a philosophical sense, this gets things precisely backward. If one believes in the moral goodness of social equity, then one should forcibly argue that point on its own, without shackling the moral worth of social equity to an empirical demonstration that it will positively impact health and/or health equity. Promotion of social justice should be the premise one starts from, not an outcome contingent on empirical demonstration of its instrumental effects.

CONCLUDING THOUGHTS ON INTERDISCIPLINARITY

I will conclude by noting that I am broadly sympathetic to many of the normative claims embedded within The Argument, and with many of the policy proposals that follow from it. For example, I believe that educational and income inequalities should be reduced, though I likely differ from proponents of The Argument like Marmot and Woolf on acceptable mechanisms for doing so. However, I believe that The Argument, and the logic that it rests on, is wrongheaded and potentially dangerous for proponents of health and social equity.

The Argument thrives in part because of some unfortunate characteristics of the contemporary environment of interdisciplinary academic research. Empirical literature in the health and social sciences is prone to exaggeration of the magnitude and clinical and policy ramifications of associations between health and other factors. Empirical researchers are incentivized to present their findings as more certain, more novel, and potentially more important than their methods warrant (Manski 2013; Prasad et al. 2013). There is considerable evidence that much empirical research, particularly the kind of observational epidemiology that supports The Argument, contains claims that are at best overstated, and potentially false (Ioannidis 2005).

Given these worries about the reliability of empirical claims, one might expect philosophers, bioethicists, and social scientists to be skeptical about their usefulness for building theoretical claims. Yet the opposite appears to be true. Scholars in the humanities and social sciences all too often cite empirical studies of suggestive associations as though they conclusively demonstrate specific causal connections and imply particular policy choices—especially when these studies appear to support preexisting theoretical or normative claims.

In her chapter in this volume, Braveman contends that I find the evidence linking social factors with health outcomes "weak," consisting "only of associations, not causal links" (39). This is not the case. My purpose is not to evaluate the overall strength of the evidence base regarding the social determinants of health but, rather, to demonstrate its complex and sometimes contested nature and to present a few reasons for scholars to be judicious while consuming this evidence. Indeed, my primary concern is that judicious skepticism is often lost in the process of cross-disciplinary translation, which is the crucible in which policies and interventions take form. Like Braveman, I believe that complete certainty is an illusory goal. My concern is with the manufacture of illusory certainty in the translation process through misunderstanding or selective citation.

In contrast to cross-disciplinary cherry-picking, we can imagine a more robust multidisciplinary engagement around health inequalities and justice that would elevate humility, transparency, and judicious skepticism as core values. Empirical researchers would present findings in a manner that does not exaggerate the findings' significance, imply causal claims when they are unwarranted, or make unjustified recommendations for policy or practice. Philosophers, bioethicists, and social scientists would approach evidence— particularly that which appears to support preexisting theoretical or normative arguments—with a more skeptical eye and a better understanding of empirical methods. Finally, scholars from multiple domains would participate in a dialogue about the appropriate role of evidence in interdisciplinary health inequalities research. Such an engagement would better prepare us to understand not only what the data show, but also what they do not show, which would in turn result in better science, better theorizing, and, ultimately, better policies.

NOTES

1. See, for example, Venkatapuram and Marmot 2009; and Kittay's claim (chapter 4, this volume) that "my own argument does not rest on the accuracy of the position. What is important for my claim is only that socioeconomic factors, such as level of income, race, ethnicity, disability, etc., *track* health disparities, not that they directly *cause* them" (131).

2. It is also worth noting that the bulk of their argument regarding the so-called income inequality thesis has been forcefully challenged. As one later commentary put it, "The evidence for a correlation between income inequality and the health of the

population is slowly dissipating" (Mackenbach 2002). Yet while the income inequality thesis is still routinely cited (see, e.g., Kittay, chapter 4, this volume), articles that complicate it (Pop, Ingen, and Oorschot 2013) or directly challenge it (Lynch et al. 2004) generally are not.

3. See Kelleher, chapter 3, this volume.

4. I should note here that this is not the same as the claim, favored by proponents of procedural justice, that "just" policies by definition result in just outcomes, regardless of what those outcomes may be. The consonances view of justice claims, rather, that justice in one domain will produce just outcomes in another, where the meaning of justice in each domain is independently defined.

REFERENCES

Adelson, Naomi. 2005. "The Embodiment of Inequity: Health Disparities in Aboriginal Canada." *Canadian Journal of Public Health* 96 suppl. 2: S45–61.

Alter, David A., Alice Chong, Peter C. Austin, Cameron Mustard, Karey Iron, Jack I. Williams, Christopher D. Morgan, Jack V. Tu, Jane Irvine, C. David Naylor, and Sesami Study Group. 2006. "Socioeconomic Status and Mortality after Acute Myocardial Infarction." *Annals of Internal Medicine* 144 (2): 82–93.

Alter, David A., Karey Iron, Peter C. Austin, and C. David Naylor. 2004. "Socioeconomic Status, Service Patterns, and Perceptions of Care among Survivors of Acute Myocardial Infarction in Canada." *Journal of the American Medical Association* 291 (9): 1100–1107.

Asada, Yukiko. 2007. *Health Inequality: Morality and Measurement.* Toronto: University of Toronto Press.

Benatar, Solomon. 1998. "Global Disparities in Health and Human Rights: A Critical Commentary." *American Journal of Public Health* 88 (2): 295–300.

Borrell, Carme, Maica Rodriguez-Sanz, M. Isabel Pasarin, M. Teresa Brugal, Patricia Garcia-de-Olalla, Marc Mari-Dell'Olmo, and Joan Cayla. 2006. "AIDS Mortality before and after the Introduction of Highly Active Antiretroviral Therapy: Does It Vary with Socioeconomic Group in a Country with a National Health System?" *European Journal of Public Health* 16 (6): 601–8.

Braveman, Paula A., and Sofia Gruskin. 2003. "Defining Equity in Health." *Journal of Epidemiology and Community Health* 57 (4): 254–58. doi:10.1136/jech.57.4.254.

Brock, Dan W. 2000. "Broadening the Bioethics Agenda." *Kennedy Institute of Ethics Journal* 10 (1): 21–38.

Callahan, Daniel. 1995. *Setting Limits: Medical Goals in an Aging Society.* New York: Simon and Schuster.

Carter-Pokras, Olivia, and Claudia Baquet. 2002. "What Is a 'Health Disparity'?" *Public Health Reports* 117 (5): 426–34.

Case, Anne, and Christina Paxson. 2011. "The Long Reach of Childhood Health and Circumstance: Evidence from the Whitehall II Study." *Economic Journal (London)* 121 (554): F183–F204.

Coburn, David. 2000. "Income Inequality, Social Cohesion, and the Health Status of Populations: The Role of Neo-liberalism." *Social Science and Medicine* 51: 135–46.

———. 2004. "Beyond the Income Inequality Hypothesis: Class, Neo-liberalism, and Health Inequalities." *Social Science and Medicine* 58 (1): 41–56.

Daniels, Norman. 1982. "Equity of Access to Health Care: Some Conceptual and Ethical Issues." *Milbank Memorial Fund Quarterly: Health and Society* 60 (1): 51–81.

———. 1983. "Health Care Needs and Distributive Justice." In *In Search of Equity: Health Needs and the Health Care System*, edited by Ronald Bayer, Arthur L. Caplan, and Norman Daniels, 1–41. The Hastings Center Series in Ethics. New York: Plenum.

———. 1985. *Just Health Care*. New York: Cambridge University Press.

———. 2006. "Equity and Population Health: Toward a Broader Bioethics Agenda." *Hastings Center Report* 36 (4): 22–35.

———. 2008. *Just Health: Meeting Health Needs Fairly*. New York: Cambridge University Press.

Daniels, Norman, Bruce Kennedy, and Ichiro Kawachi. 1999. "Why Justice Is Good for Our Health: The Social Determinants of Health Inequalities." *Daedalus* 128 (4): 215–51.

———. 2000. *Is Inequality Bad for Our Health?* Boston: Beacon.

Diez Roux, Ana. V. 2001. "Investigating Neighborhood and Area Effects on Health." *American Journal of Public Health* 91 (11): 1783–89.

Diez Roux, Ana V., Sharon Stein Merkin, Donna Arnett, Lloyd Chambless, Mark Massing, F. Javier Nieto, Paul Sorlie, Moyses Szklo, Herman A. Tyroler, and Robert L. Watson. 2001. "Neighborhood of Residence and Incidence of Coronary Heart Disease." *New England Journal of Medicine* 345 (2): 99–106.

Farmer, Paul. 2003. *Pathologies of Power: Health, Human Rights, and the New War on the Poor*. Berkeley: University of California Press.

Frolich, Katherine L., Nancy Ross, and Chantelle Richmond. 2006. "Health Disparities in Canada Today: Some Evidence and a Theoretical Framework." *Health Policy* 79: 132–43.

Gitelman, Lisa, ed. 2013. *"Raw Data" Is an Oxymoron*. Cambridge, MA: MIT Press.

Goldberg, Daniel S. 2009. "In Support of a Broad Model of Public Health: Disparities, Social Epidemiology and Public Health Causation " *Public Health Ethics* 2 (1): 70–83.

Harper, Sam, Nicholas B. King, Stephen C. Meersman, Marsha E. Reichman, Nancy Breen, and John Lynch. 2010. "Implicit Value Judgements in the Measurement of Health Inequalities." *Milbank Quarterly* 88 (1): 4–29.

Harper, Sam, and Erin C. Strumpf. 2012. "Social Epidemiology: Questionable Answers and Answerable Questions." *Epidemiology* 23 (6): 795–98.

Hausman, Daniel M. 2007. "What's Wrong with Health Inequalities?" *Journal of Political Philosophy* 15 (1): 46–66.

House, James S. 2002. "Understanding Social Factors and Inequalities in Health: 20th Century Progress and 21st Century Prospects." *Journal of Health and Social Behavior* 43 (2): 125–42.

House, James S., and David R. Williams. 2003. "Understanding and Reducing Socioeconomic and Racial/Ethnic Disparities in Health." In *Health and Social Justice: Politics, Ideology, and Inequity in the Distribution of Disease*, edited by Richard Hofrichter. San Francisco: Jossey-Bass.

Ioannidis, John P. A. 2005. "Why Most Published Research Findings Are False." *PLoS Medicine* 2 (8): e124.

James, Paul D., Russell Wilkins, Allan S. Detsky, Peter Tugwell, and Douglas G. Manuel. 2007. "Avoidable Mortality by Neighbourhood Income in Canada: 25 Years after the Establishment of Universal Health Insurance." *Journal of Epidemiology and Community Health* 61 (4): 287–96.

Kawachi, Ichiro, Bruce P. Kennedy, Kimberly Lochner, and Deborah Prothrow-Stith. 1997. "Social Capital, Income Inequality, and Mortality." *American Journal of Public Health* 87 (9): 1491–98.

Kawachi, Ichiro, S. V. Subramanian, and Naomar deAlmeida-Filho. 2002. "A Glossary for Health Inequalities." *Journal of Epidemiology and Community Health* 56 (9): 647–52.

King, Nicholas B., Sam Harper, Stephen C. Meersman, Marsha E. Reichman, Nancy Breen, and John Lynch. 2010. "We'll Take the Red Pill: A Reply to Asada." *Milbank Quarterly* 88 (4): 623–27.

King, Nicholas B., Sam Harper, and Meredith E. Young. 2012. "Use of Relative and Absolute Effect Measures in Reporting Health Inequalities: Structured Review." *British Medical Journal* 345: e5774.

Krieger, Nancy. 1994. "Epidemiology and the Web of Causation: Has Anyone Seen the Spider?" *Social Science and Medicine* 39 (7): 887–903.

———. 1999. "Sticky Webs, Hungry Spiders, Buzzing Flies, and Fractal Metaphors: On the Misleading Juxtaposition of 'Risk Factor' versus 'Social' Epidemiology." *Journal of Epidemiology and Community Health* 53 (11): 678–80.

———. 2001. "Theories for Social Epidemiology in the 21st Century: An Ecosocial Perspective." *International Journal of Epidemiology* 30 (4): 668–77.

Lantz, Paula M., James S. House, James M. Lepkowski, David R. Williams, Richard P. Mero, and Jieming Chen. 1998. "Socioeconomic Factors, Health Behaviors, and Mortality." *Journal of the American Medical Association* 279 (21): 1703–8.

LaVeist, Thomas A. 1993. "Segregation, Poverty, and Empowerment: Health Consequences for African Americans." *Milbank Quarterly* 71 (1): 41–64.

Levine, Robert S., Nathaniel C. Briggs, Barbara S. Kilbourne, William D. King, Yvonne Fry-Johnson, Peter T. Baltrus, Baqar A. Husaini, and George S. Rust. 2007. "Black White Mortality from HIV in the United States before and after Introduction of Highly Active Antiretroviral Therapy in 1996." *American Journal of Public Health* 97 (10): 1884–92.

Link, Bruce G., Mary E. Northridge, Jo C. Phelan, and Michael L. Ganz. 1998. "Social Epidemiology and the Fundamental Cause Concept: On the Structuring of Effective Cancer Screens by Socioeconomic Status." *Milbank Quarterly* 76 (3): 375–402.

Link, Bruce G., and Jo C. Phelan. 1995. "Social Conditions as Fundamental Causes of Disease." *Journal of Health and Social Behavior* 35 (extra issue): 80–94.

———. 2002. "McKeown and the Idea That Social Conditions Are Fundamental Causes of Disease." *American Journal of Public Health* 92 (5): 730–32.

Lynch, John, George Davey Smith, Sam Harper, Marianne Hillemeier, Nancy Ross, George A. Kaplan, and Michael Wolfson. 2004. "Is Income Inequality a Determinant of Population Health? Part 1. A Systematic Review." *Milbank Quarterly* 82 (1): 5–99.

Mackenbach, Johan P. 2002. "Income Inequality and Population Health." *British Medical Journal* 324: 1–2.

Manski, Charles F. 2013. *Public Policy in an Uncertain World*. Cambridge, MA: Harvard University Press.

Marchand, Sarah, Daniel Wikler, and Bruce Landesman. 1998. "Class, Health and Justice." *Milbank Quarterly* 76 (3): 449–67.

Marmot, Michael. 2004. *The Status Syndrome: How Social Standing Affects Our Health and Longevity*. New York: Henry Holt and Company.

McKeown, Thomas. 1979. *The Role of Medicine: Dream, Mirage, or Nemesis?* Princeton, NJ: Princeton University Press.

McKinlay, John B. 1986. "A Case for Refocusing Upstream: The Political Economy of Illness." In *The Sociology of Health and Illness: Critical Perspectives*, edited by Peter Conrad and Rochelle Kern, 484–98. New York: St. Martin's.

McKinlay, John B., and Sonja M. McKinlay. 1977. "The Questionable Contribution of Medical Measures to the Decline of Mortality in the United States in the Twentieth Century." *Milbank Memorial Fund Quarterly: Health and Society* 55 (3): 405–28.

McKinlay, John B., Sonja M. McKinlay, and Robert Beaglehole. 1989. "A Review of the Evidence Concerning the Impact of Medical Measures on Recent Mortality and Morbidity in the United States." *International Journal of Health Services: Planning, Administration, Evaluation* 19 (2): 181–208.

NCHS (National Center for Health Statistics). 2010. *Health, United States, 2009: With Special Feature on Medical Technology*. Hyattsville, MD: National Center for Health Statistics.

Northridge, Mary E., Elliot D. Sclar, and Padmini Biswas. 2003. "Sorting Out the Connections between the Built Environment and Health: A Conceptual Framework for Navigating Pathways and Planning Healthy Cities." *Journal of Urban Health* 80 (4): 556–68.

Peter, Fabienne, and Timothy Evans. 2001. "Ethical Dimensions of Health Equity." In *Challenging Inequities in Health: From Ethics to Action*, edited by M. Whitehead, F. Diderichsen, A. Bhuiya and M. Wirth, 25–33. New York: Oxford.

Phelan, Jo C., and Bruce G. Link. 2005. "Controlling Disease and Creating Disparities: A Fundamental Cause Perspective." *The Journals of Gerontology Series B: Psychological Sciences and Social Sciences* 60 (Special Issue 2): 27–33.

Pop, IoanaAndreea, Erik Ingen, and Wim Oorschot. 2013. "Inequality, Wealth and Health: Is Decreasing Income Inequality the Key to Create Healthier Societies?" *Social Indicators Research* 113 (3): 1025–43.

Porter, Theodore M. 1995. *Trust in Numbers: The Pursuit of Objectivity in Science and Public Life*. Princeton, NJ: Princeton University Press.

Powers, Madison, and Ruth Faden. 2000. "Inequalities in Health, Inequalities in Health Care: Four Generations of Discussion about Justice and Cost-Effectiveness Analysis." *Kennedy Institute of Ethics Journal* 10 (2): 109–27.

———. 2006. *Social Justice: The Moral Foundations of Public Health and Health Policy*. Issues in Biomedical Ethics. New York: Oxford University Press.

Prasad, Vinay, Joel Jorgenson, John P. Ioannidis, and Adam Cifu. 2013. "Observational Studies Often Make Clinical Practice Recommendations: An Empirical Evaluation of Authors' Attitudes." *Journal of Clinical Epidemiology* 66 (4): 361–66 e4.

Ross, Nancy A., Stephane Tremblay, and Katie Graham. 2004. "Neighborhood Influences on Health in Montreal, Canada." *Social Science and Medicine* 59: 1485–94.

Rubin, Marcie S., Cynthia G. Colen, and Bruce G. Link. 2010. "Examination of Inequalities in HIV/AIDS Mortality in the United States from a Fundamental Cause Perspective." *American Journal Public Health* 100 (6): 1053–59.

Sareen, Jitender, Tracie O. Afifi, Katherine A. McMillan, and Gordon J. G. Asmundson. 2011. "Relationship between Household Income and Mental Disorders: Findings from a Population-Based Longitudinal Study." *Archives of General Psychiatry* 68 (4): 419–27.

Schneider, E., M. K. Glynn, T. Kajese, and M. T. McKenna. 2006. "Epidemiology of HIV/AIDS—United States, 1981–2005." *Morbidity and Mortality Weekly Report* 55 (21): 589–92.

Schulz, Amy, David R. Williams, Barbara A. Israel, and Lora Bex Lempert. 2002. "Racial and Spatial Relations as Fundamental Determinants of Health in Detroit." *Milbank Quarterly* 80 (4): 677–707.

Segall, Shlomi. 2010. *Health, Luck and Justice*. Princeton, NJ: Princeton University Press.

Sen, Amartya K. 2002. "Why Health Equity?" *Health Economics* 11 (8): 659–66.Smedley, Brian D., Adrienne Y. Stith, and Alan R. Nelson. 2003. *Unequal Treatment: Confronting Racial and Ethnic Disparities in Health Care*. Washington, DC: National Academy Press.

Smedley, Brian D., Adrienne Y. Stith, and Alan R. Nelson. 2003. *Unequal Treatment: Confronting Racial and Ethnic Disparities in Health Care*. Washington, DC: National Academy Press.

Susser, Mervyn, and Ezra Susser. 1996a. "Choosing a Future for Epidemiology: I. Eras and Paradigms." *American Journal of Public Health* 86 (5): 668–73.

———. 1996b. "Choosing a Future for Epidemiology: II. From Black Box to Chinese Boxes and Eco-Epidemiology." *American Journal of Public Health* 86 (5): 674–77.

Temkin, Larry S. 1993. *Inequality*. New York: Oxford University Press.

Venkatapuram, Sridhar, and Michael Marmot. 2009. "Epidemiology and Social Justice in Light of Social Determinants of Health Research." *Bioethics* 23 (2): 79–89.

Walzer, Michael. 1983. *Spheres of Justice: A Defense of Pluralism and Equality*. New York: Basic Books.

Whitehead, Margaret. 1992. "The Concepts and Principles of Equity and Health." *International Journal of Health Services* 22 (3): 429–45.

WHOCSDH (World Health Organization Commission on the Social Determinants of Health). 2008. *Closing the Gap in a Generation: Health Equity through Action on the Social Determinants of Health*. Geneva: World Health Organization.

Wilkinson, Richard G. 1996. *Unhealthy Societies: The Afflictions of Inequality*. London: Routledge.

Wilkinson, Richard, and Kate Pickett. 2009. *The Spirit Level: Why More Equal Societies Almost Always Do Better*. London: Penguin Books.

Williams, David R., and Chiquita Collins. 2001. "Racial Residential Segregation: A Fundamental Cause of Racial Disparities in Health." *Public Health Reports* 116 (5): 404–16.

Williams, David R., and Pamela Braboy Jackson. 2005. "Social Sources of Racial Disparities in Health." *Health Affairs* 24 (2): 325–34.

Wolff, Jonathan. 2011. "How Should Governments Respond to the Social Determinants of Health?" *Preventive Medicine* 53 (4–5): 253–55.

Wrigley, Neil. 2002. "'Food Deserts' in British Cities: Policy Context and Research Priorities." *Urban Studies* 39 (11): 2029–40.

Young, Iris Marion. 2001. "Equality of Whom? Social Groups and Judgments of Injustice." *Journal of Political Philosophy* 9 (1): 1–18.

9

Cultural Health Capital

A Sociological Intervention into Patient-Centered
Care and the Affordable Care Act

Janet K. Shim, Jamie Suki Chang, and Leslie A. Dubbin

ABSTRACT

The landmark 2010 Patient Protection and Affordable Care Act (ACA) promulgated a number of fundamental changes to our nation's health-care system. While the lion's share of attention has been focused on its provisions to expand access to insurance, less visible and controversial aspects of the ACA included the creation of institutions and strategies to reduce health disparities and enhance the quality and patient-centeredness of health care. Patient-centered care (PCC) is now regarded as a moral and ethical imperative: a right—the right of patients to be informed, to exercise autonomy in their medical decisions—and an issue of respect—respect for patients' values, preferences, and expressed needs. Moreover, it is also seen as an economic imperative, under the rationale that when patients are more engaged and better informed, their treatment will be less costly. In this chapter, we offer the concept of cultural health capital (CHC) as a sociological intervention for analyzing these changes aimed at making health care more patient-centered, particularly for historically underserved populations. In particular, we use the notion of CHC to illustrate how PCC is accomplished or undone through complex interpersonal and interactional work that is highly dependent on access to stratified cultural resources that both patients and providers bring to health-care interactions. In so doing, we aim to contest, that racism in health care is the primary source of health inequalities. Instead we argue that patients' and providers' cultural assets and interactional styles—themselves the product of complex social, cultural, historical, political, and economic contexts—influence their abilities to communicate with and understand one another. In doing so, we problematize the embrace of individual autonomy so prevalent in discourses on patient-centered care.

INTRODUCTION

In 2010, the landmark Patient Protection and Affordable Care Act, or the ACA, promulgated a number of fundamental changes to our nation's healthcare system. While the lion's share of attention and debate was rightly placed on its provisions to expand access to insurance and to care, less visible—and much less controversial—aspects of the ACA include measures institutionalizing what has come to be known as *patient-centered care*. While there is some variability in definitions, by most accounts patient-centered care (PCC) aims to provide "care that that is respectful of and responsive to individual patient preferences, needs, and values and ensuring that patient values guide all clinical decisions" (Institute of Medicine 2001, 6).

Therefore, patient-centeredness is regarded as a right—the right of patients to be informed, to exercise autonomy in their medical decisions—and an issue of respect—respect for patients' values, preferences, and expressed needs. It is often framed as a moral and ethical imperative, regardless of whether it achieves other goals, including a more just distribution of healthcare resources (Epstein et al. 2010; Gerteis et al. 1993; Gillespie, Florin, and Gillam 2004; Institute of Medicine 2001; M. Stewart et al. 2003); at the same time, PCC is very often promoted as a means to address health disparities or inequities in care, as we discuss below (Epstein et al. 2010). It is also worth mentioning that patient-centeredness is seen as synergistic with another of the aims of high-quality care, as identified by the Institute of Medicine: equity. Equity is defined as "providing care that does not vary in quality because of personal characteristics such as gender, ethnicity, geographic location, and socioeconomic status" (Institute of Medicine 2001, 6). If care is patient-centered, then it is also likely to be equitable—that is, variable in ways that do not affect quality or safety and are not based on personal characteristics related to social status, but that reflect legitimate and justifiable differences in patient's preferences, needs, and values. There are therefore notions of fairness that are directly and indirectly embedded into PCC: taking patients as unique individuals into account can lead to fair and even beneficial variations in care that has been customized, rather than to unfair variations stemming from the improper consideration of personal characteristics unrelated to the patient's condition.

The ACA has sought to institutionalize these commitments to patient-centered care through, for example, the establishment of a Patient-Centered Outcomes Research Institute (PCORI) to compare the clinical effectiveness of medical treatments; the development of a national quality improvement strategy to improve the delivery of health-care services; the encouragement of pilot projects to test patient-centered medical homes; and the establishment of a Community-Based Collaborative Care Network Program to support consortia of coordinated services for low-income uninsured and underinsured populations. Altogether, the ACA codifies and legitimates patient-centered care as the primary means through which to pursue the "Triple Aim" of improved health outcomes, better patient care experiences, and lower costs (see, e.g., Institute for Healthcare Improvement 2013).

Yet, as this chapter argues, the codification of PCC actually leads to an imperative that patients be activated, engaged, and health literate. In what follows, we position cultural health capital (CHC) as a sociological intervention as we embark on these changes aimed at making health care more patient-centered, particularly for populations historically underserved by existing systems. Through the concept of CHC, we illustrate how patient-centered care is accomplished or undone through complex interpersonal and interactional work that is highly dependent on access to stratified cultural resources that both patients and providers bring to health-care interactions. Using data from a qualitative study, we hope to show how both patients' and providers' cultural assets, dispositions, and interactional styles influence their abilities to achieve PCC.

FROM THE PROBLEM OF PATIENT-PROVIDER INTERACTIONS TO THE SOLUTION OF PATIENT-CENTERED CARE

Researchers have been advocating for the adoption of a patient-centered approach in the delivery of medical care for the past thirty years. However, patient-provider interaction as an object of scrutiny, and the problems attendant within it—variously characterized as asymmetry, hierarchy, dominance, medicalization, and inequality—have also long been acknowledged in such fields as sociology, anthropology, and bioethics. In our own discipline, sociology, one of the core concerns that gave rise to health, illness, and medicine becoming bona fide objects of sociological inquiry was the recognition of medicine as an institution that served social functions and contributed to the structuring of society. In this vein, sociologists (e.g., Freidson 1970, 1986, 1994; Heritage and Maynard 2006; Navarro 1980, 1986; Parsons 1951, 1975; Waitzkin 1989; West 1984) began to analyze the nature of the relationship between the patient and the provider: How, institutionally speaking, is this relationship organized and sustained? How do patients and providers actually interact with one another? What social conventions and rules prevail in such encounters? What aspects of the wider social order are reflected, reproduced, and negotiated in those interactions? How do those interactions then accrete to contribute to the existing social order? By doing so, sociological approaches to analyzing patient-provider interactions take an explicitly and concertedly *social* view. The interaction is seen not as the outcome of the individual choices and behaviors of the parties involved, nor even as the product solely of the dyadic relationship. Instead, patients and providers are seen as enmeshed in social, cultural, historical, political, and economic contexts that indelibly shape—though do not determine—their interactions with one another. Thus in the sociology of health and illness, the study and problematization of patient-provider asymmetry, hierarchy, and inequality has a long history.

In the biomedical and clinical literature, however, concerns about inequality in the medical relationship have often been recast as problems of communication and as informational and interpersonal processes that appear to differentially affect providers' interactions with patients from different populations (e.g., Balsa and McGuire 2001, 2003; Balsa, McGuire, and Meredith 2005; Cooper et al. 2006; McGuire et al. 2008; A. Stewart et al. 1999; see also Rouse, chapter 10, this volume). One response to these concerns that has garnered a tremendous amount of recent support has been the notion of patient-centered care. PCC burst onto the health policy landscape in 2001, when the Institute of Medicine released its landmark report on health-care quality, titled *Crossing the Quality Chasm*. In this report, PCC was featured as one of six aims[1] to achieve high-quality health care (Institute of Medicine 2001).

In the wider biomedical and clinical literature, the constitutive domains of PCC include (1) understanding patients within their biopsychosocial context; (2) shared understanding; and (3) shared power and responsibility (Epstein et al. 2005; Mead and Bower 2000; M. Stewart et al. 2003; Wanzer,

Booth-Butterfield, and Gruber 2004). First, the biopsychosocial perspective recognizes the patient as a person who is influenced by their individual biography, their social context, and cultural norms and beliefs. Thus the meanings and significance of an illness will vary from person to person, and providers need to understand both the patient's story of illness and their expectations, feelings, and fears. Shared understanding refers to the patient and provider coming to a mutual sense of the clinical condition, and the treatment options that are concordant with the patient's values, wishes, and beliefs. Achieving this shared understanding requires that the clinician frame and customize information in response to their understanding of a patient's concerns and needs. The clinician should also take into account a patient's level of health literacy and ability to understand information and apply it to his or her clinical situation. And finally, although some proponents of PCC concede that it is still not clear how symmetrical patient-provider relationships can be, the principle of shared power and responsibility argues that the patient and provider together form a therapeutic alliance. That is, ideally the patient and provider should jointly consider the patient's needs and preferences (which may change over time) and deliberate together over future health and its consequences for quality of life and treatment choices. Thus the power and responsibility of making decisions about the course of care are shared, allowing—in theory—for a consensus on an approach to care to be reached.

Ultimately, the aim of PCC is "to improve clinical practice by building caring relationships that bridge demographic, social, and economic differences between clinicians and patients" (Epstein et al. 2010, 1490). Of particular note is that PCC is seen as a pathway to reducing health disparities: as one prominent group notes, "Patient-centered care is critical to addressing racial, ethnic, and socioeconomic disparities in care and outcomes. Patients who are ill, have low health literacy and numeracy, are members of marginalized groups, and have cognitive deficits tend to ask fewer questions and get less information than their peers without these obstacles. They are also less likely to understand technical and nontechnical language. The practice of patient-centered care helps bridge differences among physicians and patients in health beliefs, race, ethnicity, and culture and mitigates disparities in prevention and treatment" (Epstein et al. 2010, 1492).

Yet the contemporary health-care landscape in which PCC—now legislatively mandated by the ACA—is being implemented is characterized by an emphasis on time and cost efficiency, as well as a reduction in the range and availability of ancillary services. Recall that PCC is intended to address the

"Triple Aim" of improved health outcomes, better patient care experiences, and lower costs. But to accomplish this, health-care systems are increasingly interested in understanding how the *patient's* role affects their health-care experiences and how changes in *patient* behaviors can improve health and reduce cost. These incentives are driving the current emphasis on PCC in health-care policy and provision and, in particular, "activating patients to be better managers of their own health and health care" (Hibbard, Greene, and Overton 2013). Additionally, patient engagement—defined as "active patient and public involvement in health and healthcare" (Coulter 2011, 10)—has been framed as the "holy grail" of health care (Wilkins 2012) and the next "blockbuster drug of the century" (Kish 2012). Thus the activated, engaged, savvy, and health-literate patient is seen as critical to the future health of health-care systems and to the success of health-care reform.

Yet becoming and being the activated and engaged patient is no small task (see, e.g., Bernabeo and Holmboe 2013). Part of what is so consequential in health-care interactions is the expectation that cultural ideals of patienthood should be displayed, mobilized, and recognized; and although this presumption often remains unspoken, patients' relative success (or failure) in such performances in turn affects the amount, kinds, and nature of the care they receive. So we offer the concept of cultural health capital (CHC) as a way to better understand how patients and providers engage with one another, how the outcomes of such interactions are mutually achieved, and whether, when, and if these outcomes reflect a patient-centered approach. That is, CHC illuminates the complex interactional dynamics it takes to accomplish PCC, dynamics whose unfolding are highly dependent on the repertoire of specialized cultural resources and skills that patients and providers bring to the health-care interaction. In what follows, we define CHC, describe the study in which we examined its operation, and offer some arguments about what CHC points out that patient-centered care and patient activation miss.

CULTURAL HEALTH CAPITAL

The concept of cultural health capital (CHC) was introduced as a framework to help account for how the interactional dynamics of patient-provider encounters may produce unequal treatment (Shim 2010). CHC is a concept rooted in the sociologist Pierre Bourdieu's theory of cultural capital (Bourdieu 1980/1990, 1983/1986). Bourdieu defined culture not just as cultural objects, beliefs, and rituals, but also practices, dispositions, and styles, like verbal skills, ways of dress, and styles of self-presentation. Focusing his research on educational institutions, Bourdieu showed how such cultural skills and practices operated as forms of capital which, like economic capital, were important means of exchange in students' and parents' interactions. But because cultural capital is unequally distributed, not all students or parents were able to demonstrate successfully the expected styles of self-presentation. The education system's demand for cultural capital for success in school, Bourdieu showed, served to maintain and even justify inequality.

Consonant with Bourdieu, we theorize that both patients *and* providers activate, leverage, and deploy a repertoire of skills, competencies, resources, and styles—which we term cultural *health* capital—in order to effectively engage and interact with one another. For both patients and providers, possessing good communication skills, sensitivity to interpersonal dynamics, and the ability to adapt one's interactional style are key elements of CHC. For providers, important CHC elements may also include professional knowledge/expertise, the ability to understand the personal context of illness, and a nonjudgmental approach to providing care. And for patients, other CHC elements that are valued and rewarded as assets by providers include knowledge of medical topics and language, active presentation of social/economic status, and an enterprising, proactive, instrumental attitude toward one's own health (Dubbin, Chang, and Shim 2013; Shim 2010). Many of these elements of CHC include aspects of patient activation and engagement. But what the notion of CHC points out is that some patients and providers have many of these valued elements in their "toolbox" of skills, while others have fewer. And because these resources, as a form of capital, have exchange value in health-care interactions, the stratified distribution of CHC shapes the relationships particular patients have with particular providers and affects the medical care offered and received.

We therefore offer CHC as a framework that can augment the notion of patient-centered care by emphasizing the *interactional dynamics* that both shape and surround the pathways through which patient activation impacts clinical encounters and health-care outcomes. That is, CHC is a concept that can help us understand why patients and providers sometimes struggle to find a common language and common ground, and why engaging patients in their own care is a far more complicated affair than the definition of patient-centered care depicts.

To better understand the elements that comprise CHC and how they shape interactions, we recruited six physicians from three health-care facilities in the western United States, and seventeen of their patients who had a diagnosis of coronary artery disease and/or type 2 diabetes. We selected these particular diagnoses because they are common and chronic in nature and require active disease management and ongoing contact with health-care providers and institutions. One clinical interaction between each patient and their physician was digitally recorded in its entirety. In the weeks that followed, patient and physician participants were interviewed separately. All interactions and interviews were transcribed verbatim. We analyzed the data using a constructivist approach to grounded theory (Charmaz 2006). Our codes and categories in the current study were a combination of already existing codes capturing the constitutive elements of CHC and new codes that denote how CHC shaped clinical interactions.

In this chapter we share three vignettes from that study, through which we make some observations about the relationship of CHC to PCC.

VIGNETTE #1. ALMA AND DR. ALONZO: THE IMPORTANCE OF PATIENT AND PROVIDER HABITUS

One of the main arguments we levy for a more cautious consideration of PCC has to do with what Bourdieu (1980/1990) called *habitus*. We and others have argued that when faced with illness or some other health-related situation, the actions we imagine ourselves taking are almost instinctual, based on our "common sense" about what should be done in this kind of situation (Lo and Stacey 2008; Shim 2010). Bourdieu conceptualizes this with his notion of *habitus*. He views human actors not always as deliberate and strategic individuals pursuing planned goals, but as possessing habitus, or general styles, habits, dispositions, and ways of thinking about, viewing, and being in the world. He argues that our general sensibilities about how the world works are deeply embodied, rooted in our past experiences, our socialization, and the kinds of worlds in which we have traveled throughout our lives. Habitus shapes the kinds of skills, styles, competencies, and resources—that is, the cultural capital—that one possesses and acquires. And habitus, in Bourdieu's view, indelibly influences the direction, manner, and shape of people's actions.

In the health-care context, we argue that each patient and provider involved in a clinical encounter possesses a specific habitus that guides his or her general styles of acting within that encounter. We very often pursue better health in largely *habitual* ways that are rooted in our experiences, long-lasting ways of thinking and organizing action, and our general sensibilities about how the world works. As such, the ways in which patients and providers interact with one another, and the kinds of actions we take to maintain our health, are often hybrids of purposeful actions *and* habitual, embodied ways of thinking and conducting our lives. Patients' varying abilities and inclinations to engage in proactive actions and participate and be involved in their own care and clinical interactions are rooted in their understandings of how one ought to take care of one's own health, how one ought to navigate social institutions and agents, and so on. A key contribution of CHC theory is, first, to understand habitus as emerging from one's biographical experiences as stratified by complex social and historical processes. Second, we conceptualize each provider as also possessing a habitus that will affect her or his relationship with patients. Providers' habitus is rooted in their upbringing, clinical training, socialization as doctors, and clinical experiences and the organizational contexts in which they work; it then generates personal perceptions and expectations around responsibility, good doctoring, and good patienthood (Dubbin, Chang, and Shim 2013).

To illustrate these points, we offer a vignette from our study that features a provider we call Dr. Alonzo and her patient, Alma. Alma is a sixty-two-year-old African American female who had been seeing Dr. Alonzo for about eight months after having been diagnosed with coronary artery disease. It was immediately clear from early on in their clinic visit that both patient and provider were "on the same page":

> Dr. Alonzo: What a gorgeous blood pressure you have!
> Alma: Yes, it's way down, huh! It's come down from this morning. At
> 7:30 it was 122!
> Dr. Alonzo: Excellent. So let's see. So we started the hydralazine when?
> Alma: I went to see Dr. X [her primary care provider] on the 28th.
> Dr. Alonzo: And there you go. Good. Excellent. So this is a very good
> drug for you. . . . And no side effects?
> Alma: No, no problems.
> Dr. Alonzo: Dizzy? Woozy? No fainting?
> Alma: No. I haven't felt any dizziness or anything. No swelling.
> Dr. Alonzo: Excellent!

In this interaction, Alma signals that she is an active and engaged player in her health care: she measures her own blood pressure on a regular basis (and possesses the knowledge to be able to interpret the results as clinically good), knows her medical and drug history, and pays attention to the expected side effects of her prescribed medications. Elsewhere during the visit, Alma also knew, for example, to explain her shortness of breath when lying down in terms of how many pillows she needed to prop herself up in order to sleep comfortably (this is a common and useful measure of cardiac symptomatology). When asked about her depression, she offered information about her sleeping, aware that difficulty with sleeping is a symptom of depression. Finally, she knew all of her multiple other medical providers and when she was going to see them next. Alma's mobilization, display, and communication of what she knows about her medical care, and how she takes care of her health, and her ability to convey this succinctly and efficiently, help to facilitate the back-and-forth and free-flowing nature of their clinical encounter. From Dr. Alonzo's perspective, the skills Alma displays place her in a special category of patients and generate more intimate feelings on the part of her physician: "[Alma] is one of the upper echelons of our patient groups. . . . There are patients who know exactly what she knew. It's not the majority. . . . At some level she must be highly involved in her own care. And she's bright enough to have been educated appropriately about what is going on with her."

Recall that one of the main pillars of PCC is to understand the patient in her biopsychosocial context, as an "experiencing" individual rather than an object or a disease. Providers are called on to learn how the patient interprets illness and its significance, as well as the culturally determined norms and beliefs she uses to understand, explain, describe, and predict illness. Alma's and Dr. Alonzo's relationship appears to exemplify the benefits of patients and providers mutually understanding one another and working together to make decisions about health care.

But one clear barrier to this patient-centered charge is the fact that providers bring their own habitus, their own assumptions about how the world should work, into their interactions with their patients. For example, let's hear from Dr. Alonzo on her individual communication style:

> I'm very focused, very forthright. I don't get into their private lives unless I think it relates to a compliance issue. For example, "How far do you walk on a flat surface?" "Well, I don't walk." "Why?" "Well, I live in [a dangerous neighborhood], and I'm afraid to go out." So that's relevant. Otherwise, I don't get into their personal lives. If they're visibly depressed, let's say, or I don't like the way they look, I'll explore that. . . . But other than that, I am a practitioner who is there to solve

a problem. I'm not saving the world. I'm not even helping people. I'm making them feel better, and thereby, they're being helped. But I'm basically a problem solver. So I'm very direct. I have specific questions that will answer specific issues that I need to get at. . . . If I had to characterize my approach, it would be matter-of-fact. . . . I'm not a waffler. If I waffle about an issue, it's because there are no data that I can use to apply to the issue. . . . I think most patients, regardless of what they say . . . most patients really do want the doctors to be making the decisions.

Dr. Alonzo's description of her general style emerges from her habitus—in Bourdieu's parlance—which in turn is rooted in her upbringing, training, and socialization as a clinician, her own past experiences of doctoring, and the particulars of the health-care organization in which she works. That is, rather than her approach being simply about her personality, her disposition is the product of multiple social and cultural forces that permeate and shape her social position vis-à-vis race, class, and gender, her professional worlds, and the exigencies of the institution in which she practices. The notion of habitus not only extends an understanding of the origins of Dr. Alonzo's particular style or habitus, but also points to its consequences for the role she plays in her patients' care and the nature of their relationship:

I believe I will be able to get most of them better. . . . And I'll tell them up-front, I can get you better. And we do. . . . [But they have to] comply. That's it. They have to comply; they have to believe that I know what I'm talking about. They can argue. But they do have to comply. And I have actually told patients—and there are certain specific patient groups who need more telling than others—that look, if you want to do it your way, we're done. And I'll offer them another provider. And usually, that'll be enough to get 'em doing it my way.

For Alma's part, in the clinic visit we observed and our interview with her, she displayed an impressive and extremely detailed command of her medical history, from the dates of health-related events to her medications and their dosages (even to the point of catching a pharmacy labeling error), to the different disease processes that she is experiencing and their effects on her body, to the values of her various lab tests. Yet she clearly defers to Dr. Alonzo: "I would not think of challenging her perspectives at all. I think she's expert at her job, and that's what I think of her, as being the expert. . . . I haven't found a need to question her, because . . . before she changes things, I think she has put a lot of consideration into it. . . . She's not just doing things at whim. She's really looking into the changes that she's proposing, and she's not putting me in any jeopardy. I feel safe in her care."

In our study we found that all of our physician participants, like Dr. Alonzo, held highly engrained and taken-for-granted expectations of the CHC elements their patients, at minimum, should use to help move the interaction forward. We argue that these expectations around responsibility and good patienthood are generated from providers' habitus, which in turn is rooted in their stratified social experiences as racialized, classed, and gendered individuals, their clinical training and socialization, and the organizational contexts in which they work.

Alma's example shows that she clearly demonstrates some agency in her interactions with Dr. Alonzo. Yet given the extent of her health-related knowledge, attention to detail, and command of her medical history and the particulars of her medical conditions, it is also clear that she possesses the potential to exercise significantly more agency than she does. In the end, it is Dr. Alonzo who appears to exert the most control over the decisions that are made regarding medications, symptom management, and treatment. While Alma willingly defers to Dr. Alonzo's expert opinions, this deference and Dr. Alonzo's habituated expectations of her patients and their relationships with her demonstrate that the provider determines what cultural resources—what kinds of CHC— hold value for her in the first place. Through their expectations for the kinds of CHC patients need to have in order to optimize the clinical encounter, providers possess unequal power in that they set the rules of the game.

Thus there are two conceptual contributions that habitus makes to analyzing health-care interactions. The first concerns patients. The kinds of attributes that define an activated, engaged, and health-literate patient are not simply skills that people can just pick up. Habitus is the product of one's social experiences, and those social experiences are highly stratified. This in turn means that the kinds of actions people engage in, the questions they have, the kinds of information that they want and don't want when faced with illness, how they go about managing their illness, whether they even think about a disease as something to be "managed" or whether it is simply something to be borne—all of these are socially stratified as well.

Second, we argue that the existence of provider habitus, and its impact on shaping expectations about patients' responsibilities and behaviors, means that the provider possesses disproportionate power to set the rules of the interaction, that is, the kinds of CHC that are valued and the specific gains to patients who deploy them. Thus the patient-centered charge to get to know the patient in her biopsychosocial context ignores that this context is set on top of a landscape that is already shaped and structured by power and inequality.

Interactional asymmetry emerges from the power of the provider—as a representative of the medical profession and backed by its legitimacy—to define the kinds of knowledge and understandings that are seen as valid and, as importantly, to determine the relative weight of that value in terms of subsequent actions generated. As in the example of Alma and Dr. Alonzo, the attention and care that the providers offer may actually constitute rewards given in response to how well the patients have displayed and deployed their repertoire of cultural skills. That is, their interactions can be seen as social transactions, and CHC underscores the significance of the *work* that cultural resources *do* in these transactions. Having a sense of initiative, the ability to take action to manage one's health, and knowledge and health literacy—all of these resources of the activated and engaged patient operate both directly and indirectly. Patients with significant CHC can *directly* facilitate communication and appropriate treatment. But CHC also operates *indirectly*, by positively influencing providers' perceptions of patients, generating "cascades" of subsequent actions that may enhance care. In these senses, CHC functions as symbolic capital, as a form of capital that patients accrue, and that brings them approval and rewards in the form of deeper relationships with their providers and more attentive care. It is this dual nature of CHC, as an instrumental *and* symbolic form of capital, that offers a conceptual elaboration of what it takes to achieve patient-centered care.

VIGNETTE #2. DR. DEANGELO AND MARIEL: COMPLICATING SHARED UNDERSTANDING

For the second vignette, we introduce Dr. Deangelo and Mariel. Mariel immigrated to the United States late in her life and lives in one of the poorest and most dangerous neighborhoods in San Francisco. She suffers from severe congestive heart failure and has been through a number of major cardiac procedures and surgeries that led to severe postoperative complications whose long-term effects substantially impinge on her present life. Her mobility is limited, she requires oxygen to breathe, she must undergo dialysis several times a week, and she uses a wheelchair. For these reasons, she and her husband have discussed with Dr. Deangelo the risks of any further interventions. As Dr. Deangelo explained to us:

> [Mariel] and her husband and I have talked many times about how there may be times when people will bring up the notion of maybe we should do another surgery some day and how do you feel about that and we're all in absolute agreement that we're not going back there. . . . I think it's very high risk for her to consider anything like that unless there's really something very different. . . . She's just barely riding above the waves here and she's going to get splashed from time to time and one of these times she's going to die but she's okay with that and so am I, compared to putting her through another huge process that would completely mean she'd never be able to be functional again. I'm just not going to do that to her and she doesn't want it either. . . . I hope I'm not wrong but I do truly believe (a) it's what she wants, and (b) I think it's the right thing. I would make that decision in her shoes too. . . . She's great now compared to [after the surgery]. . . . She's in a very high-mortality end stage and she's doing great with what she's got and I'm not going to take that away from her.

Dr. Deangelo then mentions that Mariel's current symptoms have put her in the emergency room occasionally and that for Dr. Deangelo, the crux of the issue is to preempt the ER staff from doing additional procedures on Mariel: "So I'll get these panicked calls from [another facility's ER], . . . 'We think we ought to do an infusion study because maybe we ought to recath her and maybe we ought to—' And I'm like, 'No, no. No, don't do it. Get her feeling better and send her to me.'"

As Dr. Deangelo perceives it, Mariel's experience of such episodes is that the ER doctors "'were going to do these things and they called you [Dr. Deangelo] and then I got to go home.' And she [Mariel] was so happy." While Dr. Deangelo acknowledges that Mariel has significant cardiac problems, she resists any further diagnostic testing or interventions: "Can we control it medically without going through all this testing and stuff? I don't care. Don't do a nuclear test on her. I don't care what the results are. It's not going to change what I feel that she needs."

For her part, Mariel's understanding is that Dr. Deangelo "told me not to allow anybody to do something in my heart because I will die." Thus at one point, she was scheduled for a cardiac procedure, but then canceled it: "So

I said, no, I'm not going. I cannot accept the procedure. . . . [The hospital] called here, and I said, 'No, I am not going because my doctor, my cardiologist does not allow me to put something in my heart.'" Yet on the other hand, she related that she had had a defibrillator implanted when Dr. Deangelo was on vacation and unable to consult with her and her husband: "When they put the defibrillator, I asked the cardiologist . . . if it's okay for me to put this one, and he said, it's okay. Because Dr. Deangelo is on vacation, I cannot talk to her. . . . My husband was crying because he's scared of putting this one because he knows Dr. Deangelo don't like any procedure to be done. But I signed [the consent form allowing surgery]." At other times in our interview with her, Mariel spoke about her doctors being "the expert," of acceding to their recommendations, and also of her husband making health-care decisions on her behalf.

It is impossible to know whether, if Dr. Deangelo had been available for a consultation, she would have recommended for or against the defibrillator, and ultimately what Mariel's decision would then have been. However, it does seem that Mariel, in this case, consented to a procedure that she (and her husband) anticipated that Dr. Deangelo would not recommend. Given this, we find ourselves wondering about the extent to which Mariel and Dr. Deangelo are fully on the same page about Mariel's preferences regarding additional interventions.

We offer this vignette as an example of the complexity and often deep ambivalence that surrounds what it means to have "shared understanding," the second pillar of PCC. According to this principle, providers are to solicit and understand the patient's concerns, interests, needs, and preferences in order to come to a shared understanding of the clinical condition and the treatment options desired. On the one hand, Dr. Deangelo is clearly motivated by what she believes to be Mariel's preferences and needs, unique to who she is as an individual and to the exigencies of her current medical condition and prognosis. Dr. Deangelo clearly cares for Mariel, whom she described as "a favorite patient." Dr. Deangelo has come to know Mariel's family well. She is impressed by Mariel's positive attitude, her close social network, and her willingness to manage multiple complex health issues, especially given the barriers and limitations she faces. Dr. Deangelo frequently reminded Mariel of her commitment to support her in any way she could.

But for Mariel, this long and committed relationship she has with Dr. Deangelo, the trust that she has in her doctors' judgments, along with the intimate partnership she has with her husband—all inevitably complicate any notions of *a patient's* (in the singular) understanding of her own needs and preferences, the clinical condition, and the treatment options. Moreover, in this case as in our larger study, we also found that "shared understanding" was often equated to "shared *biomedical* understanding." Instances of and efforts to build shared understanding were most often predicated on *patients* sharing *providers' biomedical* understandings of the clinical condition and treatment options, rather than the converse or a hybridized understanding. Based on Mariel's description of the decision about the defibrillator implantation, it may be that Mariel's preferences and Dr. Deangelo's preferences were not as consonant as Dr. Deangelo believes. Indeed, in decisions that were made with Dr. Deangelo's involvement, the interpretation and rendition of Mariel's preferences that seems to predominate is Dr. Deangelo's. That is, shared understandings seem to facilitate patient-centered care when *patients* (may come to) share *providers' biomedical* understandings, and may obscure more equivocal situations in which patients may not fully agree with their providers.

Cultural health capital theory points out the transactional nature of health-care interactions, even in those that may otherwise evince characteristics of PCC. Mariel and Dr. Deangelo's relationship is only one of many patient-provider interactions we witnessed in our study that appeared to be based on a mutual understanding of the goals and methods of treatment, and therefore exemplary of patient-centered care. Yet in the history of their relationship, we found instances that seemed to belie a complete affinity, motivating questions about the extent to which understandings of an illness or condition can truly be shared among two individuals who come from different backgrounds and have unequal power in the relationship. When patients and their families appear to share providers' definition of the situation, then, CHC theory suggests that this effects both material and symbolic functions in a cyclical way, not only facilitating medical decision making and the provision of care but also causing providers to be favorably disposed toward certain patients, and in turn shaping further inclinations to provide care. Shared understanding is clearly an outcome that is sought under the PCC approach, but as we can see in the example of Maribel and Dr. Deangelo—whose apparent harmony may belie a more complicated ambivalence—it is not altogether clear how and when it can be and is achieved. Instead, "shared understanding" is a complicated interactional process to be continually orchestrated, and a quality of value that can be leveraged by patients and providers, though to unequal degrees and with often asymmetrical effects. That is, shared understanding is a negotiated process and achievement, one that takes place on an uneven playing field, making this aspect of PCC potentially difficult to realize even in "good" patient-provider relationships.

VIGNETTE #3. AHMAD AND DR. CRANE: PCC AND THE REPRODUCTION OF INEQUALITY

In our third vignette from the clinic, we turn to Ahmad and his cardiologist, Dr. Crane. Ahmad is a sixty-three-year-old man who has been seeing Dr. Crane for several years. He has a history of coronary artery disease, and on the day we met him, he had a regular cardiology appointment with Dr. Crane as part of his periodic follow-up after having some cardiac procedures done. It was obvious from the clinic visit and our separate interviews with both provider and patient that Ahmad and Dr. Crane have a congenial relationship. Dr. Crane describes him as follows: "He's a really nice guy . . . fantastic. . . . He has a nice manner. I try to take good care of everybody, but obviously there's certain personalities that are just easier and it probably depends on the provider. Every provider is going to do better with a certain kind of patient. Ahmad is very inquisitive about his condition but at the same time he doesn't let off lots of stress vibes or what have you. . . . He's very aware of himself and he's not a nervous Nellie but at the same time when he feels something he tells me about it so he's just really easy to work with." Here, Dr. Crane notes in particular that what makes Ahmad "really easy to work with" is not just the types of knowledge or expertise he has, but also his approach to solving problems, an ability to learn new ways of thinking about symptoms, and a well-calibrated awareness of himself and his symptoms.

At this particular appointment, Dr. Crane and Ahmad spent some time discussing what he was doing to maintain his cardiovascular health. They reviewed his cholesterol, which was "perfect" according to Dr. Crane; Ahmad volunteered, "Even my diet, I'm just taking care of that too"; and Dr. Crane inquired about his exercise habits, to which Ahmad replied that he worked out for thirty minutes five days a week. The majority of the appointment was taken up with their discussion of the results of a follow-up imaging test Dr. Crane had ordered to try to ascertain the source of some cardiac symptoms Ahmad was experiencing. The next steps to be taken hinged on whether he was still experiencing the symptoms or not: if he was, then additional, more aggressive testing procedures could be prescribed; but if he was not, then another, less invasive follow-up test could be done nonemergently.

At one point during their interaction, Dr. Crane asked, "You said you're still getting some symptoms there," to which Ahmad agreed, "Some symptoms, yeah." But in short order Dr. Crane explained:

> Dr. Crane: The way that I was thinking about things, coming in this morning was, if you are having symptoms right now, then probably the best thing to do is another catheterization, and just take a look at your heart arteries and see what's going on. But you said you're not, you're feeling pretty good.
>
> Ahmad: Yeah. I'm okay.
>
> Dr. Crane: So probably what we should do is, I'll get hold of them and see . . . what other tests they were thinking about doing, just to be on the safe side long-term. And then we could order one of those for you. Would you want to do that?
>
> Ahmad: Yeah. No problem, yeah.

It remains somewhat unclear from this exchange whether Ahmad was still experiencing those symptoms at the time of his visit with Dr. Crane. Ahmad may have simply been confirming that he no longer experiences symptoms, or he may have been acceding to her interpretation of the present situation, or maybe he discerned that his symptoms did not rise to the level of warranting the more immediate test. Then again, he might also have wished to have the additional testing done to give him peace of mind about his symptoms, which apparently had persisted for some time. In any case, Dr. Crane inferred that his symptoms were no longer an issue and that therefore they were justified in proceeding with the less aggressive route.

We highlight this vignette of Ahmad and Dr. Crane to reflect on the third pillar of patient-centered care, which is the notion of shared power and responsibility. Health care is envisioned as collaboration between a patient and provider rather than just the provider giving directions and the patient receiving them. Under the patient-centered construct, the health-care relationship shifts from an asymmetric "top-down" model, where patients are passive players, to one in which they are viewed as active and discerning consumers of care. And sharing power goes hand-in-hand with the promotion of greater patient involvement and responsibility in their own health.

Indeed, Ahmad and Dr. Crane's relationship can be said to be one in which they have shared power and responsibility. Dr. Crane took pains to explain her thinking with Ahmad and to ascertain that he (seemed to have) understood and agreed with this assessment and course of action. Moreover,

Dr. Crane spoke to us extensively about how she and Ahmad's other providers "taught him what things to look out for and so on . . . and then he's able to incorporate knowledge." She recounted that in turn, this enables her to go through her reasoning step by step with patients like Ahmad, rather than simply telling them what her medical recommendations are and implementing them. Dr. Crane's collaborative efforts, Ahmad's ready receptiveness to the plan, and Dr. Crane's fostering of Ahmad's knowledge about his condition all appear to evince a patient-provider relationship that is more of a partnership than a hierarchy.

On the other hand, though, Dr. Crane's actions and talk both implicitly and explicitly induce particular types of patient behaviors that the *physician* finds valuable, communicating not only the type of actor a patient *can* be, but the type of actor the patient *ought to* be. For example, she compliments him on his lowered cholesterol, his regular exercise habits, his dietary controls, and she tells us how easy it is to problem-solve and work with him. Ahmad reports his symptoms as she would like them to be reported (neither exaggerated as by "a nervous Nellie" nor downplayed), and assents or consents to her interpretation of the facts and the ways in which they dictate their future course of action. A patient-centered approach then does not necessarily relieve the asymmetry of the interaction; rather, asymmetry is being accomplished and reinforced in a different way.

Hence, the concept of CHC sheds light on how relationships of power are produced and reproduced during clinical interactions. It reminds us that, as patient-centered as these interactions may seem, the rules of the game are not necessarily being rewritten. CHC highlights how all exchanges are situated encounters between individuals endowed with socially structured and differentially distributed resources and competencies. As Kittay compellingly demonstrates (chapter 4, this volume), differently positioned individuals with distinctive forms and amounts of cultural, social, and symbolic capital are subject to different trajectories of medical care and experiences. Power relations, and the accumulation, exchange, and mobilization of capital, are endemic to all interactions, including clinical ones. Thus while PCC promotes the ideal of an egalitarian patient-provider relationship, CHC reminds us that the underlying architecture of the power relations at play structures the grounds on which interactions unfold.

CONCLUSION

In sum, customizing care to the individualized needs, preferences, and concerns of patients is fundamental to the construct of patient-centered care as a matter of moral and ethical practice, fairness, beneficence, and respect for the autonomy of the patient. These qualities make PCC not only a very attractive model but also a seemingly intuitive way to practice medicine. We believe, however, that the concept of CHC casts a wider net in illuminating the interactional power dynamics that precede, underlie, and go beyond PCC. CHC emphasizes that cultural resources and attributes influence patients' and providers' mutually shaped abilities to achieve PCC. In the examples of apparently smoothly functioning patient-provider relationships that we have described in this chapter, much is going on below the surface that is subject to power relations, and the structurally unequal distribution of CHC suffuses even these "good" interactions. Through the lens of CHC, we see that the achievement of PCC depends on the *providers'* perceptions and expectations of what counts as good patienthood. Patients appear to exercise relatively little control on this count. Providers define the kinds of resources, behaviors, and skills that have value for them, as well as the relative weight that value has, and in so doing, they exert greater control over the trajectories of subsequent care and attention their patients receive. This implicit process of "valuation" ultimately produces an encounter that maintains its asymmetric nature. By analytically defining CHC as a means of exchange—a differentially distributed resource—it becomes clear that the mileage a given person gets from CHC depends on who they are and where they are positioned in a stratified social field; how they obtained it; where, when, and how they deploy it; who receives it; and the actions that subsequently stem from it. Therefore, the effects of social inequalities such as race, class, gender, and other markers of social status may be reflected in the amount and types of CHC one has access to and is able to deploy, and its relative "purchasing power." In this way, we argue that using CHC as a lens to examine the practices of patient-centeredness brings us to a deeper appreciation of the often subtle dynamics that shape the achievement of justice in health care.

We began this chapter by pointing out the opportunities we have as we move forward with the Affordable Care Act and its many provisions that promise to expand access, improve quality—especially for our most vulnerable and sickest populations—and reduce health disparities. Yet at the same time, there are strong currents that run against the achievement of health equity. As we have discussed, some of them are embedded in the ACA itself, couched in language that cultivates and promotes a discourse of virtuous patienthood. Other currents contributing to the imperative to be the activated, engaged, and health literate patient are taking place in the wider world of medicine in the information age. The widespread impetus toward electronic health records, digital and mobile interventions, constant self-surveillance, and the notion that more knowledge equals better health—all of these are adding to the demands of patienthood.[2] All told, these lead to serious concerns about the effect of patient-centeredness—conceived of as individualized, customized, and tailor-made medicine—on displacing attention from the group-based, population-based, race-based, class-based, gender-based, and other relations of power that continue to stratify all aspects of our capacities to care, from community care, to family care, to self-care, to health care.

This coming age of precision medicine, of electronic infrastructures, of big data and data for everyone, gives the appearance of democratization, inclusion, and better health for all. Yet as this chapter attempts to illustrate, the kind of patienthood that is requisite to participate in this new health-care landscape—somewhat countered by the ACA, yet also enforced and endorsed by it—is elusive for many, and the reasons for this are both deep and hidden. Therefore we want to close with a call to interrogate the rhetoric celebrating individual autonomy (see also Kittay, chapter 4, this volume) and equality that seeks to elide and flatten asymmetries between patients and providers and among different populations of patients. Policy agendas fashioned on notions of patient centeredness, patient engagement, and patient activation partake of and gain momentum from such equalizing rhetorics. Using cultural health capital as a sensitizing concept, we hope to continue to ask questions about the extent to which calls to inclusion and solidarity belie and efface the politics of inequality.

NOTES

The authors deeply thank the physicians and patients who participated in our study and shared their thoughts and experiences with us. We also gratefully acknowledge the editors of this volume for their thoughtful comments and careful reviews of this chapter. The study on which this chapter was based was supported by the American Sociological Association Fund for the Advancement of the Discipline, and an intramural grant from the UCSF School of Nursing Research Committee. The second and third authors are listed in random order.

1. The six aims of high-quality care identified by the Institute of Medicine are safety, effectiveness, patient-centeredness, timeliness, efficiency, and equity.

2. See, for example, Topol 2012.

REFERENCES

Balsa, Ana I., and Thomas G. McGuire. 2001. "Statistical Discrimination in Health Care."
Journal of Health Economics 20 (6): 881–907.

———. 2003. "Prejudice, Clinical Uncertainty and Stereotyping as Sources of Health
Disparities." *Journal of Health Economics* 22 (1): 89–116.

Balsa, Ana I., Thomas G. McGuire, and Lisa S. Meredith. 2005. "Testing for Statistical
Discrimination in Health Care." *Health Services Research* 40 (1): 227–52.

Bernabeo, Elizabeth, and Eric S. Holmboe. 2013. "Patients, Providers, and Systems Need
to Acquire a Specific Set of Competencies to Achieve Truly Patient-Centered Care."
Health Affairs 32 (2): 250–58.

Bourdieu, Pierre. 1980/1990. *The Logic of Practice.* Stanford, CA: Stanford University
Press.

———. 1983/1986. "The Forms of Capital." In *Handbook of Theory and Research for the
Sociology of Education,* edited by J. G. Richardson, 241–58. New York: Greenwood.

Charmaz, Kathy. 2006. *Constructing Grounded Theory: A Practical Guide through
Qualitative Analysis.* Los Angeles: Sage.

Cooper, Lisa A., Mary Catherine Beach, Rachel L. Johnson, and Thomas S. Inui. 2006.
"Delving below the Surface: Understanding How Race and Ethnicity Influence
Relationships in Health Care." *Journal of General Internal Medicine* 21 (S1): S21–27.

Coulter, Angela. 2011. *Engaging Patients in Healthcare.* New York: McGraw-Hill.

Dubbin, Leslie A., Jamie Suki Chang, and Janet K. Shim. 2013. "Cultural Health Capital
and the Interactional Dynamics of Patient-Centered Care." *Social Science and Medicine*
93: 113–20.

Epstein, Ronald M., Kevin Fiscella, Cara S. Lesser, and Kurt C. Stange. 2010. "Why the
Nation Needs a Policy Push on Patient-Centered Health Care." *Health Affairs* 29 (8):
1489–95.

Epstein, Ronald M., Peter Franks, Kevin Fiscella, Cleveland G. Shields, Sean C. Meldrum,
Richard L. Kravitz, and Paul R. Duberstein. 2005. "Measuring Patient-Centered
Communication in Patient-Physician Consultations: Theoretical and Practical Issues."
Social Science and Medicine 61: 1516–28.

Freidson, Eliot. 1970. *The Profession of Medicine: A Study of the Sociology of Applied
Knowledge.* New York: Harper and Row.

———. 1986. *Professional Powers: A Study of the Institutionalization of Formal Knowledge.*
Chicago: University of Chicago Press.

———. 1994. *Professionalism Reborn: Theory, Prophecy, and Policy.* Chicago: University of
Chicago Press.

Gerteis, Margaret, Susan Edgman-Levitan, Jennifer Daley, and Thomas Delbanco. 1993.
Through the Patient's Eyes: Understanding and Promoting Patient-Centered Care. San
Francisco: Jossey-Bass.

Gillespie, Rosemarie, Dominique Florin, and Steve Gillam. 2004. "How Is Patient-
Centred Care Understood by the Clinical, Managerial and Lay Stakeholders
Responsible for Promoting This Agenda?" *Health Expectations* 7 (2): 142–48.

Heritage, John, and Douglas Maynard, eds. 2006. *Communication in Medical Care: Interactions between Primary Care Physicians and Patients.* Cambridge: Cambridge University Press.

Hibbard, Judith H., Jessica Greene, and Valerie Overton. 2013. "Patients with Lower Activation Associated with Higher Costs: Delivery Systems Should Know Their Patients' 'Scores.'" *Health Affairs* 32 (2): 216–22.

Institute for Healthcare Improvement. 2013. "The IHI Triple Aim." August 1. http://www.ihi.org/offerings/Initiatives/TripleAim/Pages/default.aspx.

Institute of Medicine. 2001. *Crossing the Quality Chasm: A New Health System for the 21st Century.* Washington, DC: National Academies Press.

Kish, Leonard. 2012. "The Blockbuster Drug of the Century: An Engaged Patient." *HL7 Standards.* August 28. http://www.hl7standards.com/blog/2012/08/28/drug-of-the-century/. Accessed 5 September 2013.

Lo, Ming-cheng M., and Clare L. Stacey. 2008. "Beyond Cultural Competency: Bourdieu, Patients and Clinical Encounters." *Sociology of Health and Illness* 30 (5): 741–55.

McGuire, Thomas G., John Z. Ayanian, Daniel E. Ford, Rachel E. M. Henke, Kathryn M. Rost, and Ala M. Zaslevsky. 2008. "Testing for Statistical Discrimination by Race/Ethnicity in Panel Data for Depression Treatment in Primary Care." *Health Services Research* 43 (2): 531–51.

Mead, Nicola, and Bower, Peter. 2000. "Patient-Centredness: A Conceptual Framework and Review of the Empirical Literature." *Social Science and Medicine* 51 (7): 1087–1110.

Navarro, Vicente. 1980. "Work, Ideology, and Science: The Case of Medicine." *International Journal of Health Services* 10 (4): 523–50.

———. 1986. *Crisis, Health and Medicine.* New York: Tavistock.

Parsons, Talcott. 1951. *The Social System.* New York: Free Press.

———. 1975. "The Sick Role and Role of the Physician Reconsidered." *The Milbank Memorial Fund Quarterly – Health and Society* 53 (3): 257–78.

Shim, Janet K. 2010. "Cultural Health Capital: A Theoretical Approach to Understanding Health Care Interactions and the Dynamics of Unequal Treatment." *Journal of Health and Social Behavior* 51 (1): 1–15.

Stewart, Anita L., Anna Napoles-Springer, Eliseo J. Perez-Stable, Samuel F. Posner, Andrew B. Bindman, Howard L. Pinderhughes, and A. Eugene Washington. 1999. "Interpersonal Processes of Care in Diverse Populations." *Milbank Quarterly* 77 (3): 305–39.

Stewart, Moira, Judith Brown, Wayne Weston, Ian McWhinney, Carol McWilliam, and Thomas Freeman. 2003. *Patient-Centered Medicine: Transforming the Clinical Method.* London: Sage.

Topol, Eric. 2012. *The Creative Destruction of Medicine: How the Digital Revolution Will Create Better Health Care.* New York: Basic Books.

Waitzkin, Howard. 1989. "Social Structures of Medical Oppression: A Marxist View." In *Perspectives in Medical Sociology,* edited by P. Brown, 166–78. Belmont, CA: Waveland Press.

Wanzer, Melissa B., Melanie Booth-Butterfield, and Kelly Gruber. 2004. "Perceptions of Health Care Providers' Communication: Relationships between Patient-Communication and Satisfaction." *Health Communication* 16 (3): 363–84.

West, Candace. 1984. *Routine Complications: Troubles with Talk between Doctors and Patients*. Indianapolis: Indiana University Press.

Wilkins, Steve. 2012. "Patient Engagement Is the Holy Grail of Health Care." *KevinMD*, January 27. http://www.kevinmd.com/blog/2012/01/patient-engagement-holy-grail-health-care.html. Accessed 5 September 2013.

10

Racial Health Disparities and Questions of Evidence

What Went Wrong with Healthy People 2010

Carolyn Moxley Rouse

ABSTRACT

The United States Healthy People 2010 initiative was directed toward the elimination of racial and ethnic health disparities. While racial and ethnic disparities are complex, the health of black Americans continues to fall short of the national average. By focusing on the presumptions embedded in the design of health disparities research, this essay addresses why Healthy People 2010 largely failed to reduce racial health inequality. Importantly, in thinking about health inequalities, researchers initially failed to consider how race is socially constructed; how data collection is never value-neutral; and, finally, the limits of randomized control trials when it comes to making sense of complex behavioral and structural data. The chapter ends by describing how ethnographic insights can help complicate the assumptions and conclusions of health disparities research.

INTRODUCTION

Healthy People initiatives began in 1979 and continues to be led by the U.S. Department of Health and Human Services. Essentially an institution-led crusade, Healthy People was designed to focus nationally funded health research and care on achieving a set of nationwide goals. Every ten years the goals of the initiative are redrafted by policy leaders. The overarching goals of Healthy People 2000, for example, included the *reduction of health disparities*, while the 2010 goals included the *elimination of racial and ethnic health disparities*. The 2020 goals, in contrast, included the *achievement of health equity*.[1] The changes to the mission statement seem on the surface to be absurdly trivial, and in many respects they are. Federal health policy mandates are generated by committees and therefore represent, particularly from the perspective of committee members, watered-down compromise positions rather than concise intellectual framings of a problem.[2] Cynically, one could dismiss U.S. health policy at the federal level as unreflexive bureaucratic folly, beholden to political power and therefore incapable of producing anything of value for the public. Less cynically, committees are composed of experts with knowledge of the newest policy concerns, data-driven analyses, and approaches to knowledge production. Individual committee members may not have the agency to shape policy, but collectively their expertise produces informed and relevant incremental changes to health policy.

This chapter highlights an emergent common wisdom, at times provisional, that altered the way health policy experts understood racial health disparities. In other words, changes in wording to Healthy People 2020 mark trivial but also substantive changes to the questions being asked, the quality and types of data collected, and the policy implications. Notably, the redrafted Healthy People 2020 dropped the *elimination of racial and ethnic health disparities* even though disparities still exist and continue to be included in the United States data (CDC 2011). Tracing the dissolution of the goal to eliminate racial and ethnic health disparities and replace it with the objective of *health equity* provides some lessons about the relational aspects of health-care justice.

After President Clinton announced that the Healthy People 2010 initiative would focus on eliminating health disparities by 2010, the number of published articles on the topic grew from 35 in 1998 to 1,550 in 2010.[3] The research necessary to produce these articles would not have been possible without the extraordinary levels of federal funding directed at health disparities research following Clinton's 1998 announcement. The amount of funding spent between 2000 and 2010 on research, reporting, and initiatives directed at reducing treatment inequities at the federal, state, and local levels would be difficult to quantify. But one could easily estimate that more than $1 billion was spent by Health and Human Services alone.[4] By some estimates the amount reached $3 billion (Sankar et al. 2004). What was gained from this enormous expenditure? This chapter argues that a decade of trial and error, and occasional brilliant research, led to improvements in how disparities data is collected, interpreted, and reported.

When we review the history of the initiative, several things stand out. In the early years, there were methodological concerns about whether organizing disparities by race and ethnicity was the best approach to ameliorating health differentials. On top of that, there were growing concerns about whether our nation's most powerful health-care institutions should be concerned with improving the health of identified groups ahead of the health of the entire nation, and, if so, who should decide which groups deserved consideration. If institutions should be focused on improving the health of the entire nation, how should we organize our data such that racial, regional, gender, and/or ethnic health disparities are not made invisible? Since Healthy People 2010 targeted groups, a postmortem of the initiative provides some insights as to whether such a focus was just or effective.

What we find is that funding for Healthy People 2010 encouraged states to organize efforts toward eliminating disparities, and between 1999 and 2009 the black-white life expectancy gap closed by about 2.7 years for men (to a difference of 5.4 years), and by about 1.7 years for women (to a difference of 3.8 years) (Harper, MacLehose, and Kaufman 2014). The numbers are impressive, but looking closely at the data one notices that states like New York showed significant improvements, whereas California did not. Epidemiologists concluded that the gap narrowed largely because of improved HIV/AIDS treatments and lower homicide rates, which significantly reduced black mortality. At the same time, white life expectancy slowed because of increased drug overdose deaths (Case and Deaton 2015; Harper, MacLehose, and Kaufman 2014). Racial disparities in cancer survival, infant mortality, rates of HIV/AIDS infection, and deaths due to cardiovascular disease, diabetes, and kidney disease persisted (Kochanek et al. 2011).

Reading the studies and reports published during those ten years, it is clear that medical researchers became increasingly aware that race and ethnicity are social constructs and that scientific data is neither ethics- nor value-neutral. Recognizing that disparities are traceable to a number of different causes, Dr. Thomas Frieden, who took over as director of the CDC in 2009, helped institute a new approach to the study and representation of disparities. Healthy People 2020 correlates state-by-state health data with other types of relevant data. Notably, *creating environments that promote health* has displaced *eliminating racial and ethnic health disparities* as one of the overarching goals. The rationale is that equity is achievable if policy experts focus on regional population health. So the question remains: Why did concerns about racial and ethnic disparities get supplanted or reframed? What went wrong, or right, such that categorizing health disparities only by race and ethnicity no longer made sense? Was a focus on race and ethnicity politically unviable given the nation's desire to be postracial? The best way to address these questions is to return to the motivations behind Healthy People 2010. Surgeon General David Satcher who, under the leadership of President Bill Clinton, helped draft the goals, wrote, "Both the life expectancy and the overall health of Americans have improved greatly over the last century, but not all Americans are benefiting equally from advances in health prevention and technology. There is compelling evidence that race and ethnicity correlate with persistent health disparities in the burden of illness and death" (Satcher 2001, 1).

In order to communicate to the public why racial and ethnic disparities should matter to all Americans, Satcher often highlighted six key disparities, including HIV/AIDS, immunization rates, cardiovascular disease, diabetes, cancer, and infant mortality. Health disparities, Satcher argued, were the canaries in the coal mine indicating that America had yet to fulfill its providence as the land of equal opportunity. But trying to convince Americans that national resources should be directed toward improving the health of minorities was no small task. In addition to selling the goals to the public, the scientific community had to convince politicians that both the problems and the solutions could be framed scientifically rather than emotionally or politically. Given this imperative, randomized control trials, metadata analyses, and other robust statistical approaches became the most valued research. While more qualitative studies (Ethical, Legal, and Social Implications approaches) continued to receive funding, the data from statistical methods were envisaged to give rise to evidence-based interventions that, if adopted, could presumably equalize health outcomes.

Healthy People 2010 had over 969 health objectives, of which 169 were specifically directed at reducing racial and ethnic disparities. The data from Healthy People 2010 are now in (NCHS 2012). According to the Centers for Disease Control (CDC), of the 969 objectives only 75.6 percent had the available tracking data necessary for proper assessment. Using these data, the CDC concluded that 23 percent of the objectives had been met or were exceeded and 49 percent were on their way to being met (NCHS 2012).

Of the 169 objectives directed specifically at eliminating racial and ethnic health disparities, 117, or 69 percent, showed no change. Of the remaining 52 objectives, about half showed increases in disparities, and the other half showed decreases, which means 16 percent of the goals were met.[5] There were some wonderful achievements, such as a substantial reduction in deaths due to coronary heart disease. Unfortunately, the successes were counterbalanced by significant failures, including persistently high rates of black infant mortality and a significant rise in new cases of diabetes for people under sixty-four years of age. Of Satcher's six primary health disparities, immunization rates showed the most improvement. Overall, the two groups that benefited the most from Healthy People 2010 were Asian or Pacific Islanders and non-Hispanic whites. Native groups and non-Hispanic blacks benefited the least. The CDC's final conclusion was that health disparities persist.

So why did over $1 billion dollars of targeted research and program funding fail to eliminate health disparities? To answer this question I begin by focusing on several key publications that offer significant lessons about statistical rhetoric in health disparities research. By statistical rhetoric, I mean the ways in which data are interpreted to make particular political points far beyond what the data legitimately can prove (Best 2012; King, chapter 8, this volume). I then use my own ethnographic research to help explain why the Healthy People 2010 data did not capture how race and racialized signifiers operate in the clinic. Finally, I discuss the Affordable Care Act (ACA) and how the demands of the ACA have forced researchers to attend to both the health of the nation and the health of communities.

THE SOCIAL CONSTRUCTION OF RACE AND HEALTH

Anthropologists and sociologists have written extensively and comparatively on the emergence of racial and ethnic groupings around the world (Barth 1968; Boas 1940; Loveman, Muniz, and Bailey 2011). From the paleontological record we know that the delineation between racial groupings has historically been gradual rather than sharp and that genetic diversity within racial groups is greater than that between groups (Cavalli-Sforza, Menozzi, and Piazza 1994). Given increasing global migration and intermarriage, understanding racial and ethnic boundaries requires complex tools of social analysis (Wimmer 2013). In multiracial and multiethnic societies, census checkboxes are simply incapable of capturing the diversity of opinions, beliefs, behaviors, and genetics even within populations. This means that the borders we draw around groups are arbitrary and often nonsensical (Fuentes 2012).

At the same time, in societies where people are organized phenotypically, for example under slavery and Jim Crow, those who look alike often experience similar treatment and as a result often develop shared values and cultural norms. Under less extreme circumstances, such as the contemporary United States, people from similar ethnic or racial groups often gravitate toward one another because of shared history, levels of wealth, and experiences with forms of exclusion tied to racial or ethnic misrecognition. It is, however, an overstatement to claim that the categories used by the U.S. census delineate distinct cultural communities or genetic populations. Cross-racial and ethnic marriages, friendships, collaborations, and even rape have been a feature of life in the United States since its founding. Notably, African Americans today include Americans whose ancestors were slaves three hundred years ago in the colonies as well as Americans whose parents recently immigrated from Africa or the Caribbean. Given this complexity, research on racial or ethnic health disparities must be sensitive to the fact that how one looks, and even where one is from, do not determine how one experiences the world.

Health, like race, is a social construct. Personal and cultural beliefs affect how biomedicine is valued, which in turn informs what drugs, therapies, and tests one willingly accepts. People's experiences with illness, expectations of wellness, access to resources, and sense of risk also shape how one uses health care. The question is, did Healthy People 2010 need to be sensitive to the social complexity of both race and health in order to be useful?

THE DATA

The article I regard as the first study within Healthy People 2010 was actually published in 1999, a year after the 2010 initiative was announced and a year before it officially began. The article received so much attention that by 2013 the article had been cited in over fourteen hundred published texts. The study, by Shulman et al. and titled "The Effect of Race and Sex on Physicians' Recommendations for Cardiac Catheterization," focused specifically on whether physicians were more or less likely to recommend patients for cardiac catheterization (Schulman et al. 1999). For public health experts this study was important because it indicated that behavior, in this case differential treatment by race, was quantitatively measurable through controlled experimentation.

In order to control the variables, the authors created scripted and chore-ographed videos of patients reporting symptoms of coronary artery disease. Participants in the study included 720 clinical physicians at two different pro-fessional meetings. Individually, they watched eight videos featuring either a fifty-five-year-old or seventy-year-old white man, black man, white woman, or black woman. The participants were told in the opening that the patients in each age group had identical health insurance, after which the patients de-scribed their symptoms of coronary artery disease. The physicians then indi-cated what treatment they would recommend for each patient.

In table 4, "Referral for Cardiac Catheterization according to Experimen-tal Factors," the authors organized their data such that we see the referral rate for men was 90.6 percent, compared to 84.7 percent for women. They also reported that the white patients were referred at a rate of 90.6 percent, com-pared to 84.7 percent for the black patients (Schulman et al. 1999, 624). How-ever, in their narrative, the authors state, "Black women were the only patients who were significantly less likely to be referred for cardiac catheterization than white men, who serve as a reference category" (ibid., 623). In other words, the way they presented their data in the table failed to capture their key finding, which was that the rates of referral were lower for *women* and *blacks* only be-cause the referral rates for *black women* were lower.

By loosely noting "racial" differences, and then reporting their findings using odds ratios in table 5, the authors obscured the fact that cardiac catheter-ization was recommended for black men at the same rate as for white men and women (ibid., 624). They also obscured the fact that all physicians, regardless of race or sex, gave similar treatment recommendations. These slippages led readers to assume that racism was to blame, which is exactly the story the news media reported (Best 2012).

These category solecisms, where race is treated as an independent varia-ble, were not the authors' alone. Federally funded research, including the U.S. census, continues to employ problematic racial and ethnic categories as if their relevance is knowable in the absence of contextual data. Healthy People 2010, a product of the common wisdom of the day, similarly reduced identities to the singular, for example black or white, and presumed that physician racism contributed more to racial disparities than health-care structures did. And this hypothesis determined the data collection for the first several years of the in-itiative (Dressler, Oths, and Gravlee 2005). The presumption so dominated discourses about disparities that the authors of the much-celebrated National Institutes of Health publication *Unequal Treatment: Confronting Racial and*

Ethnic Disparities in Health Care (Smedley, Stith, and Nelson 2003) were encouraged to only review the research highlighting the impact of race on healthcare delivery, quality of care, and physician and patient decision making.[6] In the summary the authors state, "Consistent with the charge, the study committee focused part of its analysis on the clinical encounter itself, and found evidence that stereotyping, biases, and uncertainty on the part of health-care providers can all contribute to unequal treatment. The conditions in which many clinical encounters take place—characterized by high time pressure, cognitive complexity, and pressures for cost-containment—may enhance the likelihood that these processes will result in care poorly matched to minority patients' needs" (Smedley, Stith, and Nelson 2003, 1). As with the Schulman study, the assumption behind *Unequal Treatment* was that cultural psychology was an underappreciated culprit in the reproduction of racial and ethnic health disparities. But what was meant by "culture"?

In the late 1990s, around the time President Clinton announced the goal of Healthy People 2010, culture was considered a leading cause in two respects. The first was patients' beliefs, lifestyles, diet, and health behaviors. For example, two 1998 articles funded by the Agency for Healthcare Research and Quality (AHRQ) attributed disparities in insulin use by "Hispanics" to "a fatalistic acceptance of the course of the disease" (Cook et al. 2000; Noel et al. 1998; AHRQ 2001). The second way in which culture was blamed was medical professional ignorance about patient culture. Lack of "cultural competency" was considered a significant cause of miscommunication and patient noncompliance (Brach and Fraserirector 2000). In neither instance did the use of the term "culture" map neatly onto anthropological understandings of culture.

Anthropologists who study American medicine look at what is called the culture of medicine. The culture of medicine includes medical education, professionalization, technology, beliefs about wellness, and the politics and economics of health care. The knowledge, discourses, and practices of this culture are so dominant and authoritative that in the clinic they generally overwhelm other belief systems or forms of knowledge production. The result is that black physicians treat patients using the same techniques of differential diagnosis as white physicians. It also means they develop some of the same prejudices toward particular patient-types as doctors from other racial and ethnic groups.

A subsequent article by Jersey Chen et al. entitled "Racial Difference in the Use of Cardiac Catheterization after Acute Myocardial Infarction" demonstrated that differential treatment must not be confused with worse treatment (Chen et al. 2001). The authors analyzed 75,893 discharge files of patients who experienced heart attacks. The data were gathered from the Cooperative Cardiovascular Project, which analyzed Medicare data from the Health Care Financing Administration. The authors concluded that black patients were less likely to receive cardiac catheterization after an infarction whether the physician was white or black, again casting doubt on the aversive racism hypothesis. A more surprising finding was that the black patients had lower unadjusted mortality rates at thirty days, and lower adjusted mortality rates at three years (ibid., 1446–47). There are likely many reasons that black survival was higher, but the importance of the Chen article was not that it proved why differential treatment exists. Rather, it suggested that perhaps health disparities research should focus on patient outcomes rather than access.

Following publication of the Chen article and public criticism of the Schulman article, the initial optimism around Healthy People 2010 turned into a low-level cynicism among researchers. Federal funding for health disparities research continued, but offstage, away from the political spotlight. The NIH's Center on Minority Health and Health Disparities (NCMHD) was established after President Clinton signed the Minority Health and Health Disparities Research and Education Act of 2000. But the Bush administration had a different agenda, which meant that 2002 was the last year funds were directly earmarked for the specific goal of *eliminating racial and ethnic health disparities*. After that the Office of Minority Health, with its significantly smaller budget, directed the initiative's oversight.

The research challenges with respect to how to define and therefore study health disparities presaged the political challenges. In July 2003 Health and Human Services (HHS) Secretary Tommy G. Thompson sent around a rough draft of the *National Healthcare Disparities Report*, an annual report published by the AHRQ. Thoroughly optimistic, Thompson's first draft focused on the overall improvements in life expectancy for all Americans. The report included examples such as the lower rate of cancer among Native American groups. This might have been something to celebrate if these same groups did not have some of the lowest life expectancies in the United States.

After many complaints, Thompson approved a substantial rewrite. In the final version health disparities were noted, but the authors refused to include the evidence used in *Unequal Treatment*. The authors of the HHS report claimed that the evidence for differential treatment based on race was weak. Medical policy analyst M. Gregg Bloche, who served on the committee that wrote *Unequal Treatment*, stated his dismay in the *New England Journal of Medicine*:

> The Institute of Medicine Committee on Understanding and Eliminating Racial and Ethnic Disparities in Health Care . . . identified more than 100 studies. . . . Nearly all these studies, in our judgment, contained flaws in design or data analysis. . . . Inference on our part was thus necessary. In concluding that racial and ethnic disparities in care exist, are associated with worse outcomes, and occur apart from insurance status, income, and education, we relied on the fact that most of the studies we examined supported this finding. . . . The December rewrite downplayed this conclusion recharacterizing our report as having only "provided some evidence that racial and ethnic differences in quality of health care exist." (Bloche 2004, 1568–69)

Regardless of how audacious Thompson's report was, the questions lingered. Should the nation's most powerful health-care institutions be concerned with improving the health of identified groups or the health of the entire nation? In addition, uncertainties about what constitutes a racial health disparity and how to study it began to overwhelm the Healthy People 2010 research. Even Bloche noted that many members of the IOM committee considered confounding factors such as differences in geography and insurance policy important, but the mandate was to focus on physician discretion and unequal quality of care. After repeated challenges to the emerging evidence, many researchers stopped trying to study the causes of differential treatment in the clinic and instead focused on the question of methods.

In an attempt to introduce more methodological clarity, in 2005 epidemiologists Sam Harper and John Lynch published a report, now used as a touchstone for Healthy People 2020, titled "Methods for Measuring Cancer Disparities: Using Data Relevant to Healthy People 2010 Cancer-Related Objectives" (Harper and Lynch 2005). Their goal was to create a scientific framework for monitoring and measuring cancer health disparities such that researchers were no longer speaking at cross-purposes. In the report the authors state, "Choosing measures of health disparity involves consideration of conceptual, ethical, and methodological issues" (ibid., 2). The idea that statistical data are essentially unusable unless the ethical framework is explicit must have seemed radical for many health-care experts who believed that objective meaning can be found in statistically significant data alone.

A 2006 *PLoS Medicine* article, "Eight Americas: Investigating Mortality Disparities across Races, Counties, and Race-Counties in the United States," attempted to address category fallacy with respect to race and ethnicity (Murray et al. 2006). The authors showed that Americans could be organized into eight racial and ethnic geographic categories: wealthy Asians, low-income rural whites, Middle America, low-income whites from Appalachia and the Mississippi River valley, western Native Americans, black Middle America, southern low-income rural blacks, and high-risk urban blacks. While their mapping was in many respects arbitrary and some of the data questionable, the data took seriously the intersection of social identity and geography, generating new inquiries (Deaton and Lubotsky 2009).

In keeping with this growing scientific reflexivity, in 2008 *Health Affairs* published an article titled "When Does a Difference Become a Disparity? Conceptualizing Racial and Ethnic Disparities in Health." The authors compared different definitions of a health disparity and how those definitions impact data collection and interpretation (Hebert et al. 2008). They compared *Unequal Treatment*, which excluded vital contextual information, with the WHO approach, which assumes that health disparities are the product of social injustice and inequality (King, chapter 8, this volume; Smedley, Stith, and Nelson 2003).

BRIDGING QUALITATIVE AND QUANTITATIVE DATA

The growing recognition in the medical community that health disparities research is never free from ethics, politics, or institutional pragmatics was exciting for me as a researcher. Studying racial health disparities ethnographically in the late 1990s and early 2000s, I had grown increasing frustrated with the literature. Racism and aversive racism clearly existed, but I was unconvinced by even my own data that a direct causal relationship between bias and treatment outcomes existed.

At the time, I had been conducting weekly field research on fourteen African American families caring for a child with a long-term illness and/or disability (1997–99) in three different hospitals. From 2000 to 2006, I focused on sickle cell disease treatment and racial health disparities at the national level. This required conducting interviews with patients, medical professionals, and advocates at five hospitals, national conferences, and a sickle cell camp, among other field sites (Rouse 2009). My goal was to try to understand how families with ill children were able to develop tools, gather resources, and organize home life to make room for treatment. For every family the choices were determined by a different set of personal and resource constraints.

My approach was qualitative and inductive. I did not enter the field with a hypothesis; rather, I tried to locate patterns in my emergent data. While I was open to any possible explanation for treatment disparities, my objects of study included (1) exploring the effectiveness of communication marked by patient and family understandings of the illness, treatments, and whether families were successful following through with treatment plans, (2) identifying racism by comparing physician, nurse, and social worker narratives about the families with observations made through long-term engagement with the families, and (3) testing the findings in the health disparities literature through targeted observations and interviews. Using open-ended ethnographic methods and following families and physicians to the most unlikely of places, I was able to collect data that would not have been captured through statistical sampling alone. Over the years, I conducted over fifteen hundred hours of observations in hospitals, clinics, homes, and national science meetings and collected over 250 formal and informal interviews and over two thousand pages of field notes.

In the emergent literature on health disparities, researchers were concluding that blacks had worse health outcomes because they lacked coping skills, did not understand medical information, were treated by racist physicians, or failed to adhere to treatment recommendations. In the clinic, I observed all of those things, their opposites, and more. Racism, aversive racism, and differential treatment were certainly factors in patient-physician interactions, but professionalism often obscured the rationale for treatment decisions. Physicians relied on evidence-based protocols, which meant, by definition, that they were performing best practices and not differential treatment.

With respect to the patients, I witnessed forms of agency, or cultural health capital, where patients and family members were able to alter how others initially saw them (Shim, Chang, and Dubbin, chapter 9, this volume). Parents employed creative tactics to gain access to care, and once they gained access to the clinic, they worked to humanize themselves and their child. For example, in an attempt to win sympathy, the parents of a child with spina bifida refused public health insurance. The mother told me that she chose an HMO so that health professionals would know they were employed and hard working.[7] Attempts to gain access often required more overt tactics. For example, in another case, a mother refused to leave the hospital waiting area until her daughter was seen by a neurologist. When one strategy for winning over health professionals failed, parents tried others, from dressing the child up for clinic visits to narrating stories of their children's academic achievements regardless of appropriateness. This intersubjective work played a critical role in the quality and extent of treatment.

The example that stands out the most is the father who was functionally illiterate, a former drug addict, and, of all my interlocutors, the best home nurse (Rouse 2004b). He quickly learned how to manage his daughter's complicated life-sustaining equipment and treatment regimens. His competence as a nurse, which included his compassion and commitment to his child, was cited as the only reason physicians continued to treat his daughter. In an extraordinary demonstration of his virtuoso skills, after the family was told that they should not call an ambulance if their daughter stopped breathing, he successfully resuscitated her for over four hours. He spent the first two hours waiting for the home health nurse to arrive. When the home health nurse arrived, she advised him to give up. Disgusted, the father transferred the child from the house to the car, and eventually to the hospital, resuscitating her the entire way. After that episode, the daughter survived another nine months. The intelligence of patients and physicians to negotiate care—despite prejudices, resource constraints, and knowledge asymmetries—had yet to be captured in the quantitative research on health disparities.

Demographically, the families I followed were black, the majority of the mothers and grandmothers were single or divorced, and they all were either economically lower middle class or poor. All were receiving some form of assistance, including state insurance for their children (MediCal), Social Security Disability Insurance (SSDI), and/or Aid to Families with Dependent Children (AFDC). AFDC switched over to Temporary Assistance for Needy Families (TANF) soon after I started my research. With the exception of one mother who traveled about one hundred miles to the hospital, all of the families were from different parts of the same metropolis.

Despite these demographic similarities, their diversity in terms of values and lifestyle stood out. In the case of the original fourteen families, about half regularly attended church, but only a few used their faith to rationalize their health-care choices. One well-educated mother, who had spent years receiving state aid in order to care for her child, listened to and agreed with conservative radio host Rush Limbaugh. There were three grandmothers who had custody of their grandchildren, and one aunt was raising her nephew. Most encouraged their children academically. Several of the children and their siblings were in advanced classes at school. A couple of families had opened their doors to young gay men who had nowhere else to live.

Most were conscious of what they ate and went out of their way to eat well, but some remained committed junk foodies. One very religious churchgoing grandmother had grandchildren in advanced placement classes, lived in a peaceful and integrated middle-class neighborhood, owned her home, collected Beanie Babies, and sold drugs.

Their diversity was discernable in the clinic as well. The parents of a multihandicapped child did not want her to die and asked the hospital to go to extremes to save their daughter's life. Another parent actively let go when she felt her daughter no longer had high enough quality of life. Another was confused and, basically, abdicated control toward the end. All basically followed the orders of the medical team. Some were methodical in their approach to home treatments and physical therapy, while others were not. All found ways to slightly modify and supplement home treatments to match the needs of the child and family. One advocated for an institutional change so that she would not have to be the one to subject her child to daily iron chelation therapy. Despite the occasional conflicts and disagreements with medical professionals, the families I worked with were overwhelmingly pleased with their children's care.[8]

With respect to the medical professionals, some were highly judgmental, even prejudiced, while the majority were not. Most engaged well with the families, but others talked to the families through a nurse or some other surrogate. Some made snide comments about the families with whom they worked; others described their institution as racist. Sometimes treatments did not work, and the way medical professionals narrated the causes for treatment failure, and who or what they chose to blame, offered insights into their subjective feelings about the way the world works. And while people had these feelings, it was often impossible to make the case that those feelings impacted the level of care or professionalism. All of the patients received exceptional care, from exemplary case management to advanced treatments, even in the face of futility. But while the families reported that they were happy with the quality of their care, the statistical data showed that black patients, on average, received inferior health care and had worse treatment outcomes. But my data, limited as it was, showed that there was no direct causal link between race and worse outcomes. Struggling to make sense of the contradictions, I chose to return to the literature and focus on the evidence used by researchers rather than the conclusions.[9]

I reread the available statistical data, paying closer attention to the assumptions underlying the methods and interpretation of evidence. I questioned everything, from what was meant by culture in these studies to why health disparities were organized as they were, by race and ethnicity. Basically, I noticed that the object that stayed stable in health disparities research was an unquestioned acceptance of medical authority, or, more accurately, common-sense notions of what constituted good health care and good health behaviors. It was only after I removed that assumption that patterns started to emerge and the professional, political, and financial entanglements of health dispari-ties research began to become clear.

Assumptions embedded in the Healthy People 2010 research included these three: *All preventive screenings are good and therefore more of them are bet-ter; Taking prescribed medications always improves health outcomes;* and *Lack of patient compliance is a primary contributor to worse health outcomes.* Starting from the assumption that more medicine was the sine qua non for eliminating racial health disparities, it followed that patient behavior and medical profes-sional behavior stood between patients and full access to the most efficient, most advanced, most humane, evidence-based health-care system in the world. Glaringly absent from much of the earlier literature that had galvanized Healthy People 2010 was a thorough investigation of the role insurance, hos-pitals, and pharmaceutical companies played in shaping health-care choices and outcomes.

Feeding this consumerist approach to ameliorating health disparities was the uncritical celebration of randomized control trials. The rationale was that racial health disparities could be improved if doctors treated all patients to evidence-based medicine built on randomized controlled trials (RCTs). But RCTs in medicine are problematic for two reasons: (1) the data are often flawed, and (2) bodies are complex. With respect to the first, RCT data is often tainted by researcher bias, the placebo effect, and poor research design and execution. More difficult to assess when reading pos-itive RCT data is the Food and Drug Administration (FDA) requirement that drug manufacturers compare their drug against a placebo as opposed to the best available treatment. This distorts the effectiveness of a new drug relative to, for example, an off-patent standard treatment. This is critical because elevating the cost of medicine by encouraging the adoption of expensive new drugs actually reduces treatment access. Another trick is to compare a new drug against a drug administered in lower or higher doses than normal. The older drug, by comparison, either does not work or causes horrific side effects. The most difficult issue is the witholding of trial data so that doctors who are vigilant cannot assess for themselves the value of a drug (Goldacre 2012).

Equally problematic is the fact that even the best RCTs treat diseases in isolation. In order to make sure that a researcher avoids confounding variables, the treatment and control groups are chosen for their similarities and receive extensive clinical care during the trial. For people with multiple chronic illnesses, the results of a study showing that a blood pressure medication worked on a group of patients whose single medical concern was high blood pressure may be irrelevant to their health needs. Medications can cause side effects and iatrogenic disease, particularly when a patient is taking more than one medication. Pharmaceutical companies have been able to expand their drug markets to people who do not need them based on the mistaken assumption that more access to health care is an unquestioned good and therefore an uncomplicated form of social justice (Dumit 2012).

This refusal to consider the complexity of bodies, treatments, and medical systems was not due to a failure of imagination. Looking back at the literature from the 1990s, medical experts were already questioning the overestimations of disease due to new diagnostic imaging, and the Dartmouth Atlas of Health Care was collecting evidence showing the profound influence of geography on types of care and regional health (Black and Welch 1993). In 2004, *Health Affairs* published a study that concluded that since rates of white utilization differed geographically, "for highly effective, high-value care, the objective should not be to ensure that black rates are simply set equal to white rates, since doing so could leave in place geographic disparities" (Baicker et al. 2004, 41). The article also detailed the effects of treatment overuse and its negative impacts on health and disparities.

My struggles with the Healthy People 2010 literature, it turns out, were not mine alone. During the decade, the failures were being taken seriously by medical researchers and folded into the 2020 initiative. Just before the ACA was passed in 2009, health disparities research had begun to move away from patient culture and noncompliance as primary explanatory models. For example, in 2008 AHRQ acknowledged that it needed to rethink how it collects data for its annual report on health-care quality and disparities. With recommendations from the Institute of Medicine, by 2009 AHRQ had instituted significant methodological changes in order to capture the role of administrative systems, medical knowledge production, training, and resource distribution on the quality of care (AHRQ 2013, 21–22). Equally compelling was the inclusion of information on "lifestyle" and "population health and safety."

Echoing the changes being instituted at the AHRQ, the CDC's director, Dr. Frieden, helped standardize an approach for measuring health disparities that addressed many of the earlier problems. The elegance of the Healthy People 2020 approach lies in its rhetorical simplicity. CDC publications now focus on the relative differences between groups rather than arbitrary goals to determine improvement. The 2010 initiative, for example, established rate goals, hoping that diagnoses and mortality would decline in all major disease categories. The problem with this approach was that it did not adjust for the fact that people die of something; you may reduce the rates in one disease category only to see another go up. The older approach also failed to take into consideration the fact that higher rates of diabetes among blacks may be matched by higher rates of diabetes among whites. That rates of diabetes went up among both blacks and whites during Healthy People 2010 makes the initiative seem less like a failure and more like a nationwide issue of foodways, city design, and changing tastes.

In the newer approach, the data was still organized by race and ethnicity, but race and ethnicity were rarely treated as independent variables. The 2011 CDC report on colon cancer, for example, compared screening rates to state poverty rates because geography or proximity to quality health care may be a significant factor (Ezzati et al. 2008; Rim et al. 2011). The CDC also compared the average number of healthy days, often used to reflect quality of life, with state income inequality or the Gini index because social inequality may affect quality of life. While health disparities data remained stubbornly tied to traditional race and ethnicity categories, the 2020 iteration of Healthy People attempted to capture the intersections of social identity and structures including income, geography, and availability of quality care.

2010 DATA

The largest gap in life expectancy, by race and ethnicity, was between the "Hispanic" population and the non-Hispanic black population. By 2010, Hispanic women had the highest life expectancy (83.8 years), followed by white women (81.1 years) and Hispanic men (78.8 years) (Minino and Murphy 2012). The difference was 6.6 years. Again, it was difficult to glean how culture, as articulated in the 1990s and early 2000s, could be read through the data. The fact that "Hispanic" refers to regions in Europe and South America where Spanish and Portuguese are spoken means that the disparities data tells us almost nothing about the relationship between culture, ancestry (genetics), and health. Complicating things further, during the same time period morbidity and morality increased among non-Hispanic whites between the ages of forty-five and fifty-four (Case and Deaton 2015).

Of the five diseases that blacks suffered from disproportionately compared to whites, nothing came close to heart disease, which accounted for, on average, one lost year of life. In addition to heart disease, blacks lost 7.6 months due to cancer, 6 months due to homicide, 4 months due to diabetes, and 3.7 months due to perinatal conditions. Whites had shorter life expectancies that ranged from .7 months to 2.4 months. They suffered disproportionately from chronic liver disease, Alzheimer's disease, chronic lower respiratory diseases, and suicide (Kochanek, Arias, and Anderson 2013). If we compared the extraordinary disparities in black incarceration, unemployment, and wealth, it's surprising that the disparities by disease were as low as they were (Alexander 2012). Importantly, behind those statistics were stories of incredible resilience and effective health practices despite structural racism—things I witnessed in my twenty-plus years of research in low-income black neighborhoods.

Did Healthy People 2010 contribute to narrowing the gaps? There was evidence that concerted efforts to standardize best medical practices and increase access to some prescription drugs and treatments ameliorated racial health disparities before the passage of the ACA (Trivedi et al. 2005). There was also evidence that the narrowing resulted from specific drug interventions and changing mortality demographics that were unrelated to the initiative (Harper, MacLehose, and Kaufman 2014). In the end, one could argue that the initiative largely failed if one compares the results of Healthy People 2010 with the data following Massachusetts's 2006 health reform. By 2010 the state data showed significant reductions in mortality resulting from regular health-care access, particularly among the poor (Sommers, Long, and Baicker 2014). Simple access to insurance mattered more than patient or physician behavior, culture, or affect in the clinic.

DISCUSSION

Before the ACA, the consumerist model of personalized health care had reached its peak. The promises of wellness were sold by pharmaceutical companies through an expanding market for mood enhancers, pain relief medications, and racialized drugs (Dumit 2012; Kahn 2012). But a growing list of FDA-approved drugs and treatments were showing questionable long-term efficacy, and efforts to eliminate late-stage cancers and cancer disparities with more frequent scans and aggressive early treatments did virtually nothing to reduce disparities in survival. They did, however, significantly increase our health-care costs (Emanuel 2014). These optional tests and life-enhancing interventions were marketed as if disease, disappointment, and suffering could be surgically removed from the human experience. It turns out that increasing people's consumption of health care does not translate into better health outcomes (Gawande 2015).

Far more important than sincere efforts to end health disparities have been the legislative reforms to health insurance. The ACA requires that states monitor the ethical and fair distribution of health and health-care services because citizenship is now tied to health insurance. States also have a financial incentive to focus on improving health and quality-of-life measures for specific populations as well as the state as a whole. Preventable disease clusters, or hot spots, threaten to drain what is now perceived as a common-pool resource rather than a privately held one (Ostrom 1990). These changes require new approaches to the study of disparities because health care is now recognized as a limited public good.

Healthy People 2010 tried to tackle an important social justice concern, but it did so by relying on complicated and controversial social identity categories. Racial and ethnic health disparities were real, but they were no less real than health disparities associated with geography (Fisher, Goodman, and Chandra 2008). And where people live continued to be shaped by economic class, race, and/or ethnicity (Hannah-Jones 2014; Massey 1993; Rugh and Massey 2010; Williams and Collins 2001). Healthy People 2010 tried to abstract race from a number of interrelated causal factors, and the lack of a mandate to alter health-care structures such as insurance, if insurance was found to be a contributor, meant the initiative had no teeth.

While race was often studied independently of economic class, there were a number of statistical studies, generally poor, that controlled for income and/or education. Missing from these studies was ethnographic evidence showing how racial signifiers operated in the clinic. The literature on discretion in the clinic shows that physicians make different treatment decisions based on whether they think patients can afford the prescription medications, on whether or not a test or treatment will be covered, and on what the reimbursement for their care will be (Abraham 1994; Bloche 2001). Without universal coverage, race signified class, which signified health coverage. For example, I observed doctors, nurses, occupational, and physical therapists making wild assumptions about black patient family dysfunction and job status that because I had been following those families I knew were wrong. Universal health coverage has the potential to change that calculus.

With a national health-care program, ideally insurance coverage becomes associated with citizenship rather than employment. Therefore, simply being a U.S. citizen means one deserves treatment access. Race and class continue to be factors in understandings of treatment deservedness, but the ACA has reduced some of the stigma and therefore broadened access to quality care. What we see in the case of the British National Health Service, however, is that a national health-care program only takes us partway there (Shaw 2012; Marmot Review 2010). Racism and aversive racism continue to exist. What we learn from a postmortem of Healthy People 2010 is that when studying racism's impact on care, researchers must not abstract race from structural elements that impact choice and experience. The qualitative, intersubjective, and indeterminate aspects of the clinical encounter matter and demonstrate why statistically coding by "race" cannot help us disentangle the structural issues of medical systems, money, and power from the affective issues of patient resistance to bad medicine and physician unequal treatment. Race is never an independent variable disconnected from the extant social inequalities that exist beyond the clinic.

CONCLUSION

Health care during most of the twentieth century was segregated; black people were disproportionately experimented on, and blacks often received the worst treatment or none at all (Washington 2006). The concern for equalizing health emerged in large part from a desire for restorative justice, but missing from the conversation was any meaningful engagement with the questions of the relationship between health and health care, and of whether or not health care is the best domain for attacking health disparities. Many racial revitalization movements in the United States have focused on health care as a critical part of liberation and self-determination, but not to the exclusion of demands for better education, voting rights, and more economic opportunities (Jackson 2013; Nelson 2011; Rouse 2004b). Recommendations from the medical community ignored that critical history.

Instead, the focus was on, essentially, finding ways to get patients to comply with evidence-based treatment modalities. Some of those evidence-based studies concluded that more frequent and earlier mammograms improved breast cancer survival, that cardiac catheterization improved outcomes for most patients who suffered a nonlethal heart attack, and that meticulous control of blood sugar levels reduced diabetes complications.[10] Notably, all of those findings later proved controversial. These decontextualized conclusions from hypothesis-driven short-term studies failed to tie recommendations in any meaningful way to the activism that had forced the conversation. This prior activism understood that black empowerment required far more than simply demanding submission to the latest medical advice. Racial justice struggles have always acknowledged the intersections between identities, resources, structures, ideologies, and health. In many ways health and well-being are tied to pedestrian needs, but the political barriers to creating healthy cities, foodways, and living-wage jobs are anything but pedestrian.

The ACA has also changed how we code for race and ethnicity in disparities research. Unlike Healthy People 2010, the new CDC data strives to capture the interconnections between economic inequality, pollution, urban planning, education, health, race, and ethnicity at the local level. It is impossible to know how health data will be collected in the future, but the failures of Healthy People 2010 demonstrated that ameliorating racial health disparities often requires ignoring the variable of race.

NOTES

I would like to thank a number of colleagues who helped in direct and indirect ways with the shaping and revisions of this chapter: Allison Bloom, Mara Buchbinder, Helena Hansen, Michele Rivkin-Fish, and Pamela Sankar.

1. For a thorough discussion of health equity see Shim, Chang, and Dubbin (chapter 9, this volume).

2. This analysis is based on numerous conversations with scholars with health-related expertise who have participated on committees tasked with drafting consensus statements. Rarely do they see themselves in the final documents, even though they had a hand in shaping the content and, perhaps more critically, in making sure certain content did not make it into the final draft.

3. Using the PubMed filter "Health Disparities in the United States," one finds that articles on health disparities in the United States increased from 35 in 1998 to 105 in 2000 to 624 in 2005 to 1,550 in 2010. In addition to the PubMed articles, during the same time period one could find an increasing number of online publications by major health institutions including the CDC, NIH, the Dartmouth Atlas, and the Kaiser Family Foundation report on Health Policy Research, Analysis, Polling, Facts, Data and Journalism.

4. For the $1 billion figure, I reviewed the Health and Human Services budget archives from FY2000 to FY2010. Funding directed specifically at eliminating racial and ethnic

health disparities spanned from 2000 to 2002, at which point the Healthy People 2010 initiative was folded into the Office of Minority Health (OMH). This change also marked a massive drop in funding: $158 million in 2002 vs. $47 million in 2003. Therefore, my estimate includes the first three years of earmarked funding as well as the budget for the OMH (2003–10) and the budget for Minority HIV/AIDS (2003–10). In the end, it is difficult to quantify exact spending levels on the initiative given that efforts to eliminate racial health disparities were funded under different budget headings, such as "Health Care for the Uninsured" or "Community Health Centers." In addition, the NIH funded health disparities research that was not part of the Healthy People 2010 initiative. Given that research to ameliorate health disparities became a research priority in the early 2000s, researchers claiming that their work contributed to this mandate were often more likely to receive funding. Sankar et al. (2004) include all federally funded research on health disparities in their $3 billion estimate. See USDHHS 2009.

5. The data to compare the success of the 169 objectives to eliminate racial and ethnic disparities versus the 800 objectives to improve the health of the nation as a whole were not available. Overall, about 16 to 17 percent of the objectives of Healthy People 2010 were met.

6. I refer to the primary text and not the supplemental material in *Unequal Treatment*. The supplemental articles were written by anthropologists and bioethicists, among others, and the authors were not constrained in their discussions.

7. I observed this Indian family in a spina bifida clinic. They were there for a one-time visit. The story was tragic because all of the other children in the clinic had state insurance and were receiving exceptional care. This five-year-old child had no mobility and had feet contractures because the family was regularly denied care by their HMO.

8. Admittedly, there was selection bias. Like most Americans who live in large urban centers, the patients I followed had access to some of the best medical care in the country. Also, all had some combination of private and state insurance. These families also may have been more outgoing than families who refused study participation, possibly because they felt they had nothing to hide. Similarly, the physicians who allowed access to their clinics were also disproportionately open to reflection and possible criticism. While the number of people I observed and interviewed, formally and informally, was relatively small (about one hundred), my observations were not limited to my study participants alone. There were ample opportunities to observe random interactions taking place throughout the hospital between health professionals and patient families. In addition, medical professionals felt comfortable telling me stories of things colleagues had said that came across as racist, or institutional issues that they believed reproduced unequal treatment.

9. I was not able to compare outcomes in my own data for a number of reasons, including the fact that even if I had compared across institutions, the sample size would never have been large enough to create any meaningful data. In addition, each case had its own particularities. I followed children with multiple congenital abnormalities, spina bifida, brachial plexus, brain tumors, and sickle cell.

10. That is not to say that all evidence-based modalities are ineffective. In fact, some of the cheapest and most readily available treatments for hypertension, for example, have contributed significantly to reductions in morbidity and mortality.

REFERENCES

Abraham, Laurie Kaye. 1994. *Mama Might Be Better Off Dead: The Failure of Health Care in Urban America.* Chicago: University of Chicago Press.

AHRQ (Agency for Healthcare Research and Quality). 2001. "Diabetes Disparities among Racial and Ethnic Minorities: Fact Sheet." *AHRQ Archive.* http://archive.ahrq .gov/research/findings/factsheets/diabetes/diabdisp/diabdisp.html. Accessed 26 August 2015.

———. 2013. "2012 National Healthcare Quality Report." *AHRQ Archive.* http://archive .ahrq.gov/research/findings/nhqrdr/nhqr12/index.html. Accessed 26 August 2015.

Alexander, Michelle. 2012. *The New Jim Crow: Mass Incarceration in the Age of Colorblindness.* New York: New Press.

Baicker, Katherine, Amitabh Chandra, Jonathan S. Skinner, and John E. Wennberg. 2004. "Who You Are and Where You Live: How Race and Geography Affect the Treatment of Medicare Beneficiaries." *Health Affairs,* October 2004, Supplemental Web Exclusive, 33–44. http://content.healthaffairs.org/content/early/2004/10/07/hlthaff.var.33/ suppl/DC1.

Barth, Frederik. 1968. "Introduction." In *Ethnic Groups and Boundaries: The Social Organization of Culture and Difference,* edited by Frederik Barth, 9–38. Long Grove, IL: Waveland.

Best, Joel. 2012. *Damned Lies and Statistics: Untangling Numbers from the Media, Politicians, and Activists.* Berkeley: University of California Press.

Black, William C., and H. Gilbert Welch. 1993. "Diagnostic Imaging and the Overestimations of Disease Prevalence and the Benefits of Therapy." *New England Journal of Medicine* 328 (17): 1237–43.

Bloche, M. Gregg. 2001. "Discretion in American Medicine." *Yale Journal of Health Policy, Law, and Ethics* 1 (1): 95–131.

———. 2004. "Health Care Disparities: Science, Politics, and Race." *New England Journal of Medicine* 350 (15): 1568–70.

Boas, Franz. 1940. *Race, Language, and Culture.* Chicago: University of Chicago Press.

Branch, Cindy, and Irene Fraserirector. 2000. "Can Cultural Competency Reduce Racial and Ethnic Health Disparities? A Review and Conceptual Model." *Medical Care Research and Review* 57 (S1): 181–217.

Case, Anne, and Angus Deaton. 2015. *Proceedings of the National Academy of Sciences of the United States of America* 112 (49): 15078–83.

Cavalli-Sforza, Luigi L., Paolo Menozzi, and Alberto Piazza. 1994. *The History and Geography of Human Genes.* Princeton, NJ: Princeton University Press.

CDC (Center for Disease Control and Prevention). 2011. "CDC Health Disparities and Inequalities Report: United States 2011." *Morbidity and Mortality Weekly Report S60.* http://www.cdc.gov/mmwr/pdf/other/su6001.pdf. 26 August 2015.

Chen, Jersey, Saif S. Rathore, Martha J. Radford, Yun Wang, and Harlan M. Krumholz. 2001. "Racial Differences in the Use of Cardiac Catheterization after Acute Myocardial Infarction." *New England Journal of Medicine* 344 (19): 1443–49.

Cook, Curtiss B., Diane M. Erdman, Gina J. Ryan, Kurt J. Greenlund, Wayne H. Giles, Daniel L. Gallina, Imad M. El-Kebbi, David C. Ziemer, Kris L. Ernst, Virginia G. Dunbar, and Lawrence S. Phillips. 2000. "The Pattern of Dyslipidemia among Urban African-Americans with Type 2 Diabetes." *Diabetes Care* 23 (3): 319–24.

Deaton, Angus, and Darren Lubotsky. 2009. "Income Inequality and Mortality in U.S. Cities: Weighing the Evidence." *Social Science and Medicine* 68: 1914–17.

Dressler, William W., Kathryn S. Oths, and Clarence C. Gravlee. 2005. "Race and Ethnicity in Public Health Research: Models to Explain Health Disparities." *Annual Review of Anthropology* 34: 231–52.

Dumit, Joseph. 2012. *Drugs for Life: How Pharmaceutical Companies Define Our Health.* Durham, NC: Duke University Press.

Emanuel, Ezekiel. 2014. *Reinventing American Health Care.* New York: Perseus Books.

Ezzati, Majid, Ari B. Friedman, Sandeep C. Kulkarni, and Christopher J. L. Murray. 2008. "The Reversal of Fortunes: Trends in County Mortality and Cross-County Mortality Disparities in the United States." *PLoS Medicine* 5 (4): e66.

Fisher, Elliott S., David C. Goodman, and Amitabh Chandra. 2008. "Regional and Racial Variation in Health Care among Medicare Beneficiaries." *Dartmouth Atlas Project.* http://www.dartmouthatlas.org/downloads/reports/AF4Q_disparities_Dec2008.pdf. Accessed 26 August 2015.

Fuentes, Agustin. 2012. *Race, Monogamy, and Other Lies They Told You: Busting Myths about Human Nature.* Berkeley: University of California Press.

Gawande, Atul. 2015. "Overkill: America's Epidemic of Unnecessary Care." *New Yorker,* 11 May 2015. http://www.newyorker.com/magazine/2015/05/11/overkill-atul-gawande. Accessed 26 August 2015.

Goldacre, Ben. 2013. *Bad Pharma: How Drug Companies Mislead Doctors and Harm Patients.* New York: Faber & Faber.

Hannah-Jones, Nikole. 2014. "Segregation Now: Investigating America's Racial Divide." *Propublica.* http://www.propublica.org/article/segregation-now-full-text. Accessed 26 August 2015.

Harper, Sam, and John Lynch. 2005. "Methods for Measuring Cancer Disparities: Using Data Relevant to Healthy People 2010 Cancer-Related Objectives." *NCI Cancer Surveillance Monograph Series Number 6.* NIH Publication No. 05-5777. Bethesda: National Cancer Institute, 2005.

Harper, Sam, Richard F. MacLehose, and Jay S. Kaufman. 2014. "Trends in the Black-White Life Expectancy Gap among U.S. States, 1990–2009." *Health Affairs* 33 (8): 1375–82.

Kahn, Jonathan D. 2012. *Race in a Bottle: The Story of BiDil and Racial Medicine in a Post-Genomic Age*. New York: Columbia University Press.

Kochanek, Kenneth D., Elizabeth Arias, and Robert N. Anderson. 2013. *How Did Cause of Death Contribute to Racial Differences in Life Expectancy in the United States in 2010?* NCHS Data Brief No. 125. Hyattsville, MD: National Center for Health Statistics.

Kochanek, Kenneth D., Jiaquan Xu, Sherry L. Murphy, Arialdi M. Minino, and Hsiang-Ching Kung. 2011. "Deaths: Final Data for 2009." *National Vital Statistics Report* 60 (3). http://www.cdc.gov/nchs/data/nvsr/nvsr60/nvsr60_03.pdf. Accessed 26 August 2015.

Loveman, Mara, Jeronimo O. Muniz, and Stanley Bailey. 2011. "Brazil in Black and White? Race Categories, the Census, and the Study of Inequality." *Ethnic and Racial Studies* 35 (8): 1466–83.

Marmot Review. 2015. *Fair Society, Healthy Lives*. London: Marmot Review. http://www.instituteofhealthequity.org/projects/fair-society-healthy-lives-the-marmot-review. Accessed 26 August 2015.

Massey, Douglas S. 1993. *American Apartheid: Segregation and the Making of the Underclass*. Cambridge, MA: Harvard University Press.

Minino, Arialdi M., and Sherry L. Murphy. 2012. *Death in the United States, 2010*. NCHS Data Brief No. 99. Hyattsville, MD: National Center for Health Statistics.

Murray, Christopher J. L., Sandeep C. Kulkarni, Catherine Michaud, Niels Tomijima, Maria T. Bulzacchelli, Terrell J. Iandiorio, and Majid Ezzati. 2006. "Eight Americas: Investigating Mortality Disparities across Races, Counties, and Race-Counties in the United States." *PLoS Medicine* 3 (9): e260.

NCHS (National Center for Health Statistics). 2012. *Healthy People 2010 Final Review*. Hyattsville, MD: National Center for Health Statistics.

Nelson, Alondra. 2011. *Body and Soul: The Black Panther Fight against Medical Discrimination*. Minneapolis: University of Minnesota Press.

Noel, Polly H., Anne C. Larme, Julie Meyer, Genevieve Marsh, Alicia Correa, and Jacqueline A. Pugh. 1998. "Patient Choice in Diabetes Education Curriculum." *Diabetes Care* 21 (6): 896–901. AHRQ Grant HS07397.

Ostrom, Elinor. 1990. *Governing the Commons: The Evolution of Institutions for Collective Action*. Cambridge: Cambridge University Press.

Rim, Sun Hee, Djenaba A. Joseph, C. Brooke Steele, Trevor D. Thompson, Laura C. Seeff, and CDC (Centers for Disease Control and Prevention). 2011. "Colorectal Cancer Screening: United States, 2002, 2004, 2006, and 2008." *Morbidity and Mortality Weekly Report: Surveillance Summaries* 60 (Supplement): 42–46.

Rouse, Carolyn. 2004a. *Engaged Surrender: African American Women and Sunni Islam*. Berkeley: University of California Press.

———. 2004b. "If She's a Vegetable, We'll Be Her Garden: Embodiment, Transcendence, and Citations of Competing Metaphors in the Case of a Dying Child." *American Ethnologist* 31 (4): 514–29.

———. 2009. *Uncertain Suffering: Racial Health Disparities and Sickle Cell Disease*. Berkeley: University of California Press.

Rugh, Jacob S., and Douglas S. Massey. 2010. "American Foreclosure Crisis." *American Sociological Review* 75 (5): 629–51.

Sankar, Pamela, Mildred K. Cho, Celeste M. Condit, Linda M. Hunt, Barbara Koenig, Patricia Marshall, Sandra Soo-Jin Lee, and Paul Spicer. 2004. "Genetic Research and Health Disparities." *Journal of the American Medical Association* 291 (24): 2985–89.

Satcher, David. 2001. "Our Commitment to Eliminate Racial and Ethnic Health Disparities." *Yale Journal of Health Policy, Law, and Ethics* 1 (1): 1–14.

Schulman, Kevin A., et al. 1999. "The Effect of Race and Sex on Physicians' Recommendations for Cardiac Catheterization." *New England Journal of Medicine* 340: 618–26.

Shaw, Susan. 2012. *Governing How We Care: Contesting Community and Defining Difference in U.S. Public Health Programs.* Philadelphia: Temple University Press.

Smedley, Brian D., Adrienne Y. Stith, and AlanR. Nelson. 2003. *Unequal Treatment: Confronting Racial and Ethnic Disparities in Health Care.* Washington, DC: National Academy Press.

Sommers, Benjamin D., Sharon K. Long, and Katherine Baicker. 2014. "Changes in Mortality after Massachusetts Health Care Reform: A Quasi-Experimental Study." *Annals of Internal Medicine* 160 (9): 585–93.

Tarozzi, Alessandro, and Angus Deaton. 2009. "Using Census and Survey Data to Estimate Poverty and Inequality for Small Areas." *Review of Economics and Statistics* 91 (4): 773–92.

Trivedi, Amal N., Alan M. Zaslavsky, Eric C. Schneider, and John Z. Ayanian. 2005. "Trends in the Quality of Care and Racial Disparities in Medicare Managed Care." *New England Journal of Medicine* 353: 692–700.

USDHHS (U.S. Department of Health and Human Services). 2009. "HHS Budget." *HHS.Gov Archive.* http://archive.hhs.gov/budget/docbudgetarchive.htm. Accessed 26 August 2015.

Wang, Haidong, Austin E. Schumacher, Carly E. Levitz, Ali H. Mokdad, and Christopher J. L. Murray. 2013. "Left Behind: Widening Disparities for Males and Females in U.S. County Life Expectancy, 1985–2010." *Population Health Metrics* 11 (1): 8.

Washington, Harriet. 2006. *Medical Apartheid: The Dark History of Medical Experimentation on Black Americans from Colonial Times to the Present.* New York: Doubleday.

Williams, David R., and Chiquita Collins. 2001. "Racial Residential Segregation: A Fundamental Cause of Racial Disparities in Health." *Public Health Reports* 116 (5): 404–16.

Wimmer, Andres. 2013. *Ethnic Boundary Making: Institutions, Power, Networks.* Oxford: Oxford University Press.

11

Health-Care Justice, Health Inequalities, and U.S. Health System Reform

Carla C. Keirns

ABSTRACT

Beyond implementation of the Affordable Care Act (ACA) of 2010, changes in health system financing and delivery have the potential to save thousands of lives and billions of dollars. New models of health-care delivery and payment are intended to alter incentives for patients and providers throughout the system. While most discussions of health-care reform have focused on broadening access to health insurance, other changes have the potential to be almost as wide-ranging in their impacts, including report cards for hospitals and physicians, standards for "never events" for which hospitals will be penalized, and pay-for-performance and accountable care programs that tie payment to outcomes.

The overarching value system embedded in these new models for payment reform is a rough utilitarianism with conceptual origins in economic analysis. These models largely imagine using financial incentives to change the behavior of physicians, hospitals, and patients. While these utilitarian-based innovations in insurance and payment policy have often proven to improve access and quality of care in the aggregate, they have frequently been shown to have less benefit or even cause harm to vulnerable populations. This chapter demonstrates how improvements in quality of care frequently have the unintended consequence of widening disparities, either because the populations who had the worst outcomes to start with are more difficult to reach with improved-care models, or because the mechanisms designed to increase access and quality actually destabilize

institutions that have long served the poor. Such challenges remain outside the scope of the economic-based conceptualizations that shape mainstream health-care reform models. As health reforms are implemented,
attention to their impact on poor patients and the institutions that serve
them will be essential.

INTRODUCTION

The U.S. health-care system is undergoing a major transition in financing,
intended to both improve health-care access for millions of Americans
and create structural changes to reduce cost and improve quality. We have
been here before. The last time the United States saw major new programs
that offered health-care coverage to large groups who lacked it was 1965,
when Medicare and Medicaid were passed (Marmor 1970; Oberlander
2003; R. B. Stevens and Stevens 1974). These programs offered broad new
entitlements to care for the elderly who qualified for Social Security based
on their work history, and to certain classes of poor people. They stabilized
the finances of hospitals that had previously cared for those populations
without compensation. They also catalyzed numerous changes to the
health-care delivery system and the politics of health care. The programs
were telling in who they included, predominantly single, divorced, or wid-
owed mothers with small children and the elderly, consistent with a variety of more piecemeal programs that had preceded them (Skocpol 1992).
Even more telling was who they left out—predominantly able-bodied single adults and families headed by working adults. This pattern of who is
considered worthy of public charity and who is not is so long-standing in
American welfare policy as to be almost unexamined (M. B. Katz 1986). It
also set up the crisis of the "uninsured" that this cycle of health reform is
designed to improve (if not solve), since low-income working adults and
their children remained the bulk of those without access to insurance on
the eve of implementation of the Affordable Care Act in 2010 (Smith and
Medalia 2014).

Medicare and Medicaid did something else that is underappreciated:
they changed the incentives within the health-care delivery system and
within the larger political environment. Municipal, university, and charity
hospitals had long sought tax dollars and contributions in part to pay for
their provision of care to the poor (Rosner 1982; Rosenberg 1987; R. Stevens
1999). Now that "everyone was a paying customer"—even the poor mothers

and grandmothers who had long evoked sympathy and inspired support—those hospitals reorganized their clinical services, closed their large open wards, and began billing everyone who sought care (Risse 1999; see also R. B. Stevens and Stevens 1974; Engel 2006). University hospitals began to see clinical care as a revenue stream rather than just a public obligation and opportunity to train their students (Rothstein 1987; Ludmerer 1999). Hospitals founded and supported by African American communities closed as Medicare and Medicaid provided a powerful mechanism to enforce racial integration in all clinical services (Gamble 1995; Quadagno 2000). Community health centers, a separate Great Society federal program, offered access to doctors with sliding-scale fees, drawing some of the tax subsidies that had previously gone to hospitals (Sardell 1988; Lefkowitz 2007). In many cities, municipal hospitals, always financially fragile and beholden to local politicians, started to go bankrupt or be closed. The closure of Philadelphia General in 1979 left one of the country's largest cities without a municipal hospital, and Washington, DC, Los Angeles, and many other cities were soon in the same boat (Offner 2001; Whiteis and Salmon 1991; Rice 1987; McLafferty 1982; Friedman 1987; Landry and Landry 2009).

Taken together, Medicare and Medicaid offered health-care coverage to millions of Americans who had not been able to buy insurance before, either due to absolute poverty or because an "actuarially fair" insurance premium (one calculated to cover the anticipated cost of care) for someone over sixty-five is unaffordable for almost everyone. In covering individuals who many agreed had a claim on social resources—the elderly, poor children under five, and their mothers—this expansion of coverage carried an implicit message that those left out had a lesser claim (Lynch 2006). Furthermore, the changes in the health-care safety net that Medicare and Medicaid brought about dismantled much of the charity care that had existed (inadequate as it always was) and set the scene for the problems of uninsurance and medical bankruptcy that have grown considerably over the past thirty years.

HEALTH INEQUALITIES UNDER REFORM

This chapter explores the consequences of a set of recent health reforms, quality improvement efforts, and delivery innovation projects in the U.S. health-care system, tracking how they alter benefits and burdens, with special attention to their impacts on vulnerable populations. The vulnerability model considers the overlapping health impacts of race/ethnicity,

socioeconomic position, medical need, discrimination, and social deprivation (Shi and Stevens 2005; Hofrichter 2003; Wilson 2009). Health-care
reform in Massachusetts, first implemented in 2006, which was the model for
the federal Affordable Care Act (ACA) of 2010, showed that a system of near
universal health care can expand access but still undercut the care of the most
vulnerable (Hanchate et al. 2012; Andrulis and Siddiqui 2011; Ku et al. 2011).
This happened through two mechanisms: decreasing access to insurance or
increasing copayments for individuals (Dennis et al. 2012), and decreasing
funding for the health-care institutions that serve the poor, even though they
continue to provide a disproportionate share of care to the uninsured and
underinsured (M. H. Katz 2011).

The stated goals, predicted results, and actual outcomes of these health
reform projects will be explored using public policy and legislative debates;
reviews of the medical, health policy, and economics literature; and the language and political promises used to advocate for particular changes. The
values embedded in these proposed, piloted, and enacted reforms will be
explored, along with their public justifications and their impacts on patients,
providers, and populations. This approach is part policy analysis, part content
analysis of statements, and embedded in a larger historical understanding of
how change has happened in U.S. health care in the past century.

HEALTH-CARE REFORM: BOTH NEW AND DÉJÀ VU

The existing policy literature on the development, design, and passage of
U.S. health reform in 2010 reveals both the animating ideas and ideals and
the political compromises made to pass the law (McDonough 2011; Starr
2011; Altman and Shactman 2011; Kirsch 2011). The ongoing political debate
about health-care reform reflects differing visions of the good society, but
also of what constitutes fairness. Debates between perspectives favoring
individualism and social solidarity have traditionally been decided in the
United States in favor of individualism, and as multiple scholars have shown,
the United States has a weak tradition of solidarity, particularly across class
and ethnic lines (Hochschild 1981; M. B. Katz 1996; Conley 2010; Gilens
1999). The continuing power of health-care reform as a political issue reflects
these differences in political constituencies, but also reflects (1) worldviews
about the proper relationships of government, families, and individuals, and
(2) the powerful linkage of health insurance to employment in the United
States, which is largely by historical accident (Hoffman 2012; Quadagno

2005; Pauly 1997), but set up a "path-dependent" approach to health care that is politically difficult to change.

The ongoing debate about health system reform in the United States also reflects a larger discussion about health care: What kind of good does it represent in a democratic republic with an economy based on capital markets with some government regulations, subsidies, and incentives? If health care is a commodity like any other, with no special moral significance, then its allocation either on a first-come-first-served basis or through a market-determined price system presents no particular questions of justice. If, on the other hand, health care is special—for example, under John Rawls's notion of special goods, discussed below—then its distribution largely by market mechanisms, which fail to provide health care to those who cannot pay, would be deeply problematic.

There are a number of ways of thinking about health-care justice that would be relevant to health reform. Egalitarian views focus on the equal distribution of health outcomes, health-care access, or opportunities or freedoms related to health. The simplest, a "strict egalitarian" approach, offers the same resources to everyone. The first objection to this in an American health context is presented by the political Right. This objection turns on whether provision for health care is a legitimate role for government, versus a personal responsibility of the people who need medical care and their families. The second objection, from the political Left, asks whether an equal distribution of health care is appropriate, since some people need more than others to reach the same level of health or functioning. This is most trivially true when comparing the acutely sick to everyone else but also, more importantly, applies to those with disabilities, chronic conditions, or socioeconomic disadvantages, who may need more resources to reach, or even have the opportunity to reach, a similar level of health to most who get the equal share. In part as a response to these worries about resource egalitarianism, a capabilities approach focuses instead on promoting people's equal capacities to do and be what they value (see chapter 2, this volume, by Jennifer Ruger). Both resource egalitarianism and the capabilities approach aim to correct inequalities in people's life circumstances, while a relational egalitarian approach elaborates instead on the core idea of what is required for people to relate to one another as moral equals (including political and social equality). For more on these considerations, and what they might mean for health justice, see chapter 3 in this volume by J. Paul Kelleher.

Another common approach, embodied in most economic modeling, is a utilitarian perspective which seeks the "greatest good for the greatest number," without much attention to the distribution of goods in society, or meeting some kind of absolute minimum need for everyone. This utilitarian approach may offer a good first approximation when figuring out how to collect taxes, set subsidies, and create a system of health insurance, as the Affordable Care Act does.

The challenge to a utilitarian approach to distribution of health care comes in evaluating fairness and consequences. Health insurance has long faced value trade-offs such as whether it should only cover catastrophic and unpredictable expenses, as the original Lloyds of London and other companies did when they created the first modern insurance policies to cover ships and their cargos at sea in the eighteenth century. The alternate view says that health insurance should be as comprehensive as possible, both to protect individuals from catastrophic costs and to allow them to have predictable medical expenses to ensure financial access to all beneficial treatment. The comprehensive perspective is often taken by those concerned that individuals of modest means may not be able to pay even routine medical expenses, and that cost may discourage them from services such as checkups, cholesterol tests, gynecological exams, and other preventive services that may prevent greater health problems and costs in the future. The Affordable Care Act has split the difference between comprehensive and catastrophic medical insurance, encouraging plans with relatively high deductibles that encourage their use largely for large and unanticipated expenses, while also requiring that preventive services be covered without copays and not subject to deductibles.

The American philosopher John Rawls was concerned about fairness, particularly in the distribution of what he called "primary goods," which he described as "things that any rational person would want regardless of their particular conception of the good" (Rawls 1971, 79–81). Rawls goes on to divide primary goods into "natural" goods with which an individual may be endowed, including intelligence, imagination, health, and other traits; and social primary goods, including civil and political rights, liberties, income, and wealth, the social bases of self-respect, and others. In contrast to a "strict egalitarian" perspective, under which everyone would be entitled to an equal share of all of these goods, Rawls allows for differences in the distribution, but describes a fair process for allocation, much like the strategy used by a parent: letting one child divide a cake or cookie and the other child pick the first piece. Rawls argues that an unequal distribution of primary goods is only fair to the extent that it improves the condition of the worst-off. This approach, of maximizing the welfare of those with the least, is called "maxi-min" in his framework. Norman Daniels, extending Rawls's framework to health care, argues that health care is a special good because it is fundamental to "fair equality of opportunity" in education, work, and other realms of life (Daniels 1985; see also Richards 1971).

An alternate approach to health-care justice is capabilities theory, in which economic arrangements are seen to be just to the extent that they support the freedom of individuals to be and do what need to achieve goals such as health, happiness, and economic self-sufficiency. This approach, developed by the development economist Amartya Sen and the philosopher Martha Nussbaum, and extended by many others, underlies the UN "human development index," which ranks countries by how well they perform in life expectancy, education, and income for their populations (UNDP 2014). A capabilities approach would also support viewing health care as a special good to which individuals have claims on society, more fully explored by Jennifer Ruger (Ruger 2009; Ruger, chapter 2, this volume). Both of these approaches would also support social responsibility for goods such as primary and secondary education, which are fundamental to both "equality of opportunity" in the Rawlsian framework and development of human capabilities in Sen and Nussbaum's formulation of justice (Baker and LeTendre 2005). Further, as epidemiologists have developed a richer understanding of the importance for health of other goods such as healthy food, well-designed housing, meaningful work, education, and safe neighborhoods that facilitate exercise, along with protection from violence, pollution, and other detrimental features, scholars such as Daniels have turned their concerns toward just distribution of these goods as well, both in their own right and because of their contribution to health and opportunity (Marmot and Wilkinson 2006; Krieger 2005; Daniels 2008).

Finally, health care in the United States presents numerous examples in which similarly situated individuals are treated differently. This violates the principle of formal justice that like cases should be treated alike, common to all of the more elaborated theories of justice above.

HEALTH-CARE REFORM AND THE AFFORDABLE CARE ACT

According to the Congressional Budget Office, implementation of the ACA was expected to provide health insurance to 12 million of the 54 million currently uninsured Americans in 2014, and by 2017 provide insurance to 26 million Americans who would otherwise lack it (CBO 2014). These estimates changed from the passage of the ACA through implementation, most notably after the Supreme Court, in 2012, made expansion of state Medicaid programs to everyone under 138 percent of the poverty line optional in *National Federation of Independent Business v. Sebelius.* While most discussions of health-care reform have focused on broadening access to health insurance and changing payment structures for hospitals and physicians, other recent changes have the potential to be almost as wide-ranging in their impacts. Report cards for hospitals and physicians, ranking them on their quality of care, and pay-for-performance and accountable care programs tie payment to health outcomes rather than simply reimbursing for the unit of care provided. These strategies attempt to use the payment system to reimburse better health instead of simply more service.

The overarching value system embedded in these new models for payment reform is a rough utilitarianism drawn from their origins in economic analysis and plans to use financial incentives to change the behavior of physicians, hospitals, and patients. Utilitarianism, which originated in the work of the British philosophers Jeremy Bentham (1748–1832) and John Stuart Mill (1806–73), is sometimes understood as calling for the greatest good for the greatest number. In a utilitarian scheme, units of "utility" or happiness are measured in the aggregate; each additional unit of happiness improves society as a whole, regardless of who enjoys it. In the context of health care, an action that improved the health of anyone would be good, as long as it did not reduce anyone else's health by a greater magnitude. This suggests that improving the care of heart attacks, asthma, or trauma in richer communities and among better-off individuals—as has been done over the last generation—would be laudable. From the perspective of health disparities, however, improvement for one group without increasing access to the worse-off—such as providing advanced cardiac care to urban residents on the coasts but not to residents of the Appalachian coal belt, or offering preventive asthma-attack medications to middle-class children but not to poor residents of inner cities—is a chief mechanism by which disparities grow.

New models of health-care delivery and payment—such as paying providers for outcomes instead of services, or behavioral economics–inspired wellness programs paying patients for completing wellness assessments and penalizing patients who smoke or have a high body-mass index—are intended to alter incentives for patients and providers throughout the system. While many of these incentives are designed to make care efficient and cost-effective, others are designed to reward quality of care and align incentives with clinically desirable outcomes. For instance, continuing the current practice of paying hospitals and providers more for surgeries with complications than for those without (Eappen et al. 2013), or paying obstetricians more for cesarean sections than for vaginal deliveries, appears to reduce incentives to improve clinical care, since providers are paid more for the "bad" outcome than the "good" one from the patient's perspective (Rehavi and Johnson 2013). Unless these payment practices change, they will blunt financial incentives to change practice. Many of these policy approaches are also based in other normative approaches to medical care. For example, the Affordable Care Act draws on welfare theories of economics and arguments about health as a driver of equality of opportunity most associated with John Rawls and Norman Daniels. Quality improvement programs, including pay for performance and nonpayment for complications, are based on beneficence toward patients and a consequentialist or compensatory justice approach to health-care providers.

DOES INSURANCE MEAN ACCESS TO CARE? PREMIUMS, COPAYMENTS, AND THE CADILLAC TAX

While insurance sold after implementation of the ACA promises to be more comprehensive than many policies sold to individuals and small businesses before reform, plans available in the health-care exchanges (state-based online marketplaces) often have substantially greater cost-sharing than most large group employer-based health insurance plans. "Actuarial value" for a health plan is defined by the fraction of anticipated health-care costs the plan would cover; the remainder is the responsibility of the individual. A "Bronze" plan under the health exchanges has to cover 60 percent of expected health-care costs. A "Silver" plan must cover 70 percent, "Gold" plans 80 percent, and "Platinum" plans 90 percent.[1] Income tax subsidies were calculated to make a Silver plan affordable (set for each market based on the second-lowest-price Silver plan available in the marketplace, the "benchmark" plan). Health plans may use a combination of premiums, deductibles (an amount of health-care costs the individual has to pay before insurance covers anything), copayments (fixed dollar amounts for doctor's visits, prescriptions, and other services), and coinsurance (a percentage of costs that the patient may be responsible for, commonly 10 to 20 percent) to reach that average value. This combination of patient costs makes it extremely difficult for individuals to shop for insurance based on price, because the premium figure quoted up front is only one factor in how much the patient is likely to pay for health care over the course of the year (Frakt 2014).

The finding that providing insurance does not guarantee access to services has been demonstrated repeatedly, at least since the beginning of Medicaid: not all providers accept all insurance programs, because Medicaid has traditionally provided lower reimbursements than other types of insurance. Finally, health reform carries the risk that politicians, policy makers, and the public will believe that the problem of provision of health services for the poor has been solved by the provision of health insurance. This mistaken belief has led to the dismantling of other (certainly also inadequate) approaches to charity care (R. B. Stevens and Stevens 1974) such as charity hospital wards, and after the ACA passed many hospitals changed their rules about whose debt they would write off and whose they would go to court to collect (Pearjan 2015). Receiving charity care at the discretion of a doctor or hospital is not, of course, the same as a right to health care. Charity can be withdrawn or withheld for any reason, can discriminate on the basis of almost any characteristic of the recipient, and is seldom adequate to meet needs.

Another area in the ACA that generated concern among advocates for improved health-care access was the so-called Cadillac tax on health plans. The Cadillac tax was designed to address a long-standing frustration among health economists and some policy makers about the "tax exclusion" of employer-based health insurance for both employee and employer. This preferential tax status for employer-based group health insurance originated in World War II, when wage and price caps temporarily made it impossible for businesses to recruit workers by offering them better wages. After World War II, this tax exclusion of the value of health insurance from income tax for workers was made permanent, making a dollar of health insurance, which is not taxed, more valuable to employees than a dollar in cash compensation, which is taxed. As a consequence, employees or their unions may seek more generous health insurance plans than they might otherwise. Then, insulated from the direct costs of health care at the point of service, individuals may use more health care than they would if they were paying out of pocket ("moral hazard," in the language of economists). This may be a good thing or a bad thing from the point of view of health, since patients are not very good at differentiating, or doctors at communicating, which tests or treatments their doctors recommend are essential to protect their health, and which are more discretionary. The aggregation of millions of such choices is thought to increase health-care cost inflation. Over the past two decades, the standard solution to this problem in the policy discourse has been to give patients "more skin in the game," translated as greater exposure to the costs of their health care. Again, this may be fine for sports injuries that could be repaired or not without affecting day-to-day functioning, but if increased out-of-pocket costs mean that patients stop taking cholesterol medicines or blood thinners to prevent heart attacks, it may be unwise from both a health and a cost perspective. This systematic shifting of costs from employers to patients and their families has been well documented (Claxton 2004; Hacker 2006), as has its impact on health-care access for individuals of modest incomes (Richman and Brodie 2014; Wharam et al. 2013; Schoen et al. 2010). For individuals with chronic illnesses, there has been substantial controversy about whether the increasing burden of copayments and coinsurance for outpatient visits and medications leads to preventable and costly hospital admissions (Li et al. 2014).

These findings are hardly new. The sociologist Earl Koos showed in the 1950s that patients of modest income would think twice about going to the doctor for all but the most severe symptoms, a reticence not shared by those of greater means in the same community (Koos 1954). The economists and health researchers who ran the RAND Health Insurance Experiment (HIE) in the 1970s and 1980s brought quantitative measurement and random assignment to questions about the impact of cost on how and when patients seek medical care, and the HIE findings are cited both by those who believe insurance should be more generous and by policy makers on the other side. In the HIE, families were randomized to several health insurance designs with a range of coinsurance and copayments, from no out-of-pocket care cost to patient costs of 25 or 50 percent of charges up to 5, 10, or 15 percent of income. As cost to the individual went up, health-care utilization went down. Individuals from lower-income families decreased their use of health care more than those from higher-income tiers did. Moreover, lower health-care utilization did not lead to statistically significant differences in the few health measures they were able to track across all participants (Newhouse and the Insurance Experiment Group 1993). But decreases in health-care utilization in response to cost included both services that experts deemed discretionary and those that experts ranked as essential. Furthermore, with a 2016 minimum wage of $7.25 per hour and a maximum individual health insurance deductible of $6,550, high-deductible insurance plans offered to employees or sold to individuals under the ACA can have cost sharing of 100 percent of costs up to 45 percent of a minimum-wage worker's annual income, threefold higher than anything contemplated in the RAND Health Insurance Experiment (IRS 2016).

The Cadillac tax on health insurance plans risks worsening this process of income-based rationing. Beginning in 2018, a 40 percent excise tax is scheduled to be imposed on the value of health insurance benefits exceeding $10,200 for individual coverage and $27,500 for family coverage (indexed to inflation). The law specifies that the thresholds can increase for individuals in high-risk professions and for employers that have a disproportionately older population. For employer-based plans, there are certainly "executive" health plans offered by some companies to their most highly compensated executives, including in sectors such as manufacturing, computing, and finance. But the primary determinants of a health insurance premium besides benefits are the age and health status of the covered population. Analysts and advocates for older, unionized workforces in manufacturing, transportation, and other sectors raised the concern during the health reform debate that their plans might be taxed under the Cadillac tax not because of the richness of their benefits, but because of the health of their workers. In an era of growing inequality and stagnating wages, these workers are already facing an increasing burden from their out-of-pocket health-care costs (Fletcher 2014).

THE LOT OF THE WORST-OFF: HEALTH-CARE ACCESS AND SAFETY-NET PROVIDERS

Even by the Congressional Budget Office's latest ten-year projections from April 2014, in 2016 to 2024 there will remain 29 million to 31 million non-elderly uninsured individuals in the United States. That fact alone demonstrates the ongoing need for additional systems of health-care provision. Furthermore, geographic clustering of the uninsured in urban communities where many poor residents live, and in rural areas with both low incomes and few health-care providers, will create a continued need for health institutions with a special mission to serve the disadvantaged. Rural critical-access hospitals across the plains, the rural South, and in other areas of the country continue to receive preferential payment rates from Medicare and Medicaid. These hospitals are also given other kinds of administrative flexibility, such as the ability to bill for rehabilitation and posthospitalization nursing care, generally because those services are otherwise not available in sparsely populated regions of the country and because these services contribute to the financial viability of these small facilities.

While the expansion of public and private insurance under health-care reform might appear to reduce the need for traditional safety-net institutions to provide health care, there will continue to be substantial need for low-cost providers due to the persistence of large numbers of uninsured individuals.

Those excluded from health insurance after reform include undocumented immigrants (categorically excluded under the law), and individuals under 100 percent of the poverty line who would qualify for Medicaid under reform but who live in states that have chosen not to expand Medicaid eligibility. Finally, individuals can be exempted from the individual mandate to buy insurance if there is no affordable plan available to them, defined in the law as a plan that costs less than 8 percent of annual income (Hall and Rosenbaum 2012; Hall 2011b; Hall 2011a; M. H. Katz 2010; M. H. Katz and Brigham 2011; Wang, Conroy, and Zuckerman 2009; McKethan et al. 2009). However, the IRS has followed the Congressional Joint Committee on Taxation's deliberations on this affordability provision to apply the definition of "affordable" employer-based coverage to the cost of employee-only coverage, not family coverage, which usually costs considerably more (Health Affairs 2014). Under the "family glitch," if the employee may have access to employer-based insurance, then the family is ineligible for tax credits to buy a policy through the ACA marketplaces even if family coverage costs 15 percent, 20 percent, or more of family income. Nonworking spouses, or working spouses whose employers don't offer coverage, and children are those most likely to be uninsured due to the "family glitch." As a result of all of these groups ineligible for coverage under the ACA or existing health policies and programs, community health centers for primary care, government hospitals, and mission-oriented non-profit hospitals will continue to be needed for those who remain uninsured despite health-care reform. Safety-net providers will also remain essential to those whose cost-sharing requirements remain burdensome and for services that may not be covered, such as vision, dental, and disability rehabilitation (Hall and Rosenbaum 2012). For example, Sarah Horton and Judith Barker (chapter 5, this volume) explore dental inequalities and their impact on Latino children.

The Massachusetts health reform enacted in 2006 under Governor Mitt Romney became the template for the national Affordable Care Act of 2010 (Gruber 2008). The politics in Massachusetts were quite different than nationally, as Massachusetts is not typical of the rest of the country in terms of income, demographics, or political environment; instead it represents a high–social service / high-tax state that is amenable to expansion of health programs.

Reform in Massachusetts showed that a system of near-universal health care can expand access but still undercut the care of the most vulnerable (Hanchate et al. 2012; Andrulis and Siddiqui 2011; Ku et al. 2011;

M. H. Katz 2011). Experiences in Massachusetts demonstrated some of the promise (Gruber 2008) and some of the challenges that the ACA may present to safety-net institutions. Massachusetts health-care reform increased coverage of the uninsured, but nearly bankrupted safety-net hospitals that had long served the most vulnerable because it failed to account for the clustering of the remaining uninsured at a few facilities (Himmelstein and Woolhandler 2010; Maxwell et al. 2011; Pande et al. 2011). These hospitals suffered from high levels of Medicaid insurance among their patients, which reimburses hospitals at rates below their costs. They also continued to see many patients without insurance despite health-care reform, while at the same time reform was paid for in part by withdrawing of subsidies for caring for the poor that these hospitals had long received from Massachusetts under its Free Care pool and the Medicaid Disproportionate Share program (Thompson 2012).

This dynamic is now being repeated in national health reform (Neuhausen et al. 2014). Hospitals in states that have not expanded Medicaid face a similar but even more difficult dynamic, with continued high rates of uninsured patients (Price and Eibner 2013; Glied and Ma 2013). As in Massachusetts, subsidies to care for the uninsured are scheduled to phase out over the first few years of national health reform, but unlike in Massachusetts, these hospitals will not see the same level of increases in insurance coverage for their patients, meaning they will be worse off than before reform unless there is a last-minute change in either coverage or subsidies. Furthermore, insurance coverage expansion may not benefit hospitals and other providers as much as anticipated: individuals with incomes below 100 percent of the federal poverty line are not eligible for tax subsidies on the insurance exchanges, because the drafters of the Affordable Care Act assumed all individuals under 138 percent of the poverty line would be covered by the Medicaid expansion included in the law. Finally, many exchange plans contract with only a few hospitals and doctors, using a so-called narrow network design, which is particularly likely to cause problems for regional referral hospitals to which a patient may be brought by ambulance even if their insurance does not cover that hospital.

Neither economists nor policy makers have really come to grips with the clustering of disadvantaged patients within and across the health-care system, whose insurance frequently reimburses at or below providers' costs. Just because there is enough money in the system as a whole does not mean that "it all averages out" in terms of the financial viability of health-care institutions. This is a long-standing problem and is a principal reason many health-care providers do not accept Medicaid insurance. "Payer mix" is a crucial determinant of the profitability of hospitals, doctors, and other health-care providers: in other words, a provider can afford to care for some patients with Medicaid or no insurance if they have enough other patients with private insurance to "cross-subsidize" them. As private insurers have become more and more skilled since the 1980s at negotiating with providers for discounts and reviewing expensive tests and procedures, providers have had less leeway to cross-subsidize "poor payers" such as Medicaid (Montague 1995). The calculations are complex, since each health-care provider and institution contracts with hundreds if not thousands of insurers. But usually Medicaid pays below the cost to provide the service, while Medicare pays at about cost or a little more, and most of the time private insurers pay between 150 percent and 300 percent of the Medicare rate. This varies by insurer, provider, region, and even which service the patient receives. Over the past four decades in cities like New York, Philadelphia, Washington, Los Angeles, and Detroit, hospitals have not generally closed due to a lack of patients, but due to a lack of money—usually high rates of uninsured and Medicaid patients whose care costs more to provide than the hospitals receive in reimbursements (Landry and Landry 2009, 271–72). Residential segregation by income has ensured that due to their geographic catchment areas, hospitals can be as unequal as our neighborhoods and schools. One solution to this problem, in which caring for the poor insured by Medicaid can drive a hospital to bankruptcy, is to increase Medicaid reimbursement rates to at least cover hospitals' and doctors' costs. This discretion belongs to the state-level policy makers who set Medicaid rates, and the legislatures that allocate taxpayer funds between health care and other priorities.

Finally, some patients are finding that their insurance plans under the ACA make it difficult to afford care at the point of service because of high deductibles, copayments, and coinsurance, and because of limitations in which hospitals, physicians, and pharmaceuticals are covered by the plans (Kliff 2014; Gottlieb 2014). This was also seen in Massachusetts, where the poorest patients found that copayments under the new system were scaled to the standards for private insurance, often in the range of $10–50, higher than the copayments they had previously faced, which had been scaled to the limited incomes of Medicaid recipients, on the order of $1–5 (McCormick et al. 2012; Mulvaney-Day et al. 2012; Clark et al. 2011; Zhu et al. 2010). Modifications to Massachusetts's programs have addressed these initial shortcomings of the program, but notably, problems with funding of safety-net institutions and levels of copayments and cost sharing for the poorest recipients are being repeated in many other states as they roll out national reform.

QUALITY, ACCOUNTABILITY, AND SERVING
VULNERABLE POPULATIONS

Innovations that improve access and quality of care in the aggregate have frequently been shown to have less benefit or even harm to vulnerable populations. Improvements in quality of care frequently have the ironic consequence of widening disparities, either because the populations who had the worst outcomes to start with are more difficult to reach with improved care, or because the mechanisms designed to increase access and quality destabilize institutions that have long served the poor. For instance, cardiac surgery report cards were started in New York in the 1980s, and within a decade it became clear that it was harder for patients with severe disease and multiple comorbidities to find a surgeon, because they could be predicted to have a higher risk of poor outcomes, but the physician's "grade" was not adjusted to account for the baseline risk of his or her patients (Brown, Clarke, and Oakley 2012; Shahian et al. 2011). Report cards in New York were associated with widening of racial and ethnic disparities, likely because surgeons perceived minority patients as at higher risk for poor clinical outcomes (Werner, Asch, and Polsky 2005). Under Medicare's policy of denying payment for readmissions (Naylor et al. 2012; Bhalla and Kalkut 2010) or hospital-acquired urinary tract infections and decubitus ulcers, hospitals have incentives to avoid elderly and disabled patients who are at high risk for these complications (Saint et al. 2009; Meddings, Saint, and McMahon 2010; Meddings et al. 2012; Morgan et al. 2012). Finally, variation in outcomes is frequently attributable to the quality of facilities where patients are treated rather than the characteristics of individual patients or providers (Heisler et al. 2003; Weinick and Hasnain-Wynia 2011). But the payer mix and reimbursements for a particular hospital determine the resources it has to bring to any given patient's care, including in the documentation of the quality of care provided (Millett et al. 2009).

Using payments to create incentives for high-quality health care seems simple on its face, and paying more for high-quality care is a sensible strategy, especially compared to simply paying by volume of medical procedures whether they produce good outcomes or bad ones. The challenge is whether incentives can be structured around factors within the control of the health-care provider. What is fair to providers in these schemes is highly controversial (Bogdan-Lovis, Fleck, and Barry 2012). The question of whether one should adjust, in health-care pay-for-performance, for severity of illness of the population served, income, geography, and many other factors known to affect outcomes mirrors the contentious debates over education reform (Carrier et al. 2011; Mehta et al. 2008). Are those who educate poor children, or provide health care to poor patients, responsible for those individuals' poorer-than-average outcomes, or are they due to poverty, living conditions, stress, or other factors outside of the control of those professionals? Or even more basic, is the sample size of a teacher's students or a doctor's patients too small to make meaningful distinctions in quality of care (Hofer et al. 1999; Krein et al. 2002)? This is a critical question in the design and implementation of pay-for-performance because health outcomes are known to vary with poverty.

The question remains unresolved whether one can separate the performance of service providers from the other influences on the health outcomes that are being ranked and scored in pay-for-performance programs. If we cannot, instead of providing incentives to improve health outcomes, the programs risk leading providers to cherry-pick healthier patients and possibly to "fire" their sicker, noncompliant patients (Hayward and Kent 2008). Analyses that adjust provider scores by known confounders—risk adjustment for the population served is one—can also be important in assessing health outcomes seen for physician practices or facilities such as hospitals, nursing homes, and rehabilitation centers.

In contrast, in the debates over Medicare and Medicaid's programs for payment for outcomes and nonpayment for complications, the decision has been made explicitly not to adjust for expected health of the population served. The argument that no one should receive second-class care is a reasonable one. But the simple measurement of outcomes does not address whether the outcomes are due to poor care (in which case penalizing providers financially makes sense), inadequate resources to provide the care (perhaps due to poor reimbursements from Medicaid), or risk factors present in the patients or community (which might be better addressed through individual or community public health interventions). Assessments of teachers and schools based on student outcomes face a similar problem of differentiating quality of instruction, differences in resources provided for instruction, and greater needs of poor students.

The assumption underlying some health reforms is that inefficient or low-quality providers will go out of business, just as in the private sector. But if the goal is to serve a population, not a customer base, then one has to ask who will replace these service providers. The existence of large urban and rural areas with inadequate health service access demonstrates that this problem has not yet been solved, and many of the hospital bankruptcies that have led to closures in the past thirty years have been due more to a poor payer mix (too many uninsured and Medicaid patients) than to inadequate clinical demand.

HEALTH CARE FOR UNDOCUMENTED IMMIGRANTS: THE LIMITS OF SELF-INTEREST IN HEALTH POLICY

The decision to exclude undocumented immigrants from national health reform was seen as critical to passage and is consistent with other recent legislation and policy initiatives at national, state, and local levels (Park 2011). This choice is problematic because of the long-established links between the United States and the countries of origin of the bulk of undocumented immigrants, including South America, Central America, and the Caribbean, as well as China by virtue of its size (Ngai 2004). Migrant labor is integral to many economic sectors of our economy, including agriculture, construction, and personal services. In addition to these economic ties, many undocumented immigrants are the spouses or children of U.S. citizens. Further, there are self-interest arguments in favor of universal health care, from reduced risk of infectious diseases to improved economic efficiency of workers to the de facto universal care we already provide at great expense in emergency departments and hospitals (Churchill 1994). These arguments—that it is in the interest of everyone that the entire population receive health care, to reduce the spread of disease and the direct or indirect cost of emergency care to taxpayers—have had little sway in the American political system. The universal health-care systems of Europe, as well as those of Asia, Africa, and Latin America, are fundamentally based on solidarity among citizens. Exclusion of noncitizens from health-care systems is not unique to the United States, and immigrants have become political flash points in health and welfare policy in many countries, including France, Germany, and South Africa (see, e.g., Ticktin 2011). In the United States, the burden on safety-net institutions in immigrant communities is likely to combine reduced funding, similar or increased need, and increased political vulnerability, as their patient population both appears to be and is composed of a larger fraction of undocumented immigrants than before reform (Matthew 2012).

TREATING LIKE CASES ALIKE: THE LIMITS OF STATE-BASED HEALTH-CARE REFORM

The decision to implement health-care reform through state governments draws on decades of U.S. social policy (Blau 2010; DiNitto and Cummins 2005). Health has traditionally been an area of state and local policy making in the United States, with the federal role limited to border quarantine and the health of sailors until after the U.S. Civil War in the 1860s, and with the federal government only taking a substantial role after World War II. Many recent health policy innovations have started in one or several states, including the Children's Health Insurance Program (CHIP) and the Massachusetts health reform that serves as the model for the ACA (Hackey and Rochefort 2001; Hackey 1998; Fox and Iglehart 1994; McDonough 2011). At the same time, state social and health programs have long been characterized by wide variation between the states in criteria for state-supported or subsidized services and in the nature, extent, and quality of the services offered. These divisions have frequently been on a regional basis, mapping to regional differences in levels of taxation, governing philosophy, and support for or hostility toward social spending. State Medicaid programs have been important exemplars of variability between states such as New York and California, which have traditionally supported generous social spending, at the price of relatively high tax burdens, and states such as Texas and Mississippi, which have followed a low-tax and limited social spending regime (R. B. Stevens and Stevens 1974). Governance models and political and administrative realities drove the choice to administer health reform at the state level, and to allow states substantial latitude in how it would be managed, much as in recent health policies from CHIP to Medicaid waivers (Fox and Iglehart 1994; Hackey 1998; Hackey and Rochefort 2001). States have dozens of choices to make in implementing health-care reform, most broadly about expanding Medicaid and running insurance exchanges, but within these programs there are hundreds of additional decisions that make each state's programs different from all others.

Most controversially and consequentially for many residents is the question of how and why states choose to expand their Medicaid programs (or not) and how the politics of race, ethnicity, and political climate affect these choices (Jacobs and Callaghan 2013; Andrews 2014). Arizona's decision to expand Medicaid because legal immigrants would otherwise have greater access to health care than citizens (an unintended consequence of the way the subsidy rules were written for private insurance) suggests that the politics could be more complex than expected (Brownstein 2013; Park 2011). The original plans for the ACA included standardizing the eligibility criteria for state Medicaid at 138 percent of the federal poverty line across all states for all categories of people (not just the elderly, disabled, or children). But the Supreme Court ruled in June 2012 that states could not be required to expand their Medicaid programs by the threat of removing all Medicaid funding for the state (U.S. Supreme Court 2012). Variations in the benefits and eligibility for Medicaid across state boundaries create differences in treatment among similarly situated individuals, which could be seen as an affront to formal justice.

The American federal system, however, has long accepted, and sometimes valorized, such differences between states in social policy, programs, and the taxes that support them. Recent health policy literature talks about the "laboratory of the states," which can try out approaches to health reform at scale and see what works and what doesn't (Fox and Iglehart 1994; Hackey and Rochefort 2001). Others have questioned whether states have the technical capacity, financial stability, or political will to expand health-care access, particularly whether they can do it affordably (Sparer 1996). The argument that states should have discretion or autonomy when spending state tax dollars is a strong one, but there is also a history of politicians from southeastern states seeing to it that federal programs like Social Security and the Hill-Burton Act, which paid for hospital construction in the 1950s and 1960s, did not disrupt racial segregation (Poole 2006).

JUSTICE, HEALTH INEQUALITIES, AND REFORM

The expansion of health insurance to as many as 30 million Americans who lacked it is a profound social change, one that many observers would have predicted was impossible based on our unique history with health policy (Gordon 2003; Quadagno 2005; Hoffman 2012). That it would be controversial was, given that history, completely predictable. Health care, taxes, and citizenship bring together some of the most profound fault lines in social thought and political structure in the United States.

The values driving reform include some drawn from economic modeling, including that optimizing efficiency is among the highest values, if not the highest value, and that improving aggregate outcomes is an acceptable outcome even if benefits are distributed inequitably (Frey 2009). The use of aggregate versus stratified outcomes in economic modeling and clinical assessment can distinguish impacts on the average person or family from impacts on the poor or disadvantaged. These stratified analyses—or their absence—are particularly important for documenting differential impacts of health reform by income.

Health reform also raises fundamental questions about our federated republic. Can citizens be denied, based on their state of residence, a benefit paid for with federal tax money (Medicaid expansion)? The rationale for state control is the future obligation to provide state matching funds. The consequence of these decisions, though, is that the poorest Americans in Mississippi or Texas are demonstrably worse off than similarly situated Americans in New York, Massachusetts, or California. This fails to meet the requirements of formal justice, in which like cases are treated alike.

Examining the place of equity in design and practice of health-care reform, and their impact on the most vulnerable patients and communities (in Rawlsian fashion), presents an opportunity to make explicit the values underlying health-care reform, in part so they can be better aligned with real-world policy outcomes.

NOTE

1. "Health Insurance Marketplace Calculator," Henry J. Kaiser Family Foundation, http://kff.org/interactive/subsidy-calculator/, accessed March 5, 2016. See the site's notes for explanation of plan levels. See also Ward and Johnson (2013).

REFERENCES

Altman, Stuart H., and David Shactman. 2011. *Power, Politics, and Universal Health Care: The Inside Story of a Century-Long Battle.* Amherst, MA: Prometheus.

Andrews, Christina. 2014. "Unintended Consequences: Medicaid Expansion and Racial Inequality in Access to Health Insurance." *Health and Social Work* 39 (3): 131–33.

Andrulis, Dennis P., and Nadia J. Siddiqui. 2011. "Health Reform Holds Both Risks and Rewards for Safety-Net Providers and Racially and Ethnically Diverse Patients." *Health Affairs* 30 (10): 1830–36.

Baker, David P., and Gerald K. LeTendre. 2005. *National Differences, Global Similarities: World Culture and the Future of Schooling.* Stanford, CA: Stanford Social Sciences.

Bhalla, Rohit, and Gary Kalkut. 2010. "Could Medicare Readmission Policy Exacerbate Health Care System Inequity?" *Annals of Internal Medicine* 152 (2): 114–17.

Blau, Joel. 2010. *The Dynamics of Social Welfare Policy.* 3rd ed. New York: Oxford University Press.

Bogdan-Lovis, Elizabeth, Leonard Fleck, and Henry C. Barry. 2012. "It's NOT FAIR! Or Is It? The Promise and the Tyranny of Evidence-Based Performance Assessment." *Theoretical Medicine and Bioethics* 33 (4): 293–311.

Brown, David L., Stephen Clarke, and Justin Oakley. 2012. "Cardiac Surgeon Report Cards, Referral for Cardiac Surgery, and the Ethical Responsibilities of Cardiologists." *Journal of the American College of Cardiology* 59 (25): 2378–82.

Brownstein, Ronald. 2013. "Why the GOP's Resistance to Medicaid Expansion Is Eroding." *National Journal*, February 7. http://www.nationaljournal.com/columns/political-connections/why-the-gop-s-resistance-to-medicaid-expansion-is-eroding-20130207. Accessed 29 August 2015.

Carrier, Emily R., Eric Schneider, Hoangmai H. Pham, and Peter B. Bach. 2011. "Association between Quality of Care and the Sociodemographic Composition of Physicians' Patient Panels: A Repeat Cross-Sectional Analysis." *Journal of General Internal Medicine* 26 (9): 987–94.

CBO (Congressional Budget Office). 2014. *Insurance Coverage Provisions of the Affordable Care Act: CBO's April 2014 Baseline.* 29 August 2015. https://www.cbo.gov/publication/43900.

Churchill, Larry R. 1994. *Self-Interest and Universal Health Care: Why Well-Insured Americans Should Support Coverage for Everyone.* Cambridge, MA: Harvard University Press.

Clark, Cheryl R., Jane Soukup, Usha Govindarajulu, Heather E. Riden, Dora A. Tovar, and Paula A. Johnson. 2011. "Lack of Access due to Costs Remains a Problem for Some in Massachusetts despite the State's Health Reforms." *Health Affairs* 30 (2): 247–55.

Claxton, Debra Draper Gary. 2004. "Managed Care Redux Health Plans Shift Responsibilities to Consumers." *Center for Studying Health System Change: Issue Briefs*, no. 79 (March): 1–4.

Conley, Dalton. 2010. *Being Black, Living in the Red: Race, Wealth, and Social Policy in America.* Berkeley: University of California Press.

Daniels, Norman. 1985. *Just Health Care.* New York: Cambridge University Press.

———. 2008. *Just Health: Meeting Health Needs Fairly.* New York: Cambridge University Press.

Dennis, Amanda, Kelly Blanchard, Denisse Córdova, Britt Wahlin, Jill Clark, Karen Edlund, Jennifer McIntosh, and Lenore Tsikitas. 2012. "What Happens to the Women Who Fall through the Cracks of Health Care Reform? Lessons from Massachusetts." *Journal of Health Politics, Policy and Law* 38 (2): 393–419.

DiNitto, Diana M., and Linda K. Cummins. 2005. *Social Welfare: Politics and Public Policy.* 6th ed. Boston: Pearson / Allyn and Beacon.

Eappen, Sunil, Bennett H. Lane, Barry Rosenberg, Stuart A. Lipsitz, David Sadoff, Dave Matheson, William R. Berry, Mark Lester, and Atul A. Gawande. 2013. "Relationship between Occurrence of Surgical Complications and Hospital Finances." *Journal of the American Medical Association* 309 (15): 1599–1606.

Engel, Jonathan. 2006. *Poor People's Medicine: Medicaid and American Charity Care since 1965*. Durham, NC: Duke University Press.

Fletcher, Rebecca Adkins. 2014. "Keeping Up with the Cadillacs: What Health Insurance Disparities, Moral Hazard, and the Cadillac Tax Mean to the Patient Protection and Affordable Care Act." *Medical Anthropology Quarterly*. [Epub ahead of print]. doi:10.1111/maq.12120.

Fox, Daniel M., and John K. Iglehart. 1994. *Five States That Could Not Wait: Lessons for Health Reform from Florida, Hawaii, Minnesota, Oregon, and Vermont*. New York: Milbank Memorial Fund.

Frakt, Austin. 2014. "Choosing a Health Plan Is Hard, Even for a Health Economist." *New York Times*, October 27.

Frey, Donald E. 2009. *America's Economic Moralists: A History of Rival Ethics and Economics*. Albany: State University of New York Press.

Friedman, Emily. 1987. "Public Hospitals Often Face Unmet Capital Needs, Underfunding, Uncompensated Patient-Care Costs." *Journal of the American Medical Association* 257 (13): 1698–1701.

Gamble, Vanessa Northington. 1995. *Making a Place for Ourselves: The Black Hospital Movement, 1920–1945*. New York: Oxford University Press.

Gilens, Martin. 1999. *Why Americans Hate Welfare: Race, Media, and the Politics of Antipoverty Policy*. Chicago: University of Chicago Press.

Glied, Sherry, and Stephanie Ma. 2013. "How States Stand to Gain or Lose Federal Funds by Opting In or Out of the Medicaid Expansion." *Commonwealth Fund: Issue Briefs* 32: 1–12.

Gordon, Colin. 2003. *Dead on Arrival: The Politics of Health Care in Twentieth-Century America*. Princeton, NJ: Princeton University Press.

Gottlieb, Scott. 2014. "Under Obamacare's 'Closed Formularies' Patients with Serious Chronic Diseases like MS Don't Get Access to Vital Medicines." *Forbes Business*. June 13. http://www.forbes.com/sites/scottgottlieb/2014/06/13/obamacare-shortchanges-patients-with-chronic-diseases/. Accessed 29 August 2015.

Gruber, Jonathan. 2008. "Taking Massachusetts National: Incremental Universalism for the United States." In *Who Has the Cure? Hamilton Project Ideas on Health Care*, edited by Jason Furman, 121–42. Washington, DC: Brookings Institution Press.

Hacker, Jacob S. 2006. *The Great Risk Shift: The Assault on American Jobs, Families, Health Care, and Retirement and How You Can Fight Back*. New York: Oxford University Press.

Hackey, Robert B. 1998. *Rethinking Health Care Policy: The New Politics of State Regulation*. Washington, DC: Georgetown University Press.

Hall, Mark A. 2011a. "Rethinking Safety-Net Access for the Uninsured." *New England Journal of Medicine* 364 (1): 7–9.

———. 2011b. "The Mission of Safety Net Organizations Following National Insurance Reform." *Journal of General Internal Medicine* 26 (7): 802–5.

Hall, Mark A., and Sara Rosenbaum, eds. 2012. *The Health Care Safety Net in a Post-Reform World*. New Brunswick, NJ: Rutgers University Press.

Hackey, Robert B., and David A. Rochefort, eds. 2001. *The New Politics of State Health Care Policy*. Lawrence: University Press of Kansas.

Hanchate, Amresh D., Karen E. Lasser, Alok Kapoor, Jennifer Rosen, Danny McCormick, Meredith M. D'Amore, and Nancy R. Kressin. 2012. "Massachusetts Reform and Disparities in Inpatient Care Utilization." *Medical Care* 50 (7): 569–77.

Hayward, Rodney A., and David M. Kent. 2008. "6 EZ Steps to Improving Your Performance." *Journal of the American Medical Association* 300 (3): 255–56.

Health Affairs. 2014. "The Family Glitch." *Health Policy Briefs*. November 10. http://www.healthaffairs.org/healthpolicybriefs/brief.php?brief_id=129. Accessed 29 August 2015.

Heisler, Michele, Dylan M. Smith, Rodney A. Hayward, Sarah L. Krein, and Eve A. Kerr. 2003. "Racial Disparities in Diabetes Care Processes, Outcomes, and Treatment Intensity." *Medical Care* 41 (11): 1221–32.

Himmelstein, David U., and Steffie Woolhandler. 2010. "Obama's Reform: No Cure for What Ails Us." *British Medical Journal* 340 (March). doi:10.1136/bmj.c1778.

Hochschild, Jennifer L. 1981. *What's Fair? American Beliefs about Distributive Justice*. Cambridge, MA: Harvard University Press.

Hofer, Timothy P., Rodney A. Hayward, Sheldon Greenfield, Edward H. Wagner, Sherrie H. Kaplan, and Willard G. Manning. 1999. "The Unreliability of Individual Physician 'Report Cards' for Assessing the Costs and Quality of Care of a Chronic Disease." *Journal of the American Medical Association* 281 (22): 2098–2105.

Hoffman, Beatrix. 2012. *Health Care for Some: Rights and Rationing in the United States since 1930*. Chicago: University of Chicago Press.

Hofrichter, Richard, ed. 2003. *Health and Social Justice: Politics, Ideology, and Inequity in the Distribution of Disease*. San Francisco: Jossey-Bass.

[IRS. 2016]. IRS Publication 969, "HealthSavings Accounts and Other Tax-Favored Health Plans," 3.

Jacobs, Lawrence R., and Timothy Callaghan. 2013. "Why States Expand Medicaid: Party, Resources, and History." *Journal of Health Politics, Policy and Law* 38 (5): 1023–50.

Katz, Michael B. 1986. *In the Shadow of the Poorhouse: A Social History of Welfare in America*. New York: Basic Books.

——. 1996. *In the Shadow of the Poorhouse: A Social History of Welfare in America*. 10th anniversary ed., revised and updated. New York: Basic Books.

Katz, Mitchell H. 2010. "Future of the Safety Net under Health Reform." *Journal of the American Medical Association* 304 (6): 679–80.

——. 2011. "Safety-Net Providers and Preparation for Health Reform: Staff Down, Staff Up, Staff Differently." *Archives of Internal Medicine* 171 (15): 1319–20.

Katz, Mitchell H., and Tangerine M. Brigham. 2011. "Transforming a Traditional Safety Net into a Coordinated Care System: Lessons from Healthy San Francisco." *Health Affairs* 30 (2): 237–45.

Kirsch, Richard. 2011. *Fighting for Our Health: The Epic Battle to Make Health Care a Right in the United States*. Albany, NY: Rockefeller Institute Press.

Kliff, Sarah. 2014. "Obamacare's Narrow Networks Are Going to Make People Furious— but They Might Control Costs." *Washington Post Wonkblog*, 13 January. http://www.washingtonpost.com/news/wonkblog/wp/2014/01/13/obamacares-narrow-networks-are-going-to-make-people-furious-but-they-might-control-costs/. Accessed 29 August 2015.

Koos, Earl Lomon. 1954. *The Health of Regionville: What the People Thought and Did about It*. New York: Columbia University Press.

Krein, Sarah L., Timothy P. Hofer, Eve A. Kerr, and Rodney A. Hayward. 2002. "Whom Should We Profile? Examining Diabetes Care Practice Variation among Primary Care Providers, Provider Groups, and Health Care Facilities." *Health Services Research* 37 (5): 1159–80.

Krieger, Nancy, ed. 2005. *Embodying Inequality: Epidemiologic Perspectives*. Amityville, NY: Baywood.

Ku, Leighton, Emily Jones, Peter Shin, Fraser Rothenberg Byrne, and Sharon K. Long. 2011. "Safety-Net Providers after Health Care Reform: Lessons from Massachusetts." *Archives of Internal Medicine* 171 (15): 1379–84.

Landry, Amy Yarbrough, and Robert J. Landry III. 2009. "Factors Associated with Hospital Bankruptcies: A Political and Economic Framework." *Journal of Healthcare Management* 54 (4): 252–72.

Lefkowitz, Bonnie. 2007. *Community Health Centers: A Movement and the People Who Made It Happen*. New Brunswick, NJ: Rutgers University Press.

Li, Rui, Lawrence E. Barker, Sundar Shrestha, Ping Zhang, O. Kenrick Duru, Tony Pearson-Clarke, and Edward W. Gregg. 2014. "Changes over Time in High Out-of-Pocket Health Care Burden in U.S. Adults with Diabetes, 2001–2011." *Diabetes Care* 37 (6): 1629–35.

Ludmerer, Kenneth M. 1999. *Time to Heal: American Medical Education from the Turn of the Century to the Era of Managed Care*. New York: Oxford University Press.

Lynch, Julia. 2006. *Age in the Welfare State: The Origins of Social Spending on Pensioners, Workers, and Children*. New York: Cambridge University Press.

Marmor, Theodore R. 1970. *The Politics of Medicare*. London: Routledge.

Marmot, Michael, and Richard G. Wilkinson, eds. 2006. *Social Determinants of Health*. 2nd ed. New York: Oxford University Press.

Matthew, Dayna Bowen. 2012. "Applying Lessons from Social Psychology to Repair the Health Care Safety Net for Undocumented Immigrants." In *The Health Care "Safety Net" in a Post-Reform World*, edited by Mark A. Hall and Sara Rosenbaum, 91–107. New Brunswick, NJ: Rutgers University Press.

Maxwell, James, Dharma E. Cortés, Karen L. Schneider, Anna Graves, and Brian Rosman. 2011. "Massachusetts' Health Care Reform Increased Access to Care for Hispanics, but Disparities Remain." *Health Affairs* 30 (8): 1451–60.

McCormick, Danny, Assaad Sayah, Hermione Lokko, Steffie Woolhandler, and Rachel Nardin. 2012. "Access to Care after Massachusetts' Health Care Reform: A Safety Net Hospital Patient Survey." *Journal of General Internal Medicine* 27 (11): 1548–54.

McDonough, John E. 2011. *Inside National Health Reform.* Berkeley: University of California Press.

McKethan, Aaron, Nadia Nguyen, Benjamin E. Sasse, and S. Lawrence Kocot. 2009. "Reforming the Medicaid Disproportionate-Share Hospital Program." *Health Affairs* 28 (5): w926–36.

McLafferty, Sara. 1982. "Neighborhood Characteristics and Hospital Closures: A Comparison of the Public, Private and Voluntary Hospital Systems." *Social Science and Medicine* 16 (19): 1667–74.

Meddings, Jennifer, Sanjay Saint, and Laurence F. McMahon. 2010. "Hospital-Acquired Catheter-Associated Urinary Tract Infection: Documentation and Coding Issues May Reduce Financial Impact of Medicare's New Payment Policy." *Infection Control* 31 (6): 627–33.

Meddings, Jennifer A., Heidi Reichert, Mary A. M. Rogers, Sanjay Saint, Joe Stephansky, and Laurence F. McMahon. 2012. "Effect of Nonpayment for Hospital-Acquired, Catheter-Associated Urinary Tract Infection: A Statewide Analysis." *Annals of Internal Medicine* 157 (5): 305–12.

Mehta, Rajendra H., Li Liang, Amrita M. Karve, Adrian F. Hernandez, John S. Rumsfeld, Gregg C. Fonarow, and Eric D. Peterson. 2008. "Association of Patient Case-Mix Adjustment, Hospital Process Performance Rankings, and Eligibility for Financial Incentives." *Journal of the American Medical Association* 300 (16): 1897–1903.

Millett, Christopher, Gopalakrishnan Netuveli, Sonia Saxena, and Azeem Majeed. 2009. "Impact of Pay for Performance on Ethnic Disparities in Intermediate Outcomes for Diabetes: A Longitudinal Study." *Diabetes Care* 32 (3): 404–9.

Montague, J. 1995. "Fighting the 'Vampire Effect': Is Health Care Heading for a Corporate Takeover?" *Hospitals and Health Networks* 69 (2): 66.

Morgan, Daniel J., Jennifer Meddings, Sanjay Saint, Ebbing Lautenbach, Michelle Shardell, Deverick Anderson, Aaron M. Milstone, et al. 2012. "Does Nonpayment for Hospital-Acquired Catheter-Associated Urinary Tract Infections Lead to Overtesting and Increased Antimicrobial Prescribing?" *Clinical Infectious Diseases* 55 (7): 923–29. doi:10.1093/cid/cis556.

Mulvaney-Day, Norah, Margarita Alegría, Anna Nillni, and Sabrina Gonzalez. 2012. "Implementation of Massachusetts Health Insurance Reform with Vulnerable Populations in a Safety-Net Setting." *Journal of Health Care for the Poor and Underserved* 23 (2): 884–902.

Naylor, Mary D., Ellen T. Kurtzman, David C. Grabowski, Charlene Harrington, Mark McClellan, and Susan C. Reinhard. 2012. "Unintended Consequences of Steps to Cut Readmissions and Reform Payment May Threaten Care of Vulnerable Older Adults." *Health Affairs* 31 (7): 1623–32. doi:10.1377/hlthaff.2012.0110.

Neuhausen, Katherine, Anna C. Davis, Jack Needleman, Robert H. Brook, David Zingmond, and Dylan H. Roby. 2014. "Disproportionate-Share Hospital Payment Reductions May Threaten the Financial Stability of Safety-Net Hospitals." *Health Affairs* 33 (6): 988–96.

Newhouse, Joseph P., and the Insurance Experiment Group. 1993. *Free for All? Lessons from the RAND Health Insurance Experiment.* Cambridge, MA: Harvard University Press.

Ngai, Mae M. 2004. *Impossible Subjects: Illegal Aliens and the Making of Modern America: Illegal Aliens and the Making of Modern America.* Princeton, NJ: Princeton University Press.

Oberlander, Jonathan. 2003. *The Political Life of Medicare.* Chicago: University of Chicago Press.

Offner, Paul. 2001. "Politics and the Public Hospital in Our Capital." *Health Affairs* 20 (4): 176–81.

Pande, Aakanksha H., Dennis Ross-Degnan, Alan M. Zaslavsky, and Joshua A. Salomon. 2011. "Effects of Healthcare Reforms on Coverage, Access, and Disparities: Quasi-Experimental Analysis of Evidence from Massachusetts." *American Journal of Preventive Medicine* 41 (1): 1–8.

Park, Lisa Sun-Hee. 2011. *Entitled to Nothing: The Struggle for Immigrant Health Care in the Age of Welfare Reform.* New York: New York University Press.

Pauly, Mark V. 1997. *Health Benefits at Work: An Economic and Political Analysis of Employment-Based Health Insurance.* Ann Arbor: University of Michigan Press.

Pearjan, Robert. 2015. "Rules Will Limit Tactics on Hospitals' Fee Collections." *New York Times,* January 12, p. A10 (New York edition).

Poole, Mary. 2006. *The Segregated Origins of Social Security: African Americans and the Welfare State.* Chapel Hill: University of North Carolina Press.

Price, Carter C., and Christine Eibner. 2013. "For States That Opt Out of Medicaid Expansion: 3.6 Million Fewer Insured and $8.4 Billion Less in Federal Payments." *Health Affairs* 32 (6): 1030–36.

Quadagno, Jill. 2000. "Promoting Civil Rights through the Welfare State: How Medicare Integrated Southern Hospitals." *Social Problems* 47 (1): 68–89.

———. 2005. *One Nation, Uninsured: Why the U.S. Has No National Health Insurance.* New York: Oxford University Press.

Rawls, John. 1971. *A Theory of Justice.* Cambridge, MA: Belknap Press of Harvard University Press.

Rehavi, M. Marit, and Erin M. Johnson. 2013. "Physicians Treating Physicians: Information and Incentives in Childbirth." NBER Working Paper w19242. Cambridge: National Bureau of Economic Research. http://papers.ssrn.com/sol3/papers .cfm?abstract_id=2295856. Accessed 29 August 2015.

Rice, Mitchell F. 1987. "Hospital Closures/Relocations in the Inner-City: Implications for Health Care in the Black Community." *Journal of Health and Human Resources Administration* 9 (3): 340–53.

Richards, David A. J. 1971. *A Theory of Reasons for Action.* Oxford: Clarendon.

Richman, Ilana B., and Mollyann Brodie. 2014. "A National Study of Burdensome Health Care Costs among Non-elderly Americans." *BMC Health Services Research* 14 (1): 435.

Risse, Guenter B. 1999. *Mending Bodies, Saving Souls: A History of Hospitals.* New York: Oxford University Press.

Rosenberg, Charles E. 1987. *The Care of Strangers: The Rise of America's Hospital System.* New York: Basic Books.

Rosner, David. 1982. *A Once Charitable Enterprise: Hospitals and Health Care in Brooklyn and New York, 1885–1915.* New York: Cambridge University Press.

Rothstein, William G. 1987. *American Medical Schools and the Practice of Medicine: A History.* New York: Oxford University Press.

Ruger, Jennifer Prah. 2009. *Health and Social Justice.* Oxford: Oxford University Press.

Saint, Sanjay, Jennifer A. Meddings, David Calfee, Christine P. Kowalski, and Sarah L. Krein. 2009. "Catheter-Associated Urinary Tract Infection and the Medicare Rule Changes." *Annals of Internal Medicine* 150 (12): 877–84.

Sardell, Alice. 1988. *The U.S. Experiment in Social Medicine: The Community Health Center Program, 1965–1986.* Pittsburgh: University of Pittsburgh Press.

Schoen, Cathy, Robin Osborn, David Squires, Michelle M. Doty, Roz Pierson, and Sandra Applebaum. 2010. "How Health Insurance Design Affects Access to Care and Costs, by Income, in Eleven Countries." *Health Affairs* 29 (12): 2323–34.

Shahian, David M., Fred H. Edwards, Jeffrey P. Jacobs, Richard L. Prager, Sharon-Lise T. Normand, Cynthia M. Shewan, Sean M. O'Brien, Eric D. Peterson, and Frederick L. Grover. 2011. "Public Reporting of Cardiac Surgery Performance: Part 1: History, Rationale, Consequences." *Annals of Thoracic Surgery* 92 (3): S2–11.

Shi, Leiyu, and Gregory D. Stevens. 2005. *Vulnerable Populations in the United States.* San Francisco: Jossey-Bass.

Skocpol, Theda. 1992. *Protecting Mothers and Soldiers: The Political Origins of Social Policy in the United States.* Cambridge, MA: Belknap Press of Harvard University.

Smith, Jessica C., and Carla Medalia. 2014. *Health Insurance Coverage in the United States: 2013.* Current Population Reports P60–250. Washington, DC: U.S. Census Bureau. http://www.census.gov/content/dam/Census/library/publications/2014/demo/p60-250.pdf. Accessed 29 August 2015.

Sparer, Michael S. 1996. *Medicaid and the Limits of State Health Reform.* Philadelphia: Temple University Press.

Starr, Paul. 2011. *Remedy and Reaction: The Peculiar American Struggle over Health Care Reform.* New Haven, CT: Yale University Press.

Stevens, Robert Bocking, and Rosemary Stevens. 1974. *Welfare Medicine in America: A Case Study of Medicaid.* New York: Free Press.

Stevens, Rosemary. 1999. *In Sickness and in Wealth: American Hospitals in the Twentieth Century.* Baltimore: Johns Hopkins University Press.

Thompson, Frank J. 2012. *Medicaid Politics: Federalism, Policy Durability, and Health Reform.* Washington, DC: Georgetown University Press.

Ticktin, Miriam I. 2011. *Casualties of Care: Immigration and the Politics of Humanitarianism in France.* Berkeley: University of California Press.

UNDP (United Nations Development Programme). 2014. *Human Development Report 2014: Sustaining Human Progress: Reducing Vulnerabilities and Building Resilience.* http://hdr.undp.org/en/2014-report. Accessed 29 August 2015.

U.S. Supreme Court. 2012. *Syllabus to National Federation of Independent Business (NFIB) v. Sebelius*. 567 U.S. http://www.supremecourt.gov/opinions/11pdf/11-393c3a2.pdf. Accessed 29 August 2015.

Wang, C. Jason, Kathleen N. Conroy, and Barry Zuckerman. 2009. "Payment Reform for Safety-Net Institutions: Improving Quality and Outcomes." *New England Journal of Medicine* 361 (19): 1821–23.

Ward, Andrew, and Pamela Jo Johnson. 2013. "Necessary Health Care and Basic Needs: Health Insurance Plans and Essential Benefits." *Health Care Analysis* 21 (4): 355–71.

Weinick, Robin M., and Romana Hasnain-Wynia. 2011. "Quality Improvement Efforts under Health Reform: How to Ensure That They Help Reduce Disparities—Not Increase Them." *Health Affairs* 30 (10): 1837–43.

Werner, Rachel M., David A. Asch, and Daniel Polsky. 2005. "Racial Profiling: The Unintended Consequences of Coronary Artery Bypass Graft Report Cards." *Circulation* 111 (10): 1257–63.

Wharam, J. Frank, Fang Zhang, Bruce E. Landon, Stephen B. Soumerai, and Dennis Ross-Degnan. 2013. "Low-Socioeconomic-Status Enrollees in High-Deductible Plans Reduced High-Severity Emergency Care." *Health Affairs* 32 (8): 1398–1406.

Whiteis, David G., and Jack W. Salmon. 1991. "Public Health Care Delivery in Five U.S. Municipalities: Lessons and Implications." *Henry Ford Hospital Medical Journal* 40 (1–2): 16–25.

Wilson, William J. 2009. *More than Just Race: Being Black and Poor in the Inner City*. New York: W. W. Norton and Company.

Zhu, Jane, Phyllis Brawarsky, Stuart Lipsitz, Haiden Huskamp, and Jennifer S. Haas. 2010. "Massachusetts Health Reform and Disparities in Coverage, Access and Health Status." *Journal of General Internal Medicine* 25 (12): 1356–62.

Contributors

JUDITH C. BARKER is professor of medical anthropology at the University of California, San Francisco, where she also serves as associate director of the Center to Address Children's Oral Health Disparities (CANDO). Her ethnographic research has long focused on health disparities and public health in vulnerable populations experiencing a wide range of chronic conditions. In over one hundred peer-reviewed journal articles and book chapters, in both the clinically focused and social science literatures, she presents the processes by which patients and their families understand and manage on a day-to-day basis their various chronic illnesses in contexts where social, health provider, environmental, and policy arenas intersect with, frame, and constrain individual-level care-seeking.

PAULA BRAVEMAN, MD, MPH, is professor of family and community medicine and director of the Center on Social Disparities in Health at the University of California, San Francisco. She completed her undergraduate training in philosophy, medicine (and family and community medicine), and epidemiology at, respectively, Swarthmore College, the University of California, San Francisco, and the University of California, Berkeley. For more than two decades, Dr. Braveman has studied and published extensively on the concept and measurement of health inequalities/disparities and health equity. Her empiric research has focused on documenting, understanding, and addressing socioeconomic and racial/ethnic inequalities in health and their social determinants. Throughout her career, she has collaborated with local, state, federal, and international health agencies to see rigorous research translated into practice with the goal of achieving greater equity in health. She was elected to the Institute of Medicine of the U.S. National Academy of Sciences in 2002.

PAUL BRODWIN is professor of anthropology at the University of Wisconsin–Milwaukee, and assistant adjunct professor at the Center for Bioethics and Medical Humanities at the Medical College of Wisconsin. He is the author of *Everyday Ethics: Voices from the Front Line of Community Psychiatry* (2013) and *Medicine and Morality in Haiti: The Contest for Healing Power* (1996), the editor of *Biotechnology and Culture: Bodies, Anxieties, Ethics* (2000) and the coeditor of *Pain as Human Experience: Anthropological Perspectives* (1992). He is a coeditor of the book series Anthropologies of American Medicine: Culture, Power, Practice, and is on the board of the journals *Culture, Medicine, and Psychiatry* and *Anthropological Quarterly*. His research has been supported by the National Science Foundation, the National Institute of Health, the Fulbright Foundation, and the Wenner-Gren Foundation.

MARA BUCHBINDER is associate professor of social medicine, adjunct associate professor of anthropology, and core faculty in the Center for Bioethics at the University of North Carolina at Chapel Hill, as well as a Greenwall Faculty Scholar (2015–18). She is the author of *All in Your Head: Making Sense of Pediatric Pain* (2015) and coauthor of *Saving Babies? The Consequences of Newborn Genetic Screening* (2013). Her research explores the sociocultural and ethical dimensions of clinical communication and the patient-provider relationship in the United States.

JAMIE SUKI CHANG is a sociologist and National Institutes of Drug Abuse postdoctoral fellow in substance use treatment at San Francisco General Hospital. Her current research involves drug and alcohol treatment, prescription opioid use, substance use stigma, provider-patient interactions, homelessness, and housing. She teaches social theory, works with community-based organizations, and is interested in developing qualitative methodologies.

DEBRA DEBRUIN, PhD, is associate professor at the Center for Bioethics at the University of Minnesota, where she has held the leadership positions of center director and director of education. She also served as a health policy fellow in the U.S. Senate as a consultant to the National Academy of Sciences' Institute of Medicine and the National Bioethics Advisory Commission, and as invited coauthor on a published opinion of the American College of Obstetricians and Gynecologists' Ethics Committee. She has been a member of a number of working groups relevant to public health in Minnesota and codirected the Minnesota Pandemic Ethics Project. Her scholarship and teaching focus on social justice issues related to gender, race, and poverty, especially in the areas of research ethics and the ethics of public health policy. In addition to her work analyzing the ethical implications of dominant conceptions of risk in pregnancy, she has also published on the inclusion of women—and specifically pregnant women—in clinical research; on ethical issues in pandemic planning concerning pregnant women and other at-risk social groups; on ethical issues in HIV response, especially in resource-poor settings; on the role of nurses in ensuring the ethical conduct of clinical trials; on feminist pedagogy; and on sexual harassment, among other issues. She designed and teaches courses on gender and the politics of health, and social justice and health.

LESLIE A. DUBBIN is chief integration officer for ambulatory care for the San Francisco Health Network. She is also assistant adjunct professor in nursing for the Department of Social and Behavioral Sciences at the University of California, San Francisco, where she teaches courses related to health policy. Her research explores the mechanisms of the reproduction of racial inequalities in health, the influences of the lived environment on individuals' experiences living with chronic illness, patient-provider interactions, and the relationship of life-course stress experiences of black women and their risk for preterm birth.

SARAH HORTON is associate professor of anthropology at the University of Colorado, Denver. She is the author of *They Leave Their Kidneys in the Fields: Injury, Illness, and Illegality among U.S. Farmworkers* (2015) and *The Santa Fe Fiesta, Reinvented: Staking Ethnonationalism Claims to a Disappearing Homeland* (2010). Horton's research examines the ways that multiple public policies leave their imprint on migrant farmworkers' health, and she has been conducting fieldwork in a farmworking community in California's Central Valley for over a decade. She is the author of numerous articles published in *American Ethnologist, American Anthropologist, Medical Anthropology, Medical Anthropology Quarterly,* and *Social Science and Medicine.*

CARLA C. KEIRNS is assistant professor of medicine (palliative care) and assistant professor of history and philosophy of medicine at the University of Kansas Medical Center, Kansas City, Kansas, where she teaches medical students and practices palliative medicine. She is completing a book on the history of asthma in the United States, and editing a volume on physicians as parents. Her research is at the intersection of public health and public policy, studying chronic disease, health disparities, and end-of-life care. She explores problems such as how and why different individuals and communities receive different kinds of health care across the life span, from studies of childhood asthma in urban communities to patterns of end-of-life care in different regions of the United States. She has authored articles and essays in clinical ethics, health services research, and history of medicine, with a focus on health disparities, end-of-life care, chronic disease, epidemiologic transitions, and public health ethics. She has worked, taught, and observed in health care settings in the United States, Australia, Mexico, and Botswana, and has taught public health in Jamaica.

J. PAUL KELLEHER is associate professor of bioethics and philosophy at the University of Wisconsin–Madison. He works in areas of applied ethics and political philosophy that address the health of populations. He has published on topics including the foundations of justice in health care; issues in public health ethics, such as public health paternalism, population screening for rare genetic conditions, and the tension between treatment and prevention; ethical issues in health economics and environmental economics; climate change and duties to future generations; and clinical ethics issues, such as conscientious refusal and treatment of severely disabled newborns. His work has appeared in leading philosophy and bioethics journals, including *Journal of Moral Philosophy, Utilitas, Kennedy Institute of Ethics Journal, Journal of Applied Philosophy, Journal of Medicine and Philosophy, Public Health Ethics, and Ethics,* and *Policy & Environment.* His main current project concerns the valuing of health and well-being in economic analyses of climate change, especially the issue of whether to apply a discount rate to benefits accruing to future generations.

NICHOLAS B. KING is an associate professor at McGill University, holding positions in the Biomedical Ethics Unit, the Institute for Health and Social Policy, and the Department of Epidemiology, Biostatistics, and Occupational Health. He codirects the Montreal Health Equity Research Consortium, a multidisciplinary project investigating health and health equity research and policies. Dr. King conducts research in the following areas: the role of social context, framing effects, and biases in the production and interpretation of health information; public health ethics and policy, including the ethics of biosecurity and public health preparedness; and health inequalities and the social determinants of health. He has published in the *BMJ*, *PLOS Medicine*, the *American Journal of Public Health*, and the *Bulletin of the World Health Organization*.

EVA FEDER KITTAY is Distinguished Professor of Philosophy at Stony Brook University / SUNY; a senior fellow of the Stony Brook Center for Medical Humanities, Compassionate Care and Bioethics, and an affiliate of the Women's Studies Program; and a Women's Studies Affiliate. She is the recipient of a Guggenheim Fellowship, a National Endowment for the Humanities fellowship, the American Philosophical Association book prize, and the Phi Beta Kappa Lebowitz Prize. She is the author of *Love's Labor: Essays on Women, Equality, and Dependency* (1999), *Metaphor: Its Cognitive Force and Linguistic Structure* (1985) and over eighty-five articles and essays on feminist philosophy, disability studies, and philosophy of language. She is coeditor of *Cognitive Disability and the Challenge to Moral Philosophy* (2010), *Blackwell Guide to Feminist Philosophy* (2007), and *Theoretical Perspectives on Dependency and Women* (2003), *Frames, Fields and Contrasts* (1992), and *Women and Moral Theory* (1985). She has also edited many journal issues on feminist philosophy and the philosophy of disability. She is currently writing a monograph tentatively titled "Disabled Minds and Things That Matter: Lessons for a Humbler Philosophy."

JOAN LIASCHENKO is a professor at the Center of Bioethics and the School of Nursing at the University of Minnesota. She is also a cochair of the ethics committee and directs the ethics consult service for the university hospital. She teaches ethics to graduate and doctoral students in the School of Nursing and several courses in the graduate program in bioethics. She developed and taught a course titled Morality and Risk and has published in the area of reproductive ethics on the interests of fetuses and potential children and the ethical obligations of obstetricians. Her major research interests are the morality of everyday practices in health care and clinical ethics. She is a member of the American Academy of Nursing and has been a visiting scholar in Australia, Canada, Germany, Japan, and New Zealand.

ANNE DRAPKIN LYERLY is associate professor of social medicine and associate director of the Center for Bioethics at the University of North Carolina, Chapel Hill. She is also a board-certified obstetrician-gynecologist. She is the author of *A Good Birth* (2013) and many articles addressing socially and morally complex issues in reproductive medicine. She cofounded the Obstetrics and Gynecology Risk Research Group, convening experts from medical epidemiology, anthropology, obstetrics-gynecology, philosophy, and gender theory to address how risk is assessed and managed in the context of pregnancy. She also cofounded the Second Wave Initiative, an effort to ensure that the health interests of women are fairly represented in biomedical research and drug and device policies, and is principal investigator on the National Institute of Child Health and Human Development (NICHD)–funded PHASES (Pregnancy and HIV/AIDS: Seeking Equitable Study) Project. She has been supported by the National Institutes of Health (NIH) and the Greenwall Foundation's Faculty Scholars program. She is former chair of the American College of Obstetricians and Gynecologists Committee on Ethics and former cochair of the 2009 Program Committee for the American Society of Bioethics and Humanities. She currently serves on the NIH Advisory Committee to the Director's Working Group on Stem Cell Research and the March of Dimes National Bioethics Committee.

MARY FAITH MARSHALL is director of the Program in Biomedical Ethics at the Center for Biomedical Ethics and Humanities at the University of Virginia (UVA), as well as professor of public health sciences in the School of Medicine and a professor in the School of Nursing. She cochairs the UVA Health System Ethics Committee and directs the Ethics Consult Service. With her colleague Lois Shepherd she teaches the course Reproductive Ethics and the Law, a joint UVA law and medical school course. Dr. Marshall is former associate dean and professor of family medicine and community health at the University of Minnesota Medical School and former codirector of the Center for Bioethics in the Academic Health Center. She is past president of the American Society for Bioethics and Humanities and the American Association for Bioethics. She is a member of the ethics committees of the American College of Obstetrics and Gynecology and the Society for Critical Care Medicine. She is an elected fellow of the American College of Critical Care Medicine. Dr. Marshall received the Trailblazer Award from the Charleston, South Carolina, chapter of the NAACP in 1999 for her work in policy approaches to perinatal substance abuse and has testified on this subject before Congress and in U.S. District Court in the case of *Crystal M. Ferguson et al. v. City of Charleston, South Carolina, et al.* Her research interests and publications focus on reproductive ethics (specifically coercive interventions in pregnancy and policy approaches to perinatal substance abuse), clinical ethics, human subjects protections and research ethics.

MICHELE RIVKIN-FISH is associate professor of anthropology at the University of North Carolina, Chapel Hill. Her research has examined reproductive and demographic politics, sexuality education, and health care reforms in Russia. She is most interested in the historical experiences and cultural values that underlie notions of justice in health policies in Russia and the United States. This interest also informs her research on the challenges of integrating feminism and anthropological insights for promoting change in post-Soviet Russia. Rivkin-Fish is the author of *Women's Health in Post-Soviet Russia: The Politics of Intervention* (2005) and the coeditor of *Dilemmas of Diversity after the Cold War: Analyses of "Cultural Difference" by U.S. and Russia-Based Scholars* (2010). Her articles have appeared in *Medical Anthropology Quarterly*; *Social Science and Medicine*; *Culture, Medicine, and Psychiatry*; *American Ethnologist*; *Signs*; and *American Anthropologist*. She is currently writing a book on the history of Russian efforts to replace routine abortion with a culture of family planning.

CAROLYN MOXLEY ROUSE is a professor in the Department of Anthropology and the director of the Program in African Studies at Princeton University. Her work explores the nexus between race, institutions, and social inequality. She is the author of *Engaged Surrender: African American Women and Islam* (2004) and *Uncertain Suffering: Racial Healthcare Disparities and Sickle Cell Disease* (2009). She also cowrote with John Jackson and Marla Frederick *Televised Redemption: The Media Production of Black Jews, Christians, and Muslims* (2016). In addition to being an anthropologist, Rouse is also a filmmaker. She has produced, directed, and/or edited a number of documentaries, including *Chicks in White Satin* (1994), *Purification to Prozac: Treating Mental Illness in Bali* (1998), and *Listening as a Radical Act: World Anthropologies and the Decentering of Western Thought* (2015).

JENNIFER PRAH RUGER is Amartya Sen Professor of Health Equity, Economics and Policy and associate dean for global studies at the University of Pennsylvania School of Social Policy & Practice and Perelman School of Medicine. Dr. Ruger's work is at the intersection of political economy, health policy, international relations, comparative social research, and law, crossing disciplines and reexamining the principles and values that underlie health policy and public health and applying these principles empirically. Her scholarship includes areas such as global health justice, global health governance, health and social justice, and shared health governance. She is author of *Health and Social Justice* (2010) as well as over 100 other publications. Her work has been cited by the United Nations, the World Bank, the World Health Organization, and the U.S. government. She was awarded a Guggenheim Fellowship, a Greenwall Faculty Scholar award in Bioethics, an NIH Career Development award, and a Donaghue Investigator award in ethics and economics of health disparities.

JANET K. SHIM is associate professor of sociology in the Department of Social and Behavioral Sciences at the University of California, San Francisco. Her current research focuses on analyzing the science of health disparities and the production of health care inequalities. Her publications have appeared in such journals as *Social Studies of Science, Journal of Health and Social Behavior, Social Science and Medicine,* and *Sociology of Health and Illness.* She is also the author of *Heart-Sick: The Politics of Risk, Inequality, and Heart Disease* (2014).

REBECCA L. WALKER is associate professor of social medicine, adjunct associate professor of philosophy, and core faculty at the Center for Bioethics at the University of North Carolina at Chapel Hill. Her research is at the intersection of moral theory and practical ethics and has addressed practical virtue ethics, concepts of autonomy in bioethics, human and animal subject research ethics, health justice and inequalities, and ethical issues in genomics. She has published in leading bioethics journals, including the *Kennedy Institute of Ethics Journal, American Journal of Bioethics, Journal of Medicine and Philosophy, Journal of Law, Medicine and Ethics, Journal of Theoretical Medicine and Bioethics,* and *AMA Journal of Ethics and Bioethics.* She has also published in bioethics-related disciplinary journals such as *Genetics in Medicine, Health Economics,* and *Nature Biotechnology.* She is coeditor of *Working Virtue: Virtue Ethics and Contemporary Moral Problems* (2007) and is currently working on a monograph tentatively titled "Of Mice and Primates: Virtue Ethics and Animal Research."

Index

Studies in Social Medicine

Nancy M. P. King, Gail E. Henderson, and Jane Stein, eds., *Beyond Regulations: Ethics in Human Subjects Research* (1999).

Laurie Zoloth, *Health Care and the Ethics of Encounter: A Jewish Discussion of Social Justice* (1999).

Susan M. Reverby, ed., *Tuskegee's Truths: Rethinking the Tuskegee Syphilis Study* (2000).

Beatrix Hoffman, *The Wages of Sickness: The Politics of Health Insurance in Progressive America* (2000).

Margarete Sandelowski, *Devices and Desires: Gender, Technology, and American Nursing* (2000).

Keith Wailoo, *Dying in the City of the Blues: Sickle Cell Anemia and the Politics of Race and Health* (2001).

Judith Andre, *Bioethics as Practice* (2002).

Chris Feudtner, *Bittersweet: Diabetes, Insulin, and the Transformation of Illness* (2003).

Ann Folwell Stanford, *Bodies in a Broken World: Women Novelists of Color and the Politics of Medicine* (2003).

Lawrence O. Gostin, *The AIDS Pandemic: Complacency, Injustice, and Unfulfilled Expectations* (2004).

Arthur A. Daemmrich, *Pharmacopolitics: Drug Regulation in the United States and Germany* (2004).

Carl Elliott and Tod Chambers, eds., *Prozac as a Way of Life* (2004).

Steven M. Stowe, *Doctoring the South: Southern Physicians and Everyday Medicine in the Mid-Nineteenth Century* (2004).

Arleen Marcia Tuchman, *Science Has No Sex: The Life of Marie Zakrzewska, M.D.* (2006).

Michael H. Cohen, *Healing at the Borderland of Medicine and Religion* (2006).

Keith Wailoo, Julie Livingston, and Peter Guarnaccia, eds., *A Death Retold: Jesica Santillan, the Bungled Transplant, and Paradoxes of Medical Citizenship* (2006).

Michelle T. Moran, *Colonizing Leprosy: Imperialism and the Politics of Public Health in the United States* (2007).

Karey Harwood, *The Infertility Treadmill: Feminist Ethics, Personal Choice, and the Use of Reproductive Technologies* (2007).

Carla Bittel, *Mary Putnam Jacobi and the Politics of Medicine in Nineteenth-Century America* (2009).

Samuel Kelton Roberts Jr., *Infectious Fear: Politics, Disease, and the Health Effects of Segregation* (2009).

Lois Shepherd, *If That Ever Happens to Me: Making Life and Death Decisions after Terri Schiavo* (2009).

Mical Raz, *What's Wrong with the Poor?: Psychiatry, Race, and the War on Poverty* (2013).

Johanna Schoen, *Abortion after Roe* (2015).

Nancy Tomes, *Remaking the American Patient: How Madison Avenue and Modern Medicine Turned Patients into Consumers* (2016).

Mara Buchbinder, Michele Rivkin-Fish, and Rebecca Walker, eds., *Understanding Health Inequalities and Justice: New Conversations across the Disciplines* (2016).